T0263445

Clinical Applications of MR Diffusion and Perfusion Imaging

Guest Editors

SCOTT B. REEDER, MD, PhD
PRATIK MUKHERJEE, MD, PhD

MAGNETIC RESONANCE IMAGING CLINICS OF NORTH AMERICA

www.mri.theclinics.com

May 2009 • Volume 17 • Number 2

SAUNDERS an imprint of ELSEVIER, Inc.

W.B. SAUNDERS COMPANY
A Division of Elsevier Inc.

1600 John F. Kennedy Boulevard • Suite 1800 • Philadelphia, Pennsylvania 19103-2899

http://www.theclinics.com

MRI CLINICS OF NORTH AMERICA Volume 17, Number 2
May 2009 ISSN 1064-9689, ISBN 13: 978-1-4377-0498-3, ISBN 10: 1-4377-0498-0

Editor: Barton Dudlick
Developmental Editor: Theresa Collier

Magnetic Resonance Imaging Clinics of North America (ISSN 1064-9689) is published quarterly by Elsevier Inc., 360 Park Avenue South, New York, NY 10010-1710. Months of issue are February, May, August, and November. Business and Editorial Offices: 1600 John F. Kennedy Blvd., Suite 1800, Philadelphia, PA 19103-2899. Customer Service Office: 11830 Westline Industrial Drive, St. Louis, MO 63146. Periodicals postage paid at New York, NY and additional mailing offices. Subscription prices are $276.00 per year (domestic individuals), $414.00 per year (domestic institutions), $134.00 per year (domestic students/residents), $308.00 per year (Canadian individuals), $520.00 per year (Canadian institutions), $400.00 per year (international individuals), $520.00 per year (international institutions), and $194.00 per year (international and Canadian students/residents). International air speed delivery is included in all *Clinics* subscription prices. All prices are subject to change without notice. **POSTMASTER:** Send address changes to *Magnetic Resonance Imaging Clinics*, 11830 Westline Industrial Drive, St. Louis, MO 63146. Customer Service (orders, claims, online, change of address): Elsevier Periodicals Customer Service, 11830 Westline Industrial Drive, St. Louis, MO 63146. Tel: 1-800-654-2452 (U.S. and Canada). Fax: 314-523-5170. E-mail: journalscustomerservice-usa@elsevier.com (for print support); journalsonlinesupport-usa@elsevier.com (for online support).

Reprints. For copies of 100 or more of articles in this publication, please contact the Commercial Reprints Department, Elsevier Inc., 360 Park Avenue South, New York, NY 10010-1710. Tel.: 212-633-3812; Fax: 212-462-1935; E-mail: reprints@elsevier.com.

Magnetic Resonance Imaging Clinics of North America is covered in the *RSNA Index of Imaging Literature, MEDLINE/PubMed (Index Medicus),* and *EMBASE/Excerpta Medica.*

Contributors

GUEST EDITORS

SCOTT B. REEDER, MD, PhD
Assistant Professor and Division Chief of
Magnetic Resonance Imaging, Departments of
Radiology, Medical Physics, Biomedical
Engineering, and Medicine, University of
Wisconsin, Madison, Wisconsin

PRATIK MUKHERJEE, MD, PhD
Associate Professor, Departments of
Radiology and Bioengineering, University of
California, San Francisco, San Francisco,
California

AUTHORS

ROLAND BAMMER, PhD
Assistant Professor of Radiology, Department
of Radiology, Stanford University, Lucas
Center, Stanford, California

DANIEL P. BARBORIAK, MD
Associate Professor of Radiology, Division of
Neuroradiology, Department of Radiology,
Duke University Medical Center, Durham,
North Carolina

JEFFREY BERMAN, PhD
Postdoctoral Scholar, Department of
Radiology and Biomedical Imaging, University
of California, San Francisco, San Francisco,
California

THORSTEN A. BLEY, MD
Visiting Assistant Professor of Radiology,
Department of Radiology, University of
Wisconsin, Madison, Wisconsin

B. NICOLAS BLOCH, MD
Department of Radiology, Beth Israel
Deaconess Medical Center, Boston,
Massachusetts

JONATHAN H. BURDETTE, MD
Associate Professor, Department of Radiology,
Wake Forest University School of Medicine,
Winston-Salem, North Carolina

DANIEL CORNFELD, MD
Assistant Professor, Department of Diagnostic
Radiology, Yale New Haven Hospital,
New Haven, Connecticut

SHELAGH B. COUTTS, MBChB, MD, FRCPC
Assistant Professor, Clinical Neurosciences;
and Hotchkiss Brain Institute, University of
Calgary; Calgary Stroke Program; and Seaman
Family Research Centre, Foothills Medical
Centre, Calgary, Alberta, Canada

RICHARD KINH GIAN DO, MD, PhD
Clinical Body MRI Fellow, Department of
Radiology, New York University Langone
Medical Center, New York, New York

RICHARD FRAYNE, PhD
Professor, Department of Radiology; and
Clinical Neurosciences; and Biomedical
Engineering; and Department of Electrical
Engineering; and Hotchkiss Brain Institute;
University of Calgary; Seaman Family MR
Research Centre, Foothills Medical Centre,
Calgary, Alberta, Canada

ASHLEY D. HARRIS, PhD
Post-doctoral Fellow, Department of
Radiology; and Clinical Neurosciences; and
Department of Biomedical Engineering; and
Hotchkiss Brain Institute, University of Calgary;
Seaman Family MR Research Centre, Foothills
Medical Centre, Calgary, Alberta, Canada

CHRISTOPHER P. HESS, MD, PhD
Assistant Professor, Department of Radiology
and Biomedical Imaging, University of
California, San Francisco, San Francisco,
California

SAMANTHA J. HOLDSWORTH, PhD
Department of Radiology, Stanford University, Lucas Center, Stanford, California

ROBERT A. KRAFT, PhD
Department of Biomedical Engineering, Wake Forest University, Winston-Salem, North Carolina

MENG LAW, MD, FRACR
Professor of Radiology and Neurosurgery, and Chief of Neuroradiology, Department of Radiology; and Department of Neurosurgery, University of Southern California Imaging Center, University of Southern California, Keck School of Medicine, Los Angeles County and University of Southern California Medical Center, Los Angeles, California

ROBERT E. LENKINSKI, PhD
MRI Research Division, Beth Israel Deaconess Medical Center, Boston, Massachusetts

RUSSELL N. LOW, MD
Medical Director, Sharp and Children's MRI Center; San Diego Imaging, Inc., San Diego, California

JOSEPH A. MALDJIAN, MD
Professor, Department of Radiology, Wake Forest University School of Medicine, Winston- Salem, North Carolina

COLM J. McMAHON, MB
Department of Radiology, Beth Israel Deaconess Medical Center, Boston, Massachusetts

MARIANNE MOON, MD
Radiology Resident, Department of Diagnostic Radiology, Yale New Haven Hospital, New Haven, Connecticut

MICHAEL J. PALDINO, MD
Fellow, Division of Neuroradiology, Department of Radiology, Duke University Medical Center, Durham, North Carolina

JEFFREY M. POLLOCK, MD
Department of Radiology, Wake Forest University School of Medicine, Winston-Salem; Assistant Professor, Department of Radiology, Oregon Health and Science University, Portland, Oregon

NEIL M. ROFSKY, MD
Department of Radiology, Beth Israel Deaconess Medical Center, Boston, Massachusetts

HENRY RUSINEK, PhD
Associate Professor of Radiology, Department of Radiology, New York University Langone Medical Center, New York, New York

STEFAN T. SKARE, PhD
Department of Radiology, Stanford University, Lucas Center, Stanford, California

HUAN TAN, MS
Department of Biomedical Engineering, Wake Forest University, Winston-Salem, North Carolina

BACHIR TAOULI, MD
Associate Professor of Radiology, Department of Radiology, New York University Langone Medical Center, New York, New York

MAJDA M. THURNHER, MD
Professor, Department of Radiology, Medical University of Vienna, Vienna, Austria

MARKUS UHL, MD
Associate Professor of Radiology; and Director, Division of Pediatric Radiology, Department of Diagnostic Radiology, University of Freiburg, Freiburg, Germany

WOUTER B. VELDHUIS, MD, PhD
Department of Radiology, University Medical Center Utrecht, Utrecht, The Netherlands

JEFFREY WEINREB, MD
Professor and Chief, Body Magnetic Resonance Imaging, Department of Diagnostic Radiology, Yale New Haven Hospital, New Haven, Connecticut

OLIVER WIEBEN, PhD
Assistant Professor, Department of Medical Physics; and Department of Radiology, University of Wisconsin, Madison, Wisconsin

CHRISTOPHER T. WHITLOW, MD, PhD
Department of Radiology, Wake Forest University School of Medicine, Winston-Salem, North Carolina

Contents

Considerable strides have been made by countless individual researchers in diffusion-weighted imaging (DWI) to push DWI from an experimental tool, limited to a few institutions with specialized instrumentation, to a powerful tool used routinely for diagnostic imaging. The field of DWI constantly evolves, and progress has been made on several fronts. These developments are primarily composed of improved robustness against patient and physiologic motion, increased spatial resolution, new biophysical and tissue models, and new clinical applications for DWI. This article aims to provide a succinct overview of some of these new developments and a description of some of the major challenges associated with DWI.

Diffusion MR tractography has rapidly become an important clinical tool that can delineate functionally important white matter tracts for surgical planning. One of the goals of brain surgery is to avoid damage to eloquent cortex and subcortical white matter. Diffusion tractography remains the only noninvasive method capable of segmenting the subcortical course of a white matter tract. This article reviews the technical and clinical issues surrounding presurgical diffusion tractography, including traditional diffusion tensor imaging methods and more advanced high angular resolution diffusion imaging approaches, such as q-ball imaging. An overview of the presurgical diffusion tensor imaging and q-ball tractography protocols used at our institution is also provided.

With estimates of more than 5 million people with Alzheimer's disease (AD) now living in the United States and an increasing prevalence of the disease among the aging population, there is an urgent need for the development of reliable biomarkers for early diagnosis and evaluation of potential therapeutic interventions. Structural MR imaging, the focus of the most intense research in this area to date, has identified characteristic patterns of macroscopic atrophy within larger groups of patients who have clinically probable AD, particularly within the medial temporal lobes. These changes are thought to reflect underlying neuronal cell death, and as a result are consistently demonstrated only in the late stages of the disease. Paralleling the development of new molecular markers for AD pathology in nuclear medicine are a number of encouraging results in the application of functional, perfusion, and diffusion imaging which point to a growing role for MR imaging in the evaluation of AD. This article surveys current research on the use of diffusion MR imaging for the evaluation of patients who have mild cognitive impairment and AD, and summarizes the important unifying results that are beginning to emerge on the potential role for diffusion imaging in practice.

In the brain, diffusion-weighted imaging (DWI) is an established and reliable method for the characterization of neurologic lesions. Although the diagnostic value of DWI in the early detection of ischemia has not diminished with time, many new clinical applications of DWI have also emerged. Diffusion-tensor imaging and fiber tractography have more recently been developed and optimized, allowing quantification of the magnitude and direction of diffusion along three principal eigenvectors. Diffusion-tensor imaging and fiber tractography are proving to be useful in clinical neuroradiology practice, with application to several categories of disease, and to be a powerful research tool. This article describes some of the applications of DWI and diffusion-tensor imaging in the evaluation of the diseases of the spinal cord.

Diffusion-weighted (DW) imaging provides a new contrast mechanism for evaluation of tumors of the chest, abdominal, and pelvis. By imaging microscopic motion of water molecules, DW imaging yields new qualitative and quantitative information about tumors that can be used to improve tumor detection, characterize some tumors, and monitor and predict response to treatment. DW imaging techniques provide a host of new tools for the body imager including: magnitude DW images; ADC maps with quantitative analysis; and volumetric display of data including whole body diffusion with background suppression. Experience with these DW techniques for body applications is still accumulating. However, DW imaging has already become an integral part of body MR imaging protocols at many centers.

Diffusion-weighted imaging is a noninvasive magnetic resonance technique that is capable of measuring icroscopic movement of water molecules (ie, random or Brownian motion) within biologic tissues. Diffusion weighting is achieved with a pulsed-field gradient that leaves "static" spins unaffected but causes dephasing of spin ensembles that experience different motion histories according to their diffusion paths, with respect to the direction of the gradient. This article focuses on the interesting opportunities of the use of diffusion weighted imaging in the diagnosis of musculoskeletal diseases, including trauma, tumor, and inflammation.

Quantitative analysis of dynamic contrast-enhanced MR imaging (DCE-MR imaging) has the power to provide information regarding physiologic characteristics of the microvasculature and is, therefore, of great potential value to the practice of oncology. In particular, these techniques could have a significant impact on the development of novel anticancer therapies as a promising biomarker of drug activity. Standardization of DCE-MR imaging acquisition and analysis to provide more reproducible measures of tumor vessel physiology is of crucial importance to realize this potential.

The purpose of this article is to review the pathophysiologic basis and technical aspects of DCE-MR imaging techniques.

Ashley D. Harris, Shelagh B. Coutts, and Richard Frayne

Diffusion and perfusion MR imaging have proven to be highly useful in the clinical description and understanding of acute and hyperacute ischemic stroke. In this article, the authors give a brief overview of the basic concepts of diffusion and perfusion imaging and describe some of the current developments, applications, challenges, and limitations of these techniques as applied to cerebral ischemia.

Jeffrey M. Pollock, Huan Tan, Robert A. Kraft, Christopher T. Whitlow, Jonathan H. Burdette, and Joseph A. Maldjian

Arterial spin labeling (ASL) imaging soon will be available as a routine clinical perfusion imaging sequence for a significant number of MR imaging scanners. The ASL perfusion technique offers information similar to that provided by conventional dynamic susceptibility sequences, but it does not require the use of an intravenous contrast agent, and the data can be quantified. The appearance of pathology is affected significantly by the ASL techniques used. Familiarity with the available sequence parameter options and the common appearances of pathology facilitates perfusion interpretation.

Richard Kinh Gian Do, Henry Rusinek, and Bachir Taouli

Dynamic contrast-enhanced magnetic resonance imaging (DCE-MR imaging) is emerging as a tool that can quantify changes in liver perfusion that occur in both diffuse and focal liver diseases. Recent data show promise for DCE-MR imaging of the liver in diagnosing fibrosis and cirrhosis before morphologic changes can be detected. It may also be valuable in the assessment of hepatocellular carcinoma and liver metastases. Acquisition parameters, postprocessing methods, applications, and recent results of DCE-MR imaging of the liver are also described. Finally, it reviews the limitations and future directions of DCE-MR imaging for liver applications.

Marianne Moon, Daniel Cornfeld, and Jeffrey Weinreb

This article discusses the basic principles of dynamic contrast-enhanced MR imaging (DCE-MR imaging) of the breast, including technical parameters, image acquisition, and image interpretation. Clinical DCE-MR imaging of the breast has undergone considerable growth from a once investigational technique to an important clinical tool in widespread use. Progress in MR technology and refinement of MR imaging parameters now allow for concurrent acquisition of high-spatial-resolution and adequate-temporal-resolution images, which are necessary for accurate assessment of breast lesion morphology and qualitative kinetic analysis. More advanced DCE-MR imaging techniques involving higher-temporal-resolution images and rigorous quantitative analysis of the time signal enhancement curves are currently an area of research.

Colm J. McMahon, B. Nicolas Bloch, Robert E. Lenkinski, and Neil M. Rofsky

Prostate cancer is a common tumor among men, with increasing diagnosis at an
earlier stage and a lower volume of disease because of screening with prostate-
specific antigen (PSA). The need for imaging of the prostate stems from a desire
to optimize treatment strategy on a patient and tumor-specific level. The major goals
of prostate imaging are (1) staging of known cancer, (2) determination of tumor aggressiveness, (3) diagnosis of cancer in patients who have elevated PSA but a negative biopsy, (4) treatment planning, and (5) the evaluation of therapy response. This
article concentrates on the role of dynamic contrast-enhanced MR imaging in the
evaluation of patients who have prostate cancer and how it might be used to help
achieve the above goals. Various dynamic contrast enhancement approaches
(quantitative/semiquantitative/qualitative, high temporal versus high spatial resolution) are summarized with reference to the relevant strengths and compromises of
each approach.

Magnetic Resonance Imaging Clinics of North America

THE CLINICS ARE NOW AVAILABLE ONLINE!

Access your subscription at:
www.theclinics.com

GOAL STATEMENT

The goal of *Magnetic Resonance Imaging Clinics of North America* is to keep practicing physicians up to date with current clinical practice by providing timely articles reviewing the state of the art in patient care.

ACCREDITATION

The *Magnetic Resonance Imaging Clinics of North America* is planned and implemented in accordance with the Essential Areas and Policies of the Accreditation Council for Continuing Medical Education (ACCME) through the joint sponsorship of the University of Virginia School of Medicine and Elsevier. The University of Virginia School of Medicine is accredited by the ACCME to provide continuing medical education for physicians.

The University of Virginia School of Medicine designates this educational activity for a maximum of 15 *AMA PRA Category 1 Credits*™. Physicians should only claim credit commensurate with the extent of their participation in the activity.

The American Medical Association has determined that physicians not licensed in the US who participate in this CME activity are eligible for 15 *AMA PRA Category 1 Credits*™.

Credit can be earned by reading the text material, taking the CME examination online at: http://www.theclinics.com/home/cme, and completing the evaluation. After taking the test, you will be required to review any and all incorrect answers. Following completion of the test and evaluation, your credit will be awarded and you may print your certificate.

FACULTY DISCLOSURE/CONFLICT OF INTEREST

The University of Virginia School of Medicine, as an ACCME accredited provider, endorses and strives to comply with the Accreditation Council for Continuing Medical Education (ACCME) Standards of Commercial Support, Commonwealth of Virginia statutes, University of Virginia policies and procedures, and associated federal and private regulations and guidelines on the need for disclosure and monitoring of proprietary and financial interests that may affect the scientific integrity and balance of content delivered in continuing medical education activities under our auspices.

The University of Virginia School of Medicine requires that all CME activities accredited through this institution be developed independently and be scientifically rigorous, balanced and objective in the presentation/discussion of its content, theories and practices.

All authors/editors participating in an accredited CME activity are expected to disclose to the readers relevant financial relationships with commercial entities occurring within the past 12 months (such as grants or research support, employee, consultant, stock holder, member of speakers bureau, etc.). The University of Virginia School of Medicine will employ appropriate mechanisms to resolve potential conflicts of interest to maintain the standards of fair and balanced education to the reader. Questions about specific strategies can be directed to the Office of Continuing Medical Education, University of Virginia School of Medicine, Charlottesville, Virginia.

The faculty and staff of the University of Virginia Office of Continuing Medical Education have no financial affiliations to disclose.

The authors/editors listed below have identified no professional or financial affiliations for themselves or their spouse/partner:
Roland Bammer, PhD; Jeffrey I. Berman, PhD; Daniel Cornfeld, MD; Shelagh B. Coutts, MBChB, MD, FRCPC; Richard Kinh Gian Do, MD, PhD; Eduard de Lange, MD (Test Author); Barton Dudlick (Acquisitions Editor); Richard Frayne, PhD; Ashley D. Harris, PhD; Christopher P. Hess, MD, PhD; Samantha J. Holdsworth, PhD; Robert A. Kraft, PhD; Robert E. Lenkinski, PhD; Joseph A. Maldjian, MD; Colm J. McMahon, MB; Marianne Moon, MD; Pratik Mukherjee, MD, PhD (Guest Editor); Michael J. Paldino, MD; Jeffrey M. Pollock, MD; Henry Rusinek, PhD; Stefan T. Skare, PhD; Huan Tan, MS; Majda M. Thurnher, MD; Markus Uhl, MD, PhD; Wouter B. Veldhuis, MD, PhD; Christopher T. Whitlow, MD, PhD, and Oliver Wieben, PhD.

The authors/editors listed below identified the following professional or financial affiliations for themselves or their spouse/partner:
Daniel P. Barboriak, MD is an industry funded research/investigator for Bristol-Meyers Squibb/Adnexus Therapeutics.
Thorsten Alexander Bley, MD serves on the Speakers Bureau for BRACCO, Bayer, Guerbet, and GE.
B. Nicholas Bloch, MD is a consultant for Medrad and Confirms.
Jonathan H. Burdette, MD serves on the Speakers Bureau for Bayer Healthcare Pharmaceuticals and is a consultant for Bracco Diagnostics Inc.
Meng Law, MD serves on the Speakers Bureau for Siemens Medical Solutions, owns stock in Prism Clinical Imaging, receives honoraria from Bayer Healthcare and Bracco Diagnostics, and has received a grant from Accelerate Brain Cancer Cure.
Russell N. Low, MD is a consultant for GE Medical.
Scott B. Reeder, MD, PhD (Guest Editor) receives research support from GE Healthcare and Bracco, serves on the Advisory Board for Bayer, and their spouse is employed by GE Healthcare.
Neil M. Rofsky, MD is an industry funded research/investigator for GE Healthcare, is a consultant for Epix Pharmaceuticals, and serves on the Advisory Committee for Bayer Pharmaceuticals.
Bachir Taouli, MD receives grant support from Radiological Society of North America and Bracco Diagnostics.
Jeffrey C. Weinreb, MD, FACR is an industry funded research/investigator and consultant for GE Healthcare and Bayer Pharmaceuticals and serves on the Speakers Bureau for GE Healthcare.

Disclosure of Discussion of non-FDA approved uses for pharmaceutical products and/or medical devices:
The University of Virginia School of Medicine, as an ACCME provider, requires that all faculty presenters identify and disclose any "off label" uses for pharmaceutical and medical device products. The University of Virginia School of Medicine recommends that each physician fully review all the available data on new products or procedures prior to instituting them with patients.

TO ENROLL

To enroll in the Magnetic Resonance Imaging Clinics of North America Continuing Medical Education program, call customer service at 1-800-654-2452 or visit us online at: www.theclinics.com/home/cme. The CME program is available to subscribers for an additional fee of $99.95.

Preface

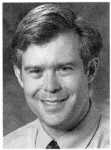

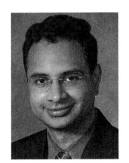

Scott B. Reeder, MD, PhD   Pratik Mukherjee, MD, PhD
Guest Editors

Conventional MR imaging of the brain and body has traditionally relied on standard contrast mechanisms, namely T1- and T2-weighted imaging. In the 1990s, the advent of contrast-enhanced imaging for advanced angiographic and perfusion-weighted imaging (PWI) led to the improved characterization of brain tumors and brain ischemia. During the early to mid 1990s, qualitative diffusion-weighted imaging (DWI) of the brain revolutionized the detection of acute ischemic stroke and the management of ischemic neurological disease.

In the first decade of the 21st century, these early DWI and PWI techniques have evolved into more advanced methodologies for clinical practice, such as diffusion tensor imaging (DTI), fiber tractography, and arterial spin labeled perfusion imaging. Furthermore, diffusion and perfusion imaging are not just for the brain anymore. Their use has exploded throughout the body, including new applications in the spinal cord, abdomen, breast, and musculoskeletal system.

In this issue of *Magnetic Resonance Imaging Clinics of North America*, we provide updates on traditional applications of diffusion and perfusion imaging to ischemic stroke and brain tumors. We also explore exciting new uses for the assessment of neurodegenerative disease, spinal cord pathology, breast tumors, liver disease, prostate cancer, whole-body metastatic disease and lymphadenopathy, and musculoskeletal disorders. The articles included in this issue have been written by leading experts in the field (including physicists and expert practitioners in neuroradiological, abdominal, breast, and musculoskeletal applications), who provide comprehensive layman explanations of advanced DWI and

PWI. It is our hope that this comprehensive body of work provides a state-of-the-art perspective on practical technical issues in DWI and PWI and new clinical applications.

Dr. Bammer and his team from Stanford University describe state-of-the-art methods in DWI and DTI, providing a comprehensive overview on the history of the development of DWI and its extension into quantitative applications. Dr. Berman from the University of California, San Francisco reviews the current methods using fiber tractography based on DTI and advanced high angular resolution diffusion imaging methods for the presurgical mapping of white matter tracts in brain tumor patients.

Dr. Hess from the University of California, San Francisco provides an overview of new findings using DTI to study Alzheimer's disease, an ever increasing public health problem in the 21st century. Then, Dr. Thurnher (of the Medical University of Vienna) and Dr. Law (of Mount Sinai Medical Center in New York) present new applications for DWI, DTI, and fiber tractography in the spinal cord: an exciting new frontier for neuroradiology.

Dr. Low from the Children's MRI Center in San Diego describes the use of DWI for whole body metastatic disease and the detection of lymphadenopathy. Dr. Bley from the University of Wisconsin describes the use of DWI for musculoskeletal applications, including examples in trauma, malignancies, and inflammatory conditions.

Switching the focus from DWI to PWI, Dr. Paladino and colleagues from Duke University provide an overview of the underlying mathematics behind quantitative perfusion weighted imaging, and how MR imaging can be used to extract

mri.theclinics.com

key parameters that describe, in a quantitative manner, the microvasculature of the various malignancies.

Dr. Harris and colleagues from the University of Calgary review the expanding uses of diffusion and perfusion imaging in acute ischemic stroke, and they include an update on recent multicenter clinical trials that use DWI and PWI to triage patients for experimental interventions. Dr. Pollock and the team at Wake Forest University report on the routine use of arterial spin labeled perfusion in a busy academic neuroradiologic practice, showing how this new technology can be helpful in evaluating a wide range of cerebrovascular and other neurological disorders.

Dr. Moon and his colleagues from Yale University review state-of-the-art methods in dynamic contrast imaging for the detection and characterization of breast tumors. Dr. Do and colleagues from New York University outline the current status of dynamic contrast-enhanced imaging in the liver for detection and characterization of liver tumors and the quantification of chronic liver disease and early stages of hepatic fibrosis. Finally, Dr. McMahon and colleagues from the Beth Israel-Deaconess Medical Center in Boston review the use of dynamic enhanced MR imaging in the evaluation of patients who have prostate cancer; they include an up-to-date review of the literature and the extensive experience of perfusion MR imaging in prostate cancer at the Beth Israel-Deaconess Medical Center.

We thank all of the authors for their excellent contributions, which make this issue an outstanding overview of state-of-the-art methods in diffusion and perfusion imaging. We also thank Barton Dudlick of Elsevier for his support. We hope that the readers of this issue find the material both interesting and worthwhile in their clinical practice.

Scott B. Reeder, MD, PhD
Departments of Radiology, Medical Physics,
Biomedical Engineering, and Medicine
University of Wisconsin
600 Highland Avenue, CSC E1/374
Madison, WI 53792, USA

Pratik Mukherjee, MD, PhD
Departments of Radiology and Bioengineering
University of California, San Francisco
San Francisco, CA, USA

E-mail addresses:
sreeder@uwhealth.org (S.B. Reeder)
pratik@radiology.ucsf.edu (P. Mukherjee)

New Methods in Diffusion-Weighted and Diffusion Tensor Imaging

Roland Bammer, PhD[a],*, Samantha J. Holdsworth, PhD[a],
Wouter B. Veldhuis, MD, PhD[b], Stefan T. Skare, PhD[a]

KEYWORDS

- Diffusion-weighted MR imaging
- Diffusion-weighted imaging
- Diffusion tensor imaging • Parallel imaging
- Diffusion-weighted whole-body imaging with background body signal suppression
- Whole-body diffusion imaging

During the past decade, diffusion-weighted imaging (DWI) has matured into a powerful and extensively used diagnostic tool and has entered the diagnostic arena mostly because of its superb sensitivity to ischemic stroke[1] during the early time window when other magnetic resonance (MR) methods and CT are still negative.[2] DWI relies on using the biophysical property of proton (self-) diffusion as a contrast-determining parameter in an MR imaging experiment. Because of the presence of restricting cellular structures, diffusion in biologic tissue is often anisotropic. That is, the diffusion coefficient is different when measured along different directions; for example, in white matter, diffusion is higher along fibers and is lower perpendicular to fibers. Thus, anisotropic diffusion can be used as a sensitive proxy measure for structural integrity of the underlying neural tissue and for noninvasive neuronal tract tracing. In muscle fibers, for example, diffusion anisotropy can be used to determine the pennation angle of muscle fibers (ie, the angle formed by the individual muscle fibers with the line of action of the muscle), allowing one to investigate biomechanical properties of muscles.

Advancements in DWI, such as q-space imaging[3] and, most importantly, diffusion tensor imaging (DTI),[4] have demonstrated great utility in furthering the diagnostic potential of MR imaging to reveal tissue features otherwise occult to conventional MR imaging; even simple variants to DWI, such as diffusion-weighted whole-body imaging with background body signal suppression (DWIBS),[5] have opened new perspectives on how DWI can be used beyond the workup on stroke.

DWI and its variants are still poised with major challenges when it comes to resolution, distortion, and operation at higher magnetic field strengths, however. The problems arise from the continued dependence on rapid single-shot echo-planar imaging (ssEPI) and DWI's motion sensitivity. In this article, the authors attempt to provide a brief overview of these challenges.

Financial support for this study was provided by the National Institutes of Health (grants 2R01EB002711, 1R01EB008706, 1R21EB006860, and P41RR09784) and the Dutch Cancer Society.

[a] Department of Radiology, Stanford University, 1201 Welch Road, Lucas Center, PS08, Stanford, CA 94305–5488, USA

[b] Department of Radiology, University Medical Center Utrecht, Room E01.132, P.O. Box 85500, 3508 GA Utrecht, The Netherlands

* Corresponding author.

E-mail address: rbammer@stanford.edu (R. Bammer).

Magn Reson Imaging Clin N Am 17 (2009) 175–204
doi:10.1016/j.mric.2009.01.011

BASIC PRINCIPLES

Diffusion is generally a three-dimensional (3D) phenomenon and can vary in magnitude depending on the direction along which it is measured. The effect of molecular diffusion in an MR experiment was first described by Torrey,[6] who noted that in the presence of a diffusive spin movement in a strong magnetic gradient field, the signal becomes attenuated. In DWI, a spin-echo sequence is generally used with a pair of strong diffusion-weighting gradients straddling the 180° refocusing pulse (Fig. 1). This sequence is known as Stejskal-Tanner pulse sequence.[7] The degree of attenuation depends on the strength (G_{Diff}) and duration (δ) of the diffusion-encoding gradients, the spacing between these gradients (Δ), the apparent diffusion coefficient (ADC), and the gyromagnetic ratio (γ) (eg, implying that hyperpolarized xenon gas experiences less attenuation from diffusion than protons because of its lower γ value). Increases in any of those parameters lead to a reduction in the MR signal intensity. The diffusion-weighting applied is represented by the diffusion attenuation factor or simply the b-value:

$$b = \gamma^2 G_{Diff^2} \delta^2 (\Delta - \delta/3) \tag{1}$$

so that the signal equation of a diffusion-weighted sequence becomes:

$$M(b) = M_0 \exp(-bADC) \tag{2}$$

where M_0 is the spin-echo signal (including proton density or any T_1/T_2 relaxation) in the absence of any diffusion weighting.

From phase-contrast MR imaging, many readers are probably familiar with the phase accrual that occurs when spins are moving along a magnetic field gradient, and might thus wonder why there is no net phase accrual associated with the diffusion process. Such phase does accumulate in spin ensembles with bulk motion, but diffusion is a random process without any coherent motion; thus, the phase accrual takes place on a per-spin basis. In other words, each diffusing spin follows its own random pathway and accrues its own phase. For an ensemble of spins, the probability displacement function (PDF) has a Gaussian distribution, and so is the PDF for the phase. Thus, when summed over all spins within a voxel, all these individual phases integrate to a net attenuation of the signal without a net phase accrual measurable to the outside world. However, in vivo examinations are frequently corrupted with bulk motion, which, unlike diffusion, is coherent and leads to unpredictable phase terms that have challenged investigators for a long time.

In pure water or cerebrospinal fluid, diffusion is unrestricted and the measured diffusion constant is independent of the direction along which the ADC was measured. If diffusion is isotropic, there is no preferred direction of water motion for these tissues. However, as mentioned previously, diffusion can be directionally dependent in biologic tissues. The directionality of diffusion is introduced because water movement in and around cellular structures is not "free" as it is in a bulk fluid; it is restricted as it comes into contact with cell membranes and other large structures. This directional dependence (ie, diffusion anisotropy) is the hallmark of another underlying diagnostic feature of DWI. It was Basser and his coworkers[4,8] who recognized that the anisotropy of measured diffusivity in tissue at each point in space ($r = [x\ y\ z]^T$) should be modeled as a second-order tensor:

$$\underline{\underline{D}}(r) = \begin{pmatrix} D(r)_{xx} & D(r)_{xy} & D(r)_{xz} \\ D(r)_{yx} & D(r)_{yy} & D(r)_{yz} \\ D(r)_{zx} & D(r)_{zy} & D(r)_{zz} \end{pmatrix} \tag{3}$$

and devised a data acquisition scheme that goes along with it. Because the diffusion tensor is symmetric (ie, $D_{ij} = D_{ji}$), only six unknown elements need to be determined in each voxel. Specifically, a diffusion tensor MR imaging (DTI) experiment in which these elements are determined on a per-pixel basis consists of acquiring a series of DWI scans, each with gradients applied along a different direction. Specifically, to estimate the tensor requires the acquisition of at least six DWI scans, together with a non–diffusion-weighted image for reference. In practice, to improve to estimation of the diffusion tensor, many more than six directions are often acquired, with the diffusion directions spread isotropically over a sphere (Fig. 2). Although this process seems intuitively trivial, this so-called "tessellation" process is

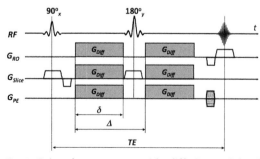

Fig. 1. Spin-echo sequence with diffusion-weighted gradients (G_{Diff}); also known as a Stejskal-Tanner sequence. TE, echo time.

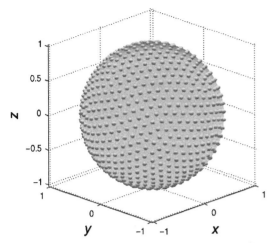

Fig. 2. Isotropic distribution of 256 diffusion-encoding directions over a sphere. Each bump on the sphere represents the point at which the diffusion-encoding vector (starting at the origin) penetrates the isosphere.

mathematically challenging.[9,10] Because any extra encoding direction adds extra time, a tradeoff is often sought between the optimum number of directions and acceptable scan time. A few tens of directions already improve the image quality of the tensor estimations and avoid orientational bias.[11] If one chooses just a minimum of six directions, care must be taken that these directions are noncollinear.

The directionality of diffusion is performed by combining the x, y, and z magnetic field gradients such that the superposition of these individual gradients leads to a net field gradient along the direction vector defined by $\mathbf{g}_{Diff} = [G_{Diff,x}\ G_{Diff,y}\ G_{Diff,z}]^T$, where $G_{Diff,i}$ ($i = x, y, z$) is the gradient strength applied along the principal direction. Assuming the aforementioned diffusion tensor model, for a particular diffusion-encoding direction, $\mathbf{g}_{Diff}$, Eq. 2 can be modified accordingly:

$$M(\underline{b}) = M_0 \exp\left[-\int_0^{TE} \mathbf{k}^T(t)\,\underline{\underline{D}}\,\mathbf{k}(t)\,dt\right] \tag{4}$$

$$= M_0 \exp(\underline{b}\ \underline{D})$$

with

$$\mathbf{k}(t) = \gamma \int_0^t \mathbf{g}_{Diff}(\tau)\,d\tau \tag{5}$$

From the six or more DWI scans acquired with the diffusion encoding along different gradient directions, the elements of $\underline{\underline{D}}\,(r)$ can be calculated by simple regression analysis.[4] Because it is normally sufficient to use a single directional DWI measurement (or, at most, three measurements along orthogonal directions to avoid confounding

signal nonuniformities from anisotropic structures) to identify regions of reduced ADC in patients who have acute stroke, one might wonder about the utility of measuring the entire tensor. By making an extra effort to measure all elements of the tensor, one can derive certain properties in each voxel, such as the extent of diffusion anisotropy or the direction in which the diffusion is highest.

To be able to interpret the tensor information, it is necessary to break down this information into single-valued measures that can be viewed as gray-scale maps readable to the radiologist. To calculate these measures, the diffusion tensor, $\underline{\underline{D}}$, is first diagonalized, which is a standard mathematic matrix operation that rotates the coordinate frame of reference independently, pixel-by-pixel, into the principal axes of the tensor. By doing so, the so-called "eigenvalues" λ_1, λ_2, and λ_3 and the orientation of the diffusion tensor are explicitly obtained by the so-called "eigenvectors" $\mathbf{e}_1$, $\mathbf{e}_2$, and $\mathbf{e}_3$. The mean diffusivity is then calculated by:

$$\langle D \rangle = (\lambda_1 + \lambda_2 + \lambda_3/3) \tag{6}$$

where the numerator of Eq. 6 is the "trace" of the matrix $\underline{\underline{D}}$ and the relative diffusion anisotropy (RA) is expressed as:

$$RA = \frac{\sigma(\lambda_1 + \lambda_2 + \lambda_3)}{\langle D \rangle} \tag{7}$$

which is the standard deviation of the eigenvalues divided by their mean. Alternatively, RA can be seen as relating the magnitude of the anisotropic portion of the tensor to the magnitude of the isotropic portion of $\underline{\underline{D}}$. Note that the eigenvectors provide information about direction of the maximum diffusion within a voxel on which fiber tracking[12,13] builds. There are other rotationally invariant scalar metrics that describe the diffusion anisotropy, most of which have different sensitivity to different ranges of diffusion anisotropy. Here, "rotationally invariant" refers to the property that such measures are independent of the orientation of the diffusion tensor. The most commonly used measure for diffusion anisotropy is fractional anisotropy (FA):

$$FA = \sqrt{\frac{1}{2}}\,\frac{\sqrt{(\lambda_1 - \lambda_2)^2 + (\lambda_2 - \lambda_3)^2 + (\lambda_3 - \lambda_1)^2}}{\sqrt{\lambda_1^2 + \lambda_2^2 + \lambda_3^2}} \tag{8}$$

where FA measures the fraction of the magnitude of $\underline{\underline{D}}$ that is anisotropic by looking at the ratio between the magnitude of the deviatoric tensor, $\underline{\underline{D}} = D - <D>$, and the full tensor.

Although the second-order diffusion tensor model served us well for almost 10 years, alternative models have become increasingly popular. Most of them address the fact that in biologic tissue, a complex interplay between different compartments and structures inside a voxel poses different amounts of hindrance to the diffusing spins. Although the second-order tensor is often illustrated as an ellipsoid (ie, the surface of the ellipsoid depicts the displacement front of protons), the true representation for a high-angular diffusion experiment, in which diffusion is measured along many directions in space, rather resembles a more wrinkled structure.

High-angular resolution diffusion-weighted imaging (HARDI)[14,15] was one of the first attempts to tackle the problem of the more complex diffusive spin displacement. Here, the 3D structure spanned by the ADC measurements was decomposed along different directions into 3D basis functions (so-called "spherical harmonics"). However, by applying directional ADC measurements, an underlying Gaussian spin displacement PDF was inherently assumed.

In fact, the complex interplay of countless structures within in a voxel renders the true spin displacement PDF to be a non-Gaussian distribution, and it may not even be symmetric. To measure the PDF or a "diffraction pattern," Callaghan and his coworkers[3,16] introduced the concept of q-space imaging. This required extremely short and strong gradients only available on small-bore experimental systems. Nevertheless, Callaghan's method was adapted for the use in neuronal tissue[17] and in vivo.[18] Realizing that the spin displacement PDF in vivo requires measurements along many directions and at many different b-values, Wedeen and colleagues[19,20] proposed a scheme to obtain an approximate measurement of the 3D displacement PDF in each voxel, known as diffusion spectrum imaging, which was then further approximated and compacted by Tuch[21] with the introduction of Q-ball imaging.

After the authors' initial discussion about how a Gaussian spin displacement PDF leads to an attenuation of the signal (and a second-order tensor) when averaged over the entire spin ensemble, the "DWI-connoisseur" should realize that for non-Gaussian PDFs, the ensemble average leads to signal contributions that can be expressed by higher order tensors (**Fig. 3**).[22] In fact, if the spin displacement PDF is asymmetric, additional phase terms exist.[22]

CURRENT PROBLEMS IN DIFFUSION-WEIGHTED MR IMAGING
Problems with Motion-induced Phase Errors

One of the greatest technical challenges for DWI is overcoming the phase effects originating from coherent macroscopic or bulk motion, although retaining its sensitivity to microscopic motion. To create diffusion-dependent contrast, DWI pulse sequences must be sensitive to incoherent molecular motion on the order of a few microns. The price for the sensitivity to motion on this microscopic scale is that even extremely small (submillimeter) displacements of tissue during the diffusion-encoding period cause signal loss and large phase changes in the resulting echo signal. The two major sources of bulk motion are (1) periodic tissue motion caused by cardiac pulsatility and (2) patient movement. Because coherent motion on this level is likely to be different during each echo acquisition, the phase of the echo in a standard spin-warp acquisition is perturbed differently and in an unpredictable fashion, ultimately leading to devastating ghosting artifacts in the final images. The additional phase impressed on the spins also challenges the phase requirements between transverse magnetization and radiofrequency (RF) pulses for fast spin-echo (FSE). For this reason, single-shot methods, such as ssEPI, must be used to avoid the phase variation from shot to shot that can cause ghost artifacts.

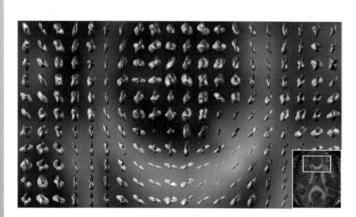

Fig. 3. Zoomed glyph visualization of spin displacement isospheres (minus isotropic component) derived from higher order diffusion tensors from a human volunteer brain (box in insert). For better contrast, a FA map is plotted underneath. Clearly, the isospheres deviate from the typically seen diffusion ellipsoids, which is most prominent in regions of merging or crossing fiber tracts.

Influence of phase errors on spatial encoding

As mentioned previously, coherent motion in the tissue sample during the diffusion preparation time leads to through-plane signal dephasing and leaves localized phase on the object being imaged before the image readout module. Even in cooperative patients, peristalsis, respiratory motion, and pulsatile flow[23,24] confound diffusion imaging and most likely corrupt image quality. To address this issue, the diffusion-weighted images are often acquired with cardiac triggering (ie, synchronized with the heart rate measured with electrocardiography or simply by a plethysmograph on a finger). In this way, imaging can be synchronized with the cardiac cycle and imaging during systole (during which motion is usually highest) can be avoided. However, this prospective triggering approach considerably cuts down the scan efficiency, because when the heart rate goes up, the quiescent time available for scanning decreases. Respiratory motion during DWI can be even more problematic, especially for body applications. In the authors' practice, breath-hold studies have proved reliable for most DWI studies outside the central nervous system (CNS).[25] In kidney studies, in which a large craniocaudal movement of the kidneys over the respiration period can be observed, breath-hold experiments are extremely useful. **Fig. 4** shows an example of such a study in a patient who has obstructive kidney disease. The tumor mass led to critically low blood flow to the kidney, as indicated by corresponding magnetic resonance angiography (MRA). The ADC reduction in the ischemic kidney was dramatic and, to the authors' knowledge, rather uncommon for tissue outside the CNS. This case suggests that DWI and ADC measurements might become useful in obstructive kidney disease to differentiate between benign renal oligemia and renal ischemia. In this context, the authors also found that ADC values correlate well with the creatinine level (**Fig. 5**).[26]

Although the through-plane dephasing results in an overall loss of signal, and thus in abnormally high ADC values, the additional spatially nonlinear phase imparted by motion conflicts with the phase terms impressed on the transverse magnetization from regular image encoding and leads to considerable ghosting artifacts if not corrected.

Before the discussion on the phase error problem for image encoding is continued, it is important to mention two other issues that need to be considered when applying DWI outside the CNS. These challenges include the presence of lipids within the tissue (eg, liver, vertebral bodies, breast) and blood flow. First, although lipids are normally suppressed to avoid large chemical shift artifacts, the presence of lipids changes with age (eg, breast, vertebral bodies) and disease (eg, metastatic infiltration, steatosis). Although lipid suppression or water-only excitation suppresses the signal of lipids, the presence of the rather rigid lipid molecules presents more or less hindrance to the diffusing water protons, and thus indirectly confounds ADC measurements. Second, although intravoxel incoherent motion was initially used for blood flow measurements, the blood volume in brain tissue is only 2% to 4%; thus, the contamination from flow on the diffusion attenuation curve (ie, MR signal over *b*-value) is rather small. However, the blood volume in other organs, such as the kidneys, can be much higher. Instead of using a b = 0 s/mm^2 scan as reference, it is often advisable to use a small *b*-value (eg, ~50 s/mm^2) as a reference point to avoid overestimating the ADC or make ADC measurements confounded by blood flow. Now, let us return to the phase problems.

In DWI, unless single-shot methods are used, k-space data are normally acquired line-by-line, or by a subset of lines after a Stejskal-Tanner diffusion preparation period. Several acquisitions ("multishot") are therefore required to form a fully encoded image. As patient physiologic and bulk motion changes from one preparation period to the next in an unpredictable fashion, so do the additional phase terms imparted on spins.[27,28] As a first-order approximation, we can assume the phase errors are only of zeroth and first order in the image domain (that is, they are constant and linear). This shifts the desired k-space trajectory by δk_x and δk_y and adds a constant phase, $\delta\varphi$, each of which differs from shot to shot (**Fig. 6**). Unaware of these additional changes to the k-space trajectory, the MR scanner incorrectly stores the acquired MR data in an equidistant data matrix for final image reconstruction; therefore, strong ghosting artifacts appear, which often render the resulting image nondiagnostic.

For single-shot examinations, these k-space shifts exist as well, but the entire trajectory itself is shifted and the k-space sampling remains consistent (ie, the originally prescribed sampling density remains; see **Fig. 6**C). However, in order to perform signal averaging or averaging over diffusion directions, magnitude images must be used (ie, the image phase needs to be cleared) unless one performs phase correction. This is because each single-shot image has its own unique phase impressed; therefore, complex averaging, normally used in MR imaging, would lead to destructive interferences in the averaged image (**Fig. 7**). Although a constant and linear phase error model can be used as a relatively good

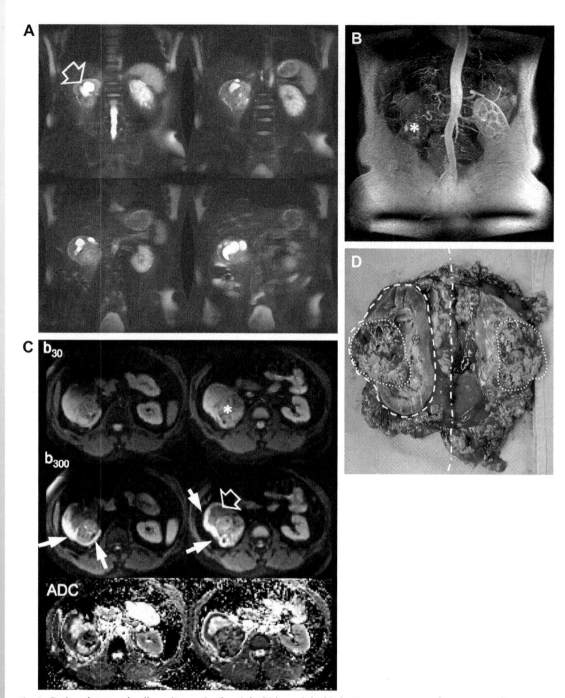

Fig. 4. Patient has renal cell carcinoma in the right kidney. (*A*) This lesion causes a significant mass effect on the adjacent renal pelvis, with resultant right-sided hydronephrosis on half-Fourier acquisition single-shot turbo spin-echo scans (*open arrow*). (*B*) Contrast-enhanced MRA (maximum intensity projection) shows that the right kidney is heavily hypoperfused. The mass (*) displaces and compresses the right renal pelvis. (*C*) Right kidney appears extremely hyperintense on the high–b-value DWI scan. The corresponding ADC values were significantly depleted (~30%–50% compared with normal tissue) (*white arrows*), which is indicative of ischemic tissue. Conversely, the hydronephrosis (*open arrow*) in this patient is characterized by an elevated ADC. The renal cell carcinoma appeared heterogeneous on ADC maps. (*D*) Kidney was surgically removed immediately after MR imaging. The specimen was cut apart in the midsagittal plane of the kidney (*dashed-dotted line*). The dashed line shows the contour of the kidney. The dotted line outlines the tumor.

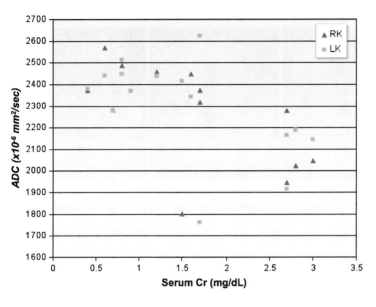

Fig. 5. Scatter-plot demonstrates the relation between serum creatinine (Cr) levels and renal ADC. Patients with elevated serum Cr have statistically significant lower renal ADCs. Two patients had unilateral renal disease, which was reflected as markedly decreased ADCs on the affected side, despite only borderline elevation of Cr and normal contralateral renal ADCs. Overall, there was a striking difference in ADCs between normal and compromised kidneys in patients who had unilateral renal disease. This technique has great potential for the evaluation of patients who have renal disease, particularly those who have unilateral disease, such as renal artery stenosis and congenital hydronephrosis, which may not be reflected in cruder measures of renal function, such as serum Cr. LK, left kidney; RK, right kidney.

approximation for the phase error problem in DWI, it is shown elsewhere in this article that a nonlinear spatial phase error model best characterizes the real situation.

Problems with violating the meiboom-gill condition in fast spin-echo

The extra phase impressed on the spins also has considerable implications on how RF pulses can be used after diffusion-contrast preparation. In particular, the authors are concerned about the spin phase relative to the RF phase of FSE refocusing pulses. FSE has become the "workhorse" for routine clinical MR imaging because of its speed, high signal-to-noise ratio (SNR), and reliability. FSE is robust, and artifacts are uncommon with this sequence. FSE often works well when many other sequences fail. However, for RF pulses in the FSE train with a poor slice profile (which produces flip angles between 0° and the nominal flip angle [180°] in the slopes of the slice profile), or when the refocusing flip angles are intentionally set below 180° (in an effort to minimize the power deposition in the subject), image artifacts can develop in cases when the transverse magnetization is not aligned with the RF axis of the FSE readout pulses.

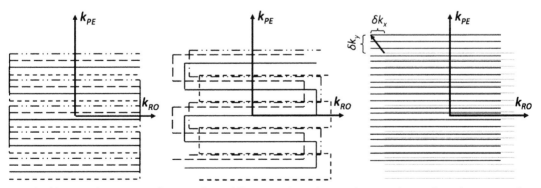

Fig. 6. (*Left*) Desired trajectory of an interleaved (four interleaves) EPI trajectory. The random phase errors from motion during diffusion-encoding produces linear phase error terms in the image domain. These can be measured with navigator methods. In the k-space domain, these linear phase errors are represented as additional shifts of the desired interleaves along k_x and k_y. (*Center*) Thus, the true interleaves are no longer situated on an equidistant grid. They are located at arbitrary positions requiring a regridding procedure onto a Cartesian grid or a discrete fourier transform-based reconstruction. (*Right*) ssEPI also experiences shifts (δk_x, δk_y), but these are the same for each line in k-space. Therefore, they do not cause ghosting artifacts. k_{PE}; phase encode direction, k_{RO}; readout direction.

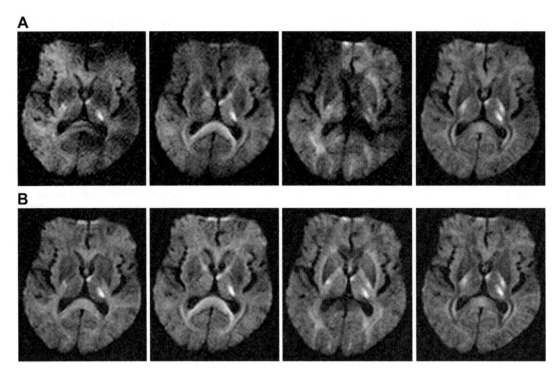

Fig. 7. (A) Conventional complex signal averaging performed in k-space using ssEPI data with diffusion weighting applied in four different diffusion-encoding directions (from left to right). The phase error for each shot leads to destructive interferences in the averaged images. (B) Averaging of the magnitude images removes the destructive interferences.

These artifacts occur because FSE relies on the amplitude stability of the Carr-Purcell-Meiboom-Gill (CPMG) sequence, which depends on the Meiboom-Gill (MG) phase condition.[29] That is, for an FSE experiment with an interecho time D, the MG condition requires the transverse magnetization at a time D/2 before the first refocusing pulse to be parallel or antiparallel to the orientation of the subsequent refocusing pulses. If, at D/2 before the FSE readout, the magnetization is 90° from the MG phase (non-MG), the emanating signal decays in amplitude and oscillates over the echo train. Thus, motion in combination with diffusion encoding might produce any phase at point D/2 with unknown amounts of the MG and the non-MG components (Fig. 8). The superposition of both components leads to unwanted fluctuation in the magnitude of the echoes within the FSE train. Each echo also incurs an additional phase term, determined by the MG and non-MG components, that competes with the desired phase encoding. As a result, diffusion preparation and FSE readouts have sometimes been deemed incompatible. Nevertheless, early on, the use of extra crusher gradients has been proposed with the intention to eliminate all but the primary refocused echo component,[30,31] because the challenges with the non-MG component develop from higher order echoes and stimulated echoes. Unfortunately, these schemes require large crusher amplitudes that increase linearly with echo number. The added time required to apply the crusher gradients generally becomes prohibitively long after only a handful of echoes. Moreover, spoiling of the CPMG sequence in this way also causes the echo amplitudes to decrease rapidly with echo number, which increases image blurring (note that much of the signal in FSE is actually from higher order echoes and stimulated echoes). In one of the following sections of this article, two avenues are discussed that allow DWI to be combined with FSE readouts.

Problems with Echo-Planar Imaging

In the previous section, it was mentioned that single-shot trajectories are relatively immune against phase errors, and therefore minimize or even entirely avoid "ghosting artifacts." For that reason, they have been established as the backbone sequences for DWI. In particular, ssEPI[32] and spiral imaging[33–36] (Fig. 9) have been used quite extensively. Until recently, single-shot imaging techniques (especially ssEPI) were almost

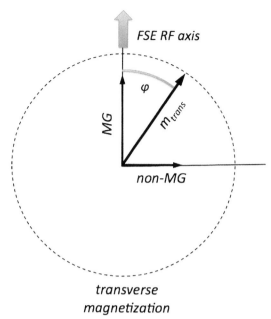

Fig. 8. Transverse magnetization after diffusion preparation demonstrates an unpredictable phase ϕ relative to the phase of the subsequent FSE refocusing pulses. The component of the transverse magnetization that is normal to the RF phase of the FSE pulses is called the non–Meiboom-Gill (MG) component and causes artifacts, whereas the component parallel or antiparallel to the FSE pulse is the "good" or MG component.

exclusively used in the clinical routine. Of particular relevance here is not only ssEPI's robustness against phase perturbations but its extremely fast (for MR standards) image formation capability. For example, using ssEPI, each image is acquired within the time frame of 0.1 second. This is especially advantageous when thousands of images need to be acquired for DTI or for even more complex acquisition schemes (eg, generalized diffusion tensor imaging,[37,38] HARDI,[14,15,39] q-space[3,17,21,40]) or for data acquisitions requiring completion within less than 20-25 seconds (eg, breath-hold examinations).

However, EPI has its own challenges. EPI is limited to low spatial resolution ($\sim 128 \times 128$) and has effects, such as image blurring, localized signal loss, and image distortions.[41] Image blurring occurs because of the T_2^*-based weighting of k-space data around the spin-echo, which becomes increasingly pronounced for short T_2^* tissues or in poorly shimmed regions. Geometric distortions and signal loss occur predominantly at boundaries between tissue and air because of the local susceptibility differences that lead to an inhomogeneous magnetic field. Over small regions, these field changes act as local gradients that

compete with the relatively weak spatial-encoding gradients along the phase encode dimension (**Fig. 10**). The extent of these distortions depends on hardware and on how quickly k-space is traversed along the phase encode dimension, because distortions and blurring are proportional to the k-space velocity, $v_{ky} = dk_y/dt$. With increasing field strength, these artifacts become more pronounced (**Fig. 11**). Two ssEPI acquisitions can be used, with one acquisition traversing k-space in the opposite direction along the phase encode direction. This enables one to process a distortion field and compute a less distorted image.[42,43]

Another effect that impairs image quality in DWI acquired using EPI is the distortions caused by eddy currents. Eddy currents are unwanted currents in conducting elements of the MR machine counteracting the rapid switching of the strong and lengthy diffusion-encoding gradients. Depending on the direction along which the diffusion-encoding gradient was applied, the local field changes induced by these eddy currents cause the images to be hampered by shearing, scaling, translation, or a combination thereof. The net consequence is that individual diffusion-weighted images are misregistered with each other. This is particularly challenging when diffusion tensor information must be processed on a per-pixel basis. It often causes scalar maps, such as the diffusion anisotropy, to have errors (**Fig. 12**).

Because the *b*-value increases quadratically with the gradient strength, more than one gradient axis is often applied simultaneously to boost the net diffusion-encoding gradient for a given echo time. An effective encoding scheme is tetrahedral encoding, which uses four encoding directions ($g_1 = [G_x\ G_y\ G_z]^T$, $g_2 = [-G_x\ G_y\ G_z]^T$, $g_3 = [G_x\ -G_y\ G_z]^T$, and $g_4 = [G_x\ G_y\ -G_z]^T$). Here, all three gradient axes are turned on simultaneously, leading to an effective gradient that is $\sqrt{3}G_i$ ($i = x, y, z$). This scheme has proved useful to compute isotropically diffusion-weighted images with little extra time but much improved SNR compared with scans with encoding applied just along the principal gradient direction (ie, along x, y, and z). However, because more effective gradients are involved, tetrahedral encoding usually demonstrates more eddy current effects than unidirectional encoding. Thus, when DWI scans with diffusion encoding along different directions are combined to compute an isotropically diffusion-weighted image, the resultant image is blurred if the eddy current-induced distortions are not compensated for. Thus, an anatomically consistent DTI data set and derivations thereof (eg, <D>, RA) and a sharp isotropically diffusion-weighted image require examinations in which the

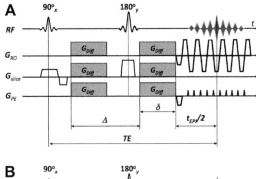

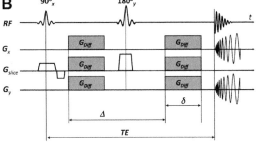

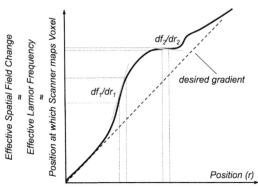

Fig. 10. With EPI, the relatively weak net gradients applied along the phase-encode direction are offset by local field changes because of susceptibility gradients of comparable magnitude. Thus, the effective field deviates from the desired linear change put on by the gradient. Local gradients are stronger (df_1/dr_1) or weaker (df_2/dr_2) than the desired gradient, leading to stretched and compressed mapping of voxels, respectively.

Fig. 9. (A) Diffusion-weighted spin-echo sequence with an EPI readout. Note that the EPI readout shown here is simplified. Typically, many more echoes are acquired for an ssEPI scan. G_{PE}, gradient in the phase encode direction; G_{RO}, gradient in the readout direction; G_{slice}, gradient in the slice select direction; t_{EPI}, duration of the EPI readout train; TE, echo time. (B) Diffusion-weighted spiral sequence.

effects from eddy currents are minimized. This can be achieved by specific modifications to the standard DWI pulse sequence (eg, by means of a dual–spin-echo preparation;[44] Fig. 13) or by registration-based postprocessing solutions.[27,45–47] Notice that with the dual–spin-echo preparation, the minimum echo time (TE) increases (and thus

SNR decreases), because a second 180° refocusing pulse is added to the sequence. The exact duration of the four diffusion gradient lobes depends on the time constants of the eddy currents[44] but can be set once by a service procedure.

NEW PRACTICAL CONCEPTS FOR DIFFUSION–WEIGHTED MR IMAGING
New Sampling Strategies to Improve Diffusion-Weighted Imaging

Parallel imaging
With the recent introduction of parallel imaging,[48–50] the quality of EPI scans in terms of reduced blurring and geometric distortions can be significantly

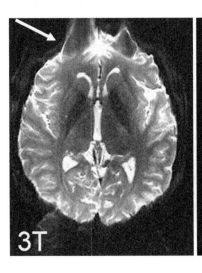

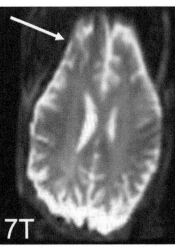

Fig. 11. Example for characteristic distortions (arrow) seen with ssEPI in adult volunteers at 3 T (left) and at 7 T (right).

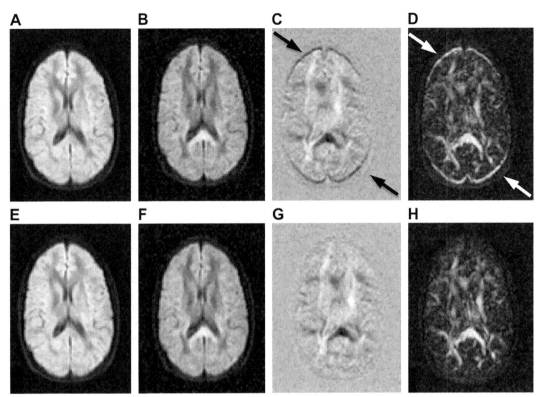

Fig. 12. Images before eddy current distortion correction (*A–D*) and images after correction (*E–H*). The reference image is the average over all diffusion-weighted images (*A, E*), distorted diffusion-weighted image before correction (*B*) and afterward (*F*), and difference between images *A* and *B* (*C*); the spatial distortion is seen best around the frontal and posterior cortex (*arrows*). (*D*) This is also seen in a map of pixel standard deviation over all diffusion-weighted images as a surrogate measure for diffusion anisotropy. After distortion correction, the difference image between images *E* and *F* (*G*) and the standard deviation map (*H*) demonstrate that the distortions from eddy currents can be removed.

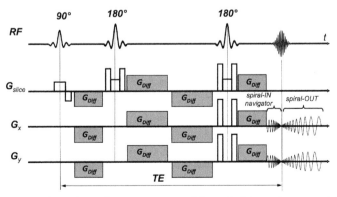

Fig. 13. Diffusion-weighed interleaved spiral-OUT sequence with a spiral-IN navigator and dual spin-echo preparation. More aggressive crusher gradients are used for the second 180° refocusing pulse to destroy the influence from stimulated echoes on the b = 0 scans. The timing of the diffusion-encoding gradient lobes depends on the time constants of the most problematic eddy currents. The dual spin-echo preparation offers almost the same diffusion attenuation (ignoring the time for the extra 180° pulse) as conventional Stejskal-Tanner preparation but has considerably diminished eddy currents because of the opposing polarity of successive diffusion gradient lobes. The eddy current reduction is of importance mostly for EPI and spiral sequences but should not underestimated for FSE. TE, echo time.

improved.[51,52] In addition to conventional gradient encoding to form an MR image, parallel imaging capitalizes on the distinct sensitivities of individual elements of receiver coil arrays that allow one to sample k-space more sparsely, and thus more quickly. The acceleration of k-space traversal along the phase encode dimension, and therefore the distortion and blurring reduction, is directly related to the reduction factor, R, used in parallel imaging (Fig. 14). Here, R is the ratio between the number of phase-encoding steps in the normally encoded image and the number of phase-encoding steps used in a parallel imaging examination.

Because fewer phase-encode lines are acquired in parallel imaging, parallel imaging-enhanced scans come with a SNR penalty that is proportional to $\sqrt{R}$ plus an extra geometry-related factor,[48] which depends on the number, size, and orientation of the individual receiver coils of the array relative to the prescribed field of view (FOV). Because of the geometry factor, or "g" factor, the SNR becomes spatially varying. Moreover, with increasing R, the chances increase for residual aliasing artifacts and excessive local SNR enhancement. The extent to which this occurs depends on the individual design of the array coil. Some of the SNR penalty of parallel imaging-enhanced diffusion-weighted EPI is compensated for by the shortened EPI train, which, in turn, affords a shorter echo time and less T_2-related signal loss.[53] Because of EPI's fast acquisition capacity, the remaining SNR loss can be regained by adding extra averages. Note that parallel imaging-enhanced DWI scans also demonstrate much less T2 shine-through effect than regular DWI scans. This is useful for identifying acute stroke lesions among preexisting subacute lesions. Subacute lesions become less conspicuous than with conventional EPI but, overall, in a recent study performed at the authors' institution in 40 patients, a clear preference for the use of parallel imaging in concert with parallel imaging was demonstrated (Fig. 15).

Parallel imaging reconstruction can be performed in the image domain (eg, sensitivity encoding[48]), in the k-space domain (eg, generalized autocalibrating partially parallel acquisitions [GRAPPA][49]), or in the hybrid domain (eg, autocalibrating reconstruction for cartesian imaging[54,55]). Initially, the authors started their parallel imaging efforts for DWI with sensitivity encoding; however, lately, their group has switched to a hybrid domain approach,[54] mainly because the hybrid approach and GRAPPA have more benign residual reconstruction artifacts, are more robust against motion, and are more compatible with partial Fourier reconstruction.[56] Initially, a variable-density k-space EPI sampling scheme was acquired to provide the intrinsic calibration information required for GRAPPA,[49] with the region around the center of k-space sampled at the Nyquist sampling rate. However, as discussed in the previous section geometric distortions in EPI depend on the v_{ky}. Thus, with a variable-density sampling scheme, different regions of k-space would contribute different amounts of distortion depending on their local v_{ky}. That is, around the center of k-space, wherein data are sampled at the Nyquist rate (ie, without any acceleration), a low spatial frequency image component with distortions equal to a normal EPI acquisition is formed, whereas a high spatial frequency image component is generated from the accelerated outer portion of k-space with considerably less distortion (Fig. 16). To avoid this artifact, it is beneficial to begin the DWI examination with a matching interleaved EPI scan (ie, the number of interleaves should match R) and with the diffusion gradients turned off (b = 0 s/mm^2) or to use a calibration scheme, as suggested by Newbould and colleagues.[57]

Phase correction

An inherent problem of ssEPI is the limited spatial resolution that can be achieved. Because all k-space data are acquired with a single readout train, T_2*-related signal loss occurs. Thus, conventional EPI is typically performed with acquisition matrices up to 128 × 128 (192 × 192 at most) with the help of parallel imaging. Achieving higher spatial resolutions to become competitive with regular structural MR imaging requires the use of multishot sequences. However, as discussed elsewhere in this article multishot acquisitions bring back the problem of shot-to-shot phase variations caused by motion. To correct these phase variations, multi-shot sequences usually have to acquire additional navigator data from which these phase terms can be estimated and used to correct for the imaging data. Such navigator data can be obtained from an extra navigator image before or after acquiring the imaging data (see Fig. 13) or by using some specially designed readout trajectories that fully sample the center of the k-space at each acquisition, such as periodically rotated overlapping parallel lines (PROPELLER)[58–60] or self-navigated interleaved spiral (SNAILS) (Fig. 17).[35] Typically, the navigator image is a low-resolution image that samples k-space at the Nyquist sampling rate or even higher. In the past, phase correction with the navigator images (in addition to previous methods that used navigator projections in one[61,62] or two[28] dimensions) was performed in the k-space

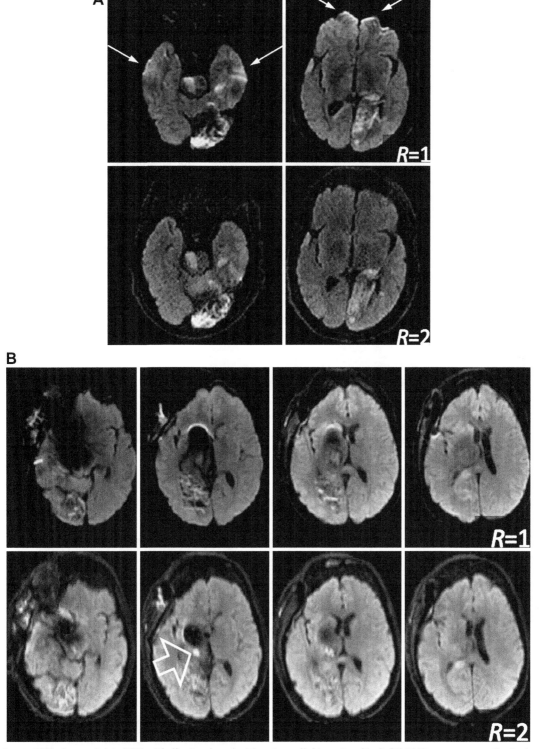

Fig. 14. Diffusion-weighted EPI with (*bottom*) and without parallel imaging (*top*). (*A*) DWI scans on a patient who has multiple stroke lesions and hemorrhagic transformation. Without parallel imaging, considerable pile-up artifacts are visible in the forebrain (*arrows*) in addition to signal hyperintensities in the temporal lobes. Parallel imaging removes these confounding artifacts. (*B*) DWI on a patient who has a coiled aneurysm. Considerable metal artifacts can be seen on conventional EPI. Although not completely eliminated, parallel imaging (*R* = 2 with partial left-to-right field of view of 75% effectively leading to threefold acceleration) could reduce the artifacts and reveal an ischemic lesion (*open arrow*).

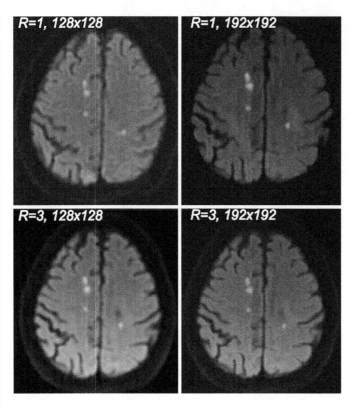

Fig. 15. Comparison of resolution (128 × 128 versus 192 × 192) and parallel imaging ($R = 1$ versus $R = 3$) is shown in a patient who has multiple tiny infarctions. The higher spatial resolution and reduced distortion reduction using $R = 3$ were clearly preferred by three independent readers. Overall, 192 × 192 $R = 3$ was the preferred option in all cases. Lesion conspicuity on the $R = 1$ scans is generally higher for subacute infarcts because of TEs of approximately 80 to 90 milliseconds instead of approximately 60 milliseconds for $R = 3$ scans and the associated higher T_2–shine-through effect.

domain[63] instead of the preferred image domain, and this was only partially successful.

Because different regions within the FOV most likely move differently, the corresponding phase impressed on the spins after the diffusion preparation is nonlinear in space. It is important to note that even if there is just a linear phase variation impressed on the spins, when the readout method

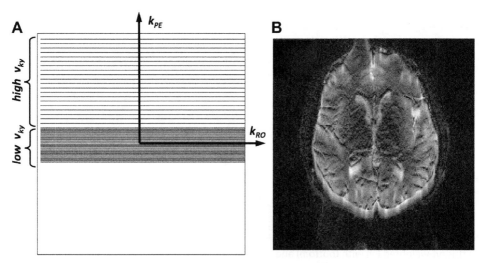

Fig. 16. (A) ssEPI partial Fourier trajectory with variable-density sampling. The region around the center of k-space is sampled at the Nyquist rate. Because of the low k-space velocity, v_{ky}, equal to that of regular EPI, no distortion reduction can be achieved for these spatial frequencies. k_{PE}, phase encode direction; k_{RO}, readout direction. (B) Corresponding EPI image. There is a misregistration between low-frequency image information content and the contour-determining high-spatial frequency components of the image because of the variable-density sampling and the resulting variable amount of distortions.

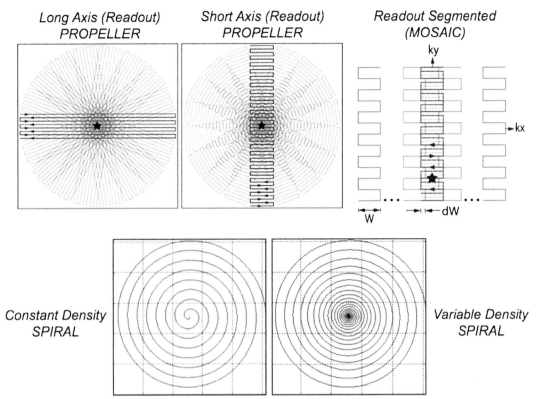

Fig. 17. (*Top*) Long-axis PROPELLER (*left*), short-axis PROPELLER (*center*), and readout-segmented (*right*) trajectories. (*Bottom*) Constant-density spiral (*left*) and variable-density spiral (*right*). W, blade width; dW, blade overlap. With long-axis PROPELLER (*top, left*), the frequency encode direction is along the long axis of the "blade," whereas phase encoding is along the short axis of the blade. With short-axis PROPELLER (*top, center*) and readout-segmented EPI (*top, right*), the readout and phase-encode axis are swapped so that the phase-encoding direction is along the long axis of the blade. (*Bottom, right*) Variable-density spiral samples the origin of k-space with greater density than peripheral portions of k-space. How quickly the spiral moves outward in a radial direction is controlled by a pitch-factor variable.

used is susceptible to geometric distortions (even to a lesser extent), this "phase tag" is squeezed or stretched in the acquired image, which effectively leads to a nonlinear phase distribution in the resultant image.[64] As a consequence, although a linear phase shift in the image domain causes a simple shift in k-space, a nonlinear phase causes additional dispersion of the k-space data (**Fig. 18**). For an accurate correction of phase errors, it is thus important that the distortion properties of the navigator image match those of the multishot diffusion image. This is typically the case for most self-navigated trajectories but can become somewhat difficult to achieve for trajectories that require an extra navigator image.

For self-navigating trajectories that allow one to reconstruct unaliased intermediate images acquired in each repetition time (TR), such as PROPELLER,[58] the simplest way to phase-correct DWI data is (1) to appodize the high-spatial frequency components to get a low-pass filtered

intermediate image that mostly contains the unwanted phase errors attributable to motion or (2) to multiply the original intermediate image by the complex conjugate of the low-pass filtered phase image. After this, the phase-corrected intermediate images can be combined (or gridded) in k-space, followed by an inverse fast Fourier transform into the image domain to get the final diffusion-weighted image.[59]

For a more generalized form of phase correction which works on arbitrary k-space data, the nonlinear phase correction proposed by Miller and Pauly[65] or the more elaborate version of Liu and Bammer[66] and Liu and colleagues[35,67] is recommended. The latter approach considers multichannel coils, parallel imaging, and off-resonances and demonstrates a better SNR than the former approach. **Fig. 19** (phase correction demonstration) shows the performance of phase correction on diffusion-weighted multishot data. For interested readers, the authors recommend an extension of

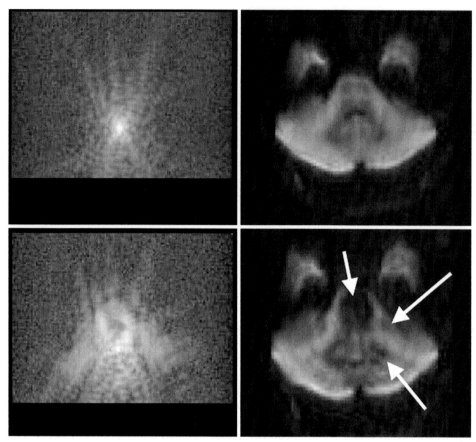

Fig. 18. Partial Fourier-encoded k-space data (*left*) and corresponding images (*right*). The top row shows a single-shot EPI scan with typical quality, whereas the bottom row shows a poor-quality shot with considerable k-space dispersion. Arrows indicate regions of profound signal distortion.

Liu's approach by Aksoy and colleagues,[68] which simultaneously corrects for subject movement between shots.

Even with navigator correction, with some trajectory types (eg, interleaved EPI), one has to be careful with local violations of the Nyquist criterion (ie, regional undersampling of k-space). This is because the linear component of the image domain phase errors shifts the trajectories at arbitrary positions away from their desired positions in k-space (see **Figs. 6** and **19**). To ameliorate this problem, Atkinson and colleagues[69] recommended oversampling of k-space and signal averaging. This is another reason the PROPELLER[58] trajectory is appealing, because the sampling within the PROPELLER blade remains consistent. PROPELLER avoids many of these problems, because k-space shifts affect the trajectory, similar to ssEPI, en bloc.

Periodically rotated overlapping parallel lines
The PROPELLER[58] technique has been introduced as a novel method that incorporates two-dimensional navigation information with the benefits of a radial-type acquisition. This multishot technique covers a thin strip or "blade" of k-space with each acquisition (see **Fig. 17**). As discussed in more detail later, by phase-cycling the RF refocusing pulses, the FSE train is stabilized and avoids phase errors that lead to a violation of the MG condition.

PROPELLER's inherent oversampling near the origin of k-space allows the removal of blades that contain uncorrectable errors from motion during diffusion encoding, such as excessive through-plane dephasing or k-space shifts that move the center of k-space outside the sampling of the blade. Because of the radial-type acquisition of this trajectory and the redundant sampling around the origin, the missing k-space data in

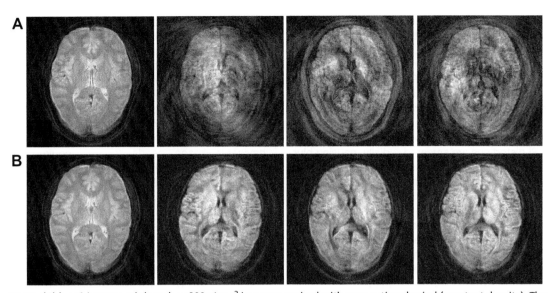

Fig. 19. (A) b = 0 image and three b = 900-s/mm^2 images acquired with conventional spiral (constant density). The three diffusion gradient directions are: $(0\ 1\ -1)^T$, $(-1\ 1\ 0)^T$, and $(0\ 1\ 1)^T$. (B) Images acquired with variable-density spiral. Nonlinear phase correction was applied to both data sets. Clearly, the oversampling of the origin of k-space allows one to calculate a much better phase error estimate. Moreover, because of the central oversampling, the chances of violating the Nyquist criterion from k-space shifts are considerably lowered.

the peripheral k-space regions cause only some benign streaking artifacts.[70]

FSE-based PROPELLER DWI has been demonstrated to be useful when higher spatial resolution is needed or in areas with severe susceptibility distortions, such as areas close to the base of the skull or metallic material,[59] wherein single-shot EPI demonstrates strong image degradation. Like other multishot techniques, the scan time of diffusion-weighted FSE PROPELLER (which is exacerbated by excessive k-space oversampling, the FSE RF pulses, and gradient balancing) is substantially longer than that of conventional ssEPI. This may limit PROPELLER's use in acute stroke or for breath-hold studies, for which scan time is critical. Because of the requirement of relatively large flip angles to cope with the non-MG issues, diffusion-weighted FSE PROPELLER becomes particularly specific absorption rate (SAR)-intense and depends on homogeneous RF transmission fields. All that is less problematic at 1.5 T but can be challenging at 3 T. To reduce SAR and boost scan efficiency, Pipe and Zwart[71] recently introduced the turboPROP method, which is based on a gradient spin-echo (GRASE)[72] readout rather than on a conventional FSE train. In GRASE, more than one gradient echo is acquired between two subsequent refocusing pulses in the FSE train and thus speeds up the readout while using fewer SAR-intense refocus-ing pulses. In GRASE, more than one gradient

echo is acquired between two subsequent refocusing pulses in the FSE train, and thus speed up the readout while using fewer SAR-intense refocusing pulses. TurboPROP provides a good tradeoff between fast data acquisition schemes, such as EPI, and low-distortion acquisition methods, such as FSE, as was demonstrated recently for fiber-tracking applications by Arfanakis and colleagues.[73]

Short-axis (readout) periodically rotated overlapping parallel lines echo-planar imaging

Skare and colleagues[60] leveraged on the great navigation capability and k-space data consistency of individual blades of the PROPELLER trajectory and paired them with the minimum-SAR and short-scan-time features of EPI. Here, the dimensions of the trajectory were transposed relative to the original PROPELLER trajectory (see Fig. 17). This serves to accelerate the traversal through k-space, and thus to reduce EPI-related distortions. Rather than using the long axis of the PROPELLER blade for the readout, the readout was placed along the short axis of the PROPELLER blade (with the phase encoding along the long axis). For a 256 × 256 acquisition matrix using 32 × 256 blades, an eight-fold reduction of EPI-related distortions theoretically can be achieved. Distortions can be diminished further by parallel imaging (additional approximately three-fold reduction) and post-processing methods using the B0-field map obtained from reversed gradient polarity methods[42] Note that transposing the PROPELLER axes is crucial to benefit from the distortion reduction capability of the short-axis readout PROPELLER blade.[60] If the long-axis PROPELLER version is used in concert with EPI,[74,75] there is no geometric distortion benefit over conventional Cartesian EPI. In fact, because of the radial nature of PROPELLER, EPI distortions are smeared radially, causing blurring in the final image. This is illustrated in **Fig. 20**, showing a comparison between short-axis and long-axis PROPELLER EPI. In addition to CNS studies, diffusion-weighted PROPELLER FSE[76–78] has recently been applied to abdominal imaging. Adding moderate diffusion attenuation helps to reduce the high signal from vessels in the liver and to improve lesion conspicuity. As shown in **Fig. 21**, the rapid imaging capacity of short-axis PROPELLER EPI makes the sequence well-suited for breath-hold studies, and the technique also has potential for DWIBS.

Readout-segmented echo-planar imaging

In the previous section, we have seen that reading out echoes with a length only a fraction of that of the nominal readout resolution shortens the echo spacing dramatically and allows one to traverse k-space much faster. In this fashion, artifacts can be significantly reduced but multiple shots are required to cover the entire k-space fully. One way to cover k-space is by using the short-axis EPI PROPELLER approach. Alternatively, one can shift the blades along the readout dimension without rotating the blade.[79] When combined with diffusion-weighting, an additional navigator image needs to be acquired,[80,81] because every blade no longer goes through the center of k-space (a prerequisite for self-navigation). Typically, this can be done by adding another 180° refocusing pulse, followed by an additional short-axis readout located at the center of k-space.[82,83] A similar phase correction as discussed elsewhere in this article can be used, except that the phase reversal of the extra 180° refocusing pulse must be considered. Again, parallel imaging can be used to reduce distortions further.[82,83] Compared with the short-axis readout PROPELLER EPI version, the need for extra navigator data cuts down slightly on scan efficiency, and the overlapped sampling of central regions of k-space also leaves PROPELLER with an SNR advantage over the readout-segmented (RS) EPI version, given the

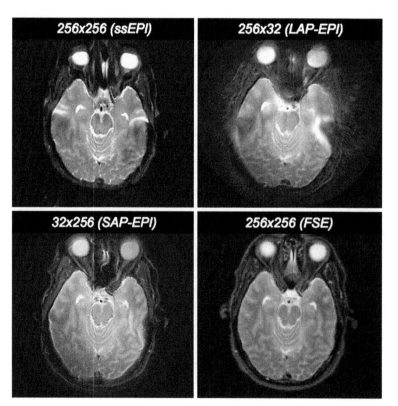

Fig. 20. Comparison of ssEPI (*top*, *left*) with long-axis PROPELLER EPI (*top*, *right*) and short-axis PROPELLER EPI (*bottom*, *left*). All blades were 32 × 256 (short-axis PROPELLER [SAP]) and 256 × 32 (long-axis PROPELLER [LAP]). Distortions with SAP EPI are markedly reduced. For each method, 25 blades were used and were swept over a range between 0° and 180°. For reference, a matching T$_2$-weighted FSE image is shown as well (*bottom, right*).

A B C

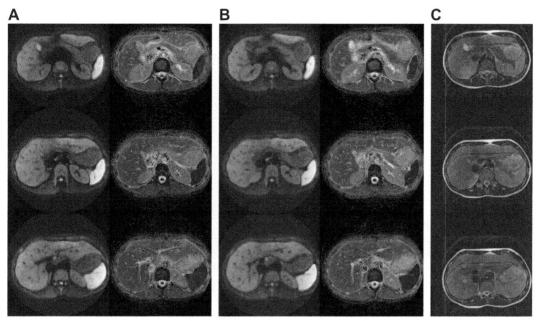

Fig. 21. Short-axis PROPELLER EPI of the abdomen with 30 8-mm slices (1-mm gap) using 10 64 × 256 blades with b = 500 s/mm². Non–breath-hold acquisition shows three isotropic DWI (*left*) and mean ADC (*right*) images located 18 mm apart (*A*), breath-hold acquisition (*B*), and corresponding free-breathing FSE acquisition (*C*).

right choice of scan parameters.[84] However, the overlapping causes structural image noise (ie, nonwhite noise), which essentially lowers the effective resolution of any PROPELLER method. Lastly, because motion can be detected from the navigator image as well, RS-EPI is also well suited to correct for motion (**Fig. 22**).

Spirals
A few studies have recently explored the self-navigating capability of the spiral readout trajectory in multishot DWI.[34–36,85] Previously, MR imaging using the spiral readout (see **Fig. 17**) was effective in such applications as functional neuroimaging[86,87] and spectroscopy.[88–91] The spiral trajectory has the merit of moment-nulling motion compensation and efficient use of gradient power.[33] Nevertheless, it turns out that conventional (constant density) spiral readout trajectories have limited potential for self-navigation because of the lack of data in the central k-space. This effectively allows zero-order and (to some extent) first-order compensation only.[63] To improve the navigating capability, one can increase the sampling density at the center of the k-space. With a recently developed analytic variable-density spiral design technique,[88] the k-space sampling density can easily be increased around the origin of k-space. This leads to

a diffusion-weighted, multishot, variable-density, spiral sequence design, which is a self-navigated technique and a promising alternative for high-resolution DWI.[35] With the analytic, variable-density, spiral design technique, the k-space sampling density can be easily manipulated and prescribed on the scanner hardware in real time. Here, each spiral interleaf oversamples the central region of the k-space and undersamples the outer region of the k-space (see **Fig. 17**). The sampling density is circularly symmetric and decreases smoothly as the radius increases in k-space. For each spiral interleaf, the phase error in image space can be estimated from the fully sampled center of k-space and used for subsequent phase correction.[35,68,92] Compared with constant density spirals, the image quality is improved dramatically with variable-density spirals. Oversampling the origin of k-space also helps to reduce the aforementioned artifacts from the linear phase error terms that lead to local undersampling of k-space (see **Fig. 19**).

Coping with the Non-Meiboom-Gill Component in Fast Spin-Echo

Phase cycling
For their original diffusion-weighted PROPELLER FSE work, Pipe and colleagues[59] suggested mitigating signal instability present in FSE-based

Reference

without motion correction

with motion correction

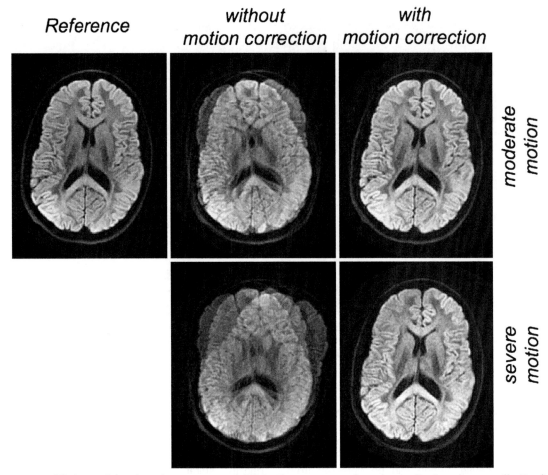

moderate motion

severe motion

Fig. 22. Diffusion-weighted readout-segmented EPI in the presence of moderate (*top*) and severe (*bottom*) patient motion. Before (*top, middle*) and after (*top, right*) motion correction. (*Top, left*) Reference image, for which the volunteer was asked to remain stationary.

DWI by varying the phase of the refocusing pulses between the x-axis and y-axis (ie, $180°_x - 180°_y - 180°_x - 180°_y$ and so forth) in the fashion of well-known phase cycling schemes.[93–95] This produces a relatively stable echo train for refocusing angles near 180°, but the echo amplitudes begin to fall off significantly for refocusing angles down to 140° (Fig. 23). Although robust in general, this approach can be problematic in the presence of poor slice profiles (ie, when the transition band is a large fraction of the overall slice thickness) or at higher magnetic field strengths, wherein more nonuniform transmit RF fields occur in the presence of B1 inhomogeneities. The requirement to keep the refocusing angles much greater than 140° might become problematic for high-field applications, primarily because of SAR concerns. However, such methods as variable-rate selective excitation[96] or turboPROP[71] have been suggested to lower SAR.

A similar approach to that of Pipe and colleagues[59] has been introduced recently by Le Roux.[31] It differs by being able to sustain echo trains for a larger number of echoes, allowing for a larger acceptable nonuniformity of the transmit RF (ie, variations down to an effective refocusing flip angle of 115°). Unlike Pipe and colleagues[59] XY phase cycling approach, Le Roux suggests a quadratic phase modulation scheme[94] to set the RF phase of the refocusing pulses within the FSE train.

Eliminating the non–Meiboom-Gill component
Norris and colleagues[97] have shown that for a CPMG train, the echoes formed by magnetization that has spent an odd number of inter-refocusing pulse periods in the transverse plane add coherently to form a single odd-parity echo, whereas an even-parity echo forms analogously. Moreover, they belong to two separate echo

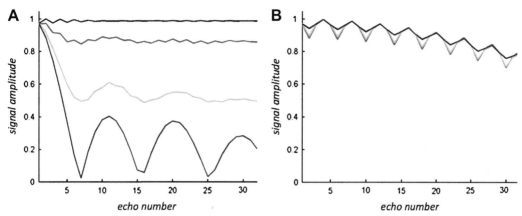

Fig. 23. Bloch simulations of multiecho readout with spin phase of 0° (black = CPMG component), 30° (red), 60° (green), and 90° (blue = non-CPMG component) relative to RF axis of the FSE train. Relaxation effects were neglected. The flip angle for all refocusing pulses was reduced from 180° to 150°. (*A*) RF phase remained constant over the FSE train. This results in considerable signal loss and oscillations of the individual echoes of the FSE train if the phase of the transverse magnetization deviates from the MG phase condition. (*B*) With the XY phase, cycling oscillates slightly but the signal amplitude remains independent of the initial phase of the transverse magnetization.

families: (1) family A, that occurring simultaneously with the repeated direct refocusing of the first spin-echo A_1, and (2) family B, that occurring simultaneously with the direct refocusing of the first stimulated echo B_1. Refocusing flip angles differing from pure 180° leads to an intermingling of the two families. The odd and even echoes in each acquisition period come alternatively from the A and B families. By creating a significant enough imbalance between the readout dephaser gradient and the readout gradient (ie, the dephaser gradient area is considerably different from half of the readout gradient area), Norris and colleagues[97] determined that the two echo parities occur temporally disseminated in the readout window (**Fig. 24**). With this method, also known as

displaced ultra fast low angle rapid acquisition with relaxation enhancement (U-FLARE), one echo parity (typically the odd one) is pushed out of the window when each echo is acquired at the price of half the available SNR and the need for several dummy echoes to stabilize the signal in the FSE train. Recently, Norris[98] improved his original approach by means of selective parity imaging. Again, displacing gradients were used; however, in contrast to displaced U-FLARE, the odd and even parity echoes were selected within a single echo train, whereby the echo parity was chosen that gave the desired signal strength at the lowest refocusing angle. Furthermore, the first echo was a 180° refocusing pulse to boost signal amplitude, and a central-out phase-encoding

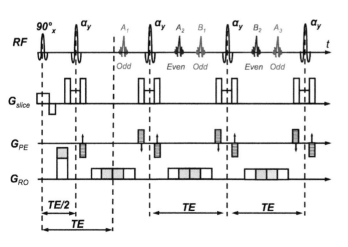

Fig. 24. U-FLARE sequence with imbalanced dephasing and readout gradients (shaded area), as originally suggested by Norris, et al.[97] The graph shows the formation of the echoes for the first three cycles of an FSE train using these imbalanced gradients. Here, the readout dephasing gradient area is too big, as shown by the gray area. This generates two echo families, *A* and *B*. The odd (*red*) and even (*blue*) parities are made up by both families, as shown in the figure. In the original displaced U-FLARE approach, the gradient imbalance was made so strong that one of the echo parities was pushed outside of the sampling window. G_{PE}, gradient in the phase encode direction; G_{RO}, gradient in the readout direction; G_{slice}, gradient in the slice select direction.

scheme was used to minimize TE. Lastly, a recursive application of the Bloch equations was used to generate smooth signal decay over the FSE train to minimize image blurring.

Also p[99] introduced a preparation method for non-CPMG FSE (again, at the cost of half the signal), in which a dephasing gradient followed by a 90° pulse was applied before the FSE train. By applying a dephasing gradient before the formation of the diffusion-weighted spin-echo, each voxel has equal components of MG and non-MG signal. The 90° echo-reset pulse, played out along the same axis as the subsequent FSE pulses, rotates the non-MG component to the longitudinal axis, wherein it is invisible in the subsequent sequence (**Fig. 25**). In addition, rephasing gradients of opposite polarity (but with an identical gradient area as the dephaser gradient) must be added after each refocusing pulse and before the acquisition of each echo and must then be rewound after each acquisition and before the next refocusing pulse to maintain the MG condition. To permit acquisition of data from the first echo without artifact, Alsop[99] ramped down the flip angles of the FSE train from 142.2° to 94.9°, 69.2°, and 63.0° and with remaining pulses set to 60°.

OUTSIDE THE BOX
Diffusion-Weighted Steady-State Free Precession

3D imaging is extremely cumbersome with conventional spin-echo Stejskal-Tanner sequences, because the long TEs and TRs render conventional DWI sequences prohibitively long. An alternative technique that allows rapid image formation suitable for 3D imaging is steady-state free precession (SSFP). In SSFP, a train of

equidistant RF pulses with flip angle α and a TR less than T_2 is applied, and a condition of SSFP develops after a few TRs. SSFP imaging is also known for its high sensitivity to flow and diffusion in the presence of magnetic field gradients.[100] Together with its 3D imaging capabilities, diffusion-weighted SSFP is therefore an attractive alternative to conventional DWI.

By adding a single short diffusion gradient within the TR interval between successive RF pulses and before the gradient echo readout, the diffusion sensitivity of the sequence can be boosted (**Fig. 26**). SSFP has therefore received attention from several researchers.[92,101–103] In contrast to the commonly used Stejskal-Tanner preparation, the signal formation in SSFP is a complex superposition of numerous spin and stimulated echoes, each of which may be formed through a multitude of coherence pathways,[104,105] limited only by the natural decay times T_1 and T_2. Contributions from any of these coherence pathways to an echo might have experienced various amounts of diffusion-encoding gradients and may have spent more or less time stored as longitudinal (T_1 decay) or transverse (T_2 decay) magnetization. This complex signal formation renders the quantification of diffusion-weighted SSFP difficult, and diffusion-weighted SSFP methods are currently mostly limited to qualitative applications. Thus, the diffusion attenuation (b-value) may vary from tissue to tissue. In contrast to Stejskal-Tanner DWI sequences, one therefore has to deal not only with "T_2–shine-through" effects but with the fact that b-values are weighted by the underlying relaxation times and other confounding factors. Recently, McNab and Miller[106] have introduced a formalism to describe the contributions from relaxation and flip angle to the diffusion-weighted SSFP signal and assessed the contributions. This is a promising step, and it

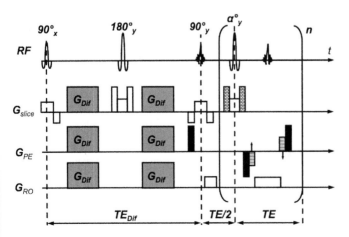

Fig. 25. Diffusion-weighted FSE sequence as suggested by Alsop. Before $t = TE$, a dephasing gradient is applied (*solid fill*) that distributes the spins evenly in the transverse plane into MG and non-MG components. The non-MG component is then aligned longitudinally by an echo reset pulse at $t = TE$. For each echo readout, the dephasing of the MG component must be first undone and then reapplied after echo sampling. G_{PE}, gradient in the phase encode direction; G_{RO}, gradient in the readout direction; G_{slice}, gradient in the slice select direction; TE_{Dif}, echo time relevant for diffusion-encoding.

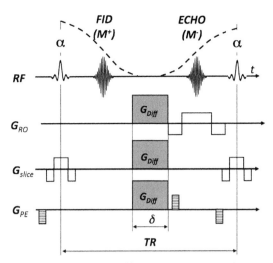

Fig. 26. One cycle of a diffusion-weighted steady-state free precession (SSFP) sequence. The ECHO component is generally quite sensitive to diffusion. Except for the diffusion-encoding gradient, all other gradients are completely balanced, and the total effective gradient is equal in each cycle to establish a steady state. FID, free induction decay; G_{PE}, gradient in the phase encode direction; G_{RO}, gradient in the readout direction; G_{slice}, gradient in the slice select direction.

potentially opens a viable avenue for 3D diffusion imaging, a technique much sought after, especially for DTI and associated fiber-tracking methods.

Diffusion-Weighted Whole-Body Imaging with Background Body Signal Suppression

The low ADC of lymph nodes and their metastatic infiltrates in addition to that of many malignant primary tumors has recently led to an increased interest in using DWI for DWIBS.[5,107,108] DWIBS has received a lot of acclaim and has caused considerable excitement in the community because it has become an important contributor to the diagnostic value of whole-body MR imaging, which, in turn, has become a serious competitor for positron emission tomography (PET) and PET-CT.[109-111]

Different variants of DWIBS exist, but the basic idea is common to all of them. First, low ADC lipids are suppressed; second, DWI of the entire body or a region of interest is performed with considerable (for tissue outside the CNS) diffusion attenuation to make the low ADC structures stand out (eg, 500–1000 s/mm^2), whereas the remainder of the other tissues are suppressed; third, maximum intensity projections (MIPs) are computed at different projection angles to improve lesion visibility and facilitate diagnostic utility; and, fourth, an inverted

gray scale is applied to the MIPs. That is, low ADC structures appear hypointense, whereas regular background appears bright to resemble scintigraphic images. The latter step is cosmetic and can be used depending on the preference of the interpreting radiologist.

DWIBS offers images that are similar in appearance to PET images, but the diagnostic potential of DWIBS awaits head-to-head comparison in large patient cohorts. When using DWIBS for the staging of patients who have lymphoma, it may aid in the detection of lymph nodes. After detection, additional judgment is still required using morphologic criteria, such as size and shape of the lymph nodes.

Fig. 27 demonstrates DWIBS performed on a patient who has lymphoma. The widespread disease is clearly visible on this coronal MIP. For whole-body applications or adipose patients with large girth sizes, achieving fat suppression based on frequency-selective methods (eg, chemical shift selective, spectral inversion recovery, spectral spatial excitation) often fails because of the homogeneity of the magnet across such a large FOV. This leaves regions of incompletely suppressed and low ADC fat behind that appear hyperintense on DWIBS and impair automatic MIP processing. Although incomplete fat suppression is not problematic for most sequences, the extremely low ADC makes even small fractions of remaining fat stand out on the MIPs. STIR-based nulling of lipids has been suggested.[5] However, the penalty of using STIR is a considerable SNR loss, because all other tissue is also inverted and only partially recovered at inversion times of approximately 160 to 200 milliseconds. Moreover, at 3 T, STIR can be somewhat challenging (even with adiabatic inversion pulses) and, at least on the authors' system, has occasionally failed to nullify fat entirely. Furthermore, the STIR preparation decreases the scan efficiency considerably.

In situations when fat suppression fails, cut-out MIPs are a good option (Fig. 28). In the authors' experience, cut-out MIPs of smaller areas can better reveal abnormalities and are less affected by surrounding clutter. The benefit of cut-out MIPs is well known from MRA and can often be useful (John Houston, personal communication, 2008). When only crude cut-out MIPs are used, superficial lymph nodes (eg, the inguinal lymph nodes in Fig. 28) are cut off, which, if only reviewing the MIP, is easily overlooked. Another problem is that the bright fatty layers are often on the ventral and lateral sides of a patient (ie, if the patient were a cube, the bright fat is on two faces of the cube, making it nearly impossible to "look behind

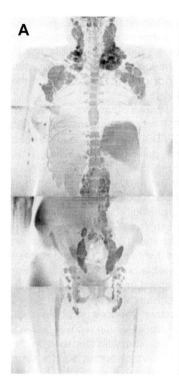

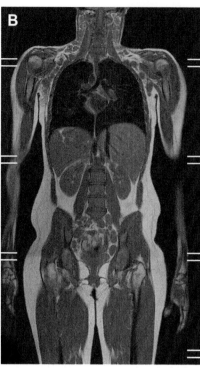

Fig. 27. Female patient who has lymphoma. (*A*) Whole-body DWIBS examination clearly reveals numerous disseminated lesions throughout the body. In the right hip region, the chemical shift selective fat suppression failed to work. (*B*) Corresponding whole-body T1-weighted FSE scan. (Patient raw data set, *courtesy of* R.A.J. Nievelstein, MD, PhD and T.C. Kwee, MD, Utrecht, The Netherlands.)

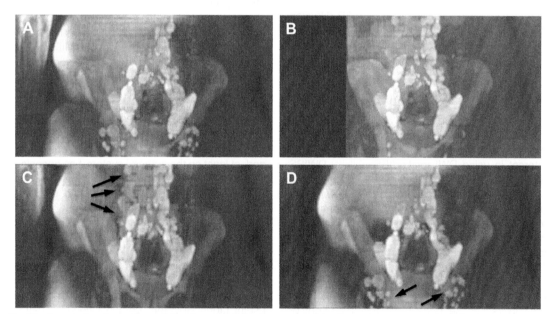

Fig. 28. One station from the multistation whole-body examination shown in Fig. 27, in which fat suppression on the patient's right side was incomplete. (*A*) Because of the low ADC of fat, it appears hyperintense on DWI scans, thus affecting the MIP procedure. Some of the diseased lymphatic tissue is poorly visualized on the MIP. (*B*) Crude cut-out MIP can get rid of some of the fat but is still not fully satisfying. Ideally, the 3D shaped cut-outs offered by some advanced image processing workstations would be more suitable. (*C*) Thinner slab MIPs help to reveal the lymph nodes in the abdomen (*arrows*), but the inguinal nodes were outside of the slab and were missed. (*D*) Changing the slab location brings back those nodes, but unsuppressed fat comes back in the abdominal region, masking nodes. This example demonstrates the importance of good fat suppression or the availability of cut-out MIP tools.

it," even by rotating the volume MIP). If fat suppression fails only on one side of "the cube", it is less aesthetically pleasing but less of a clinical problem, because rotating the MIP allows the reader to look "behind" the superimposing bright fat. An easier solution is the use of thin-slab MIPs (see **Fig. 28**C and D), although, as shown in the example, caution must also be exercised and, as with MRA, the thin-source images should always be reviewed.

It is also the authors' experience that for certain regions, non-adiabatic fat suppression works equally well (as can be seen from **Fig. 27**). This, of course, has a tremendous advantage because it boosts scan performance (ie, more slices per TR) and SNR. Without the concern about fat suppression, and consequently reduced SNR, one can focus on resolution and thinner sections. **Fig. 29** shows an example of such a study on a male pelvis, which clearly reveals the morphologic structure of inguinal lymph nodes in much better detail. However, as mentioned previously, the read-out time for conventional ssEPI lengthens with increasing resolution to the point that blurring

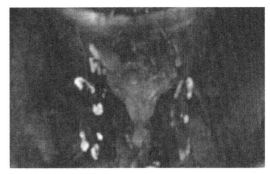

Fig. 29. Thin-section (3-mm/0-mm gap) DWIBS of the male pelvis (without gray-scale inversion) using spectral-spatial water-only excitation. The inguinal lymph nodes and their morphologic structure are well visualized.

and geometric distortions impair image acquisition. Parallel imaging ameliorates this problem to some extent, but for certain applications, such as (sentinel) node screening in the axilla, the coil sensitivity variation and coverage provided by the coil elements are suboptimal and parallel imaging soon reaches its limits. At the authors'

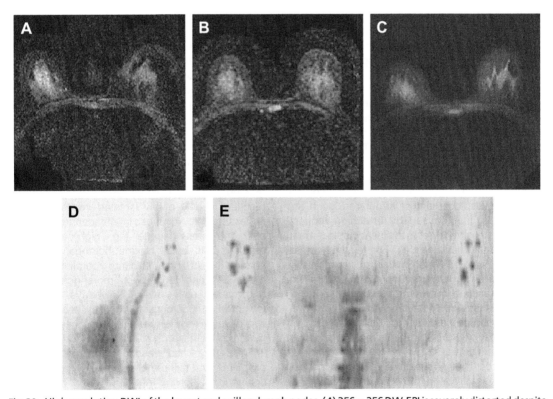

Fig. 30. High-resolution DWI of the breast and axillary lymph nodes. (A) 256 × 256 DW-EPI is severely distorted despite the use of parallel imaging (array spatial sensitivity encoding technique). (B) 128 × 128 ASSET-DW-EPI scan. (C) 256 × 256 multishot SNAILS-DWI scan reveals much better detail and is less distorted. High-resolution SNAILS data set allows multiplanar reformats for DWIBS processing and clearly shows axillary lymph nodes on unilateral sagittal MIP (D) and coronal chest-wall MIP (E). The SNAILS acquisition time was 5 minutes for both breasts and axillas.

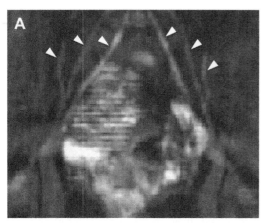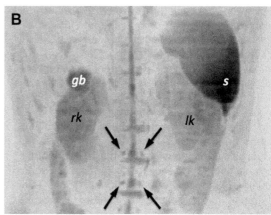

Fig. 31. (*A*) Visualization of the lumbar nerves in a patient (*arrowheads*) using DWIBS (without inverted gray scale). (*B*) DWIBS in another patient clearly reveals the spinal cord and the nerve roots and ganglions (*arrows*). gb, gallbladder; s, spleen; rk, right kidney; lk, left kidney.

institution, a switch has therefore been made to multishot techniques, such as SNAILS.[35] Fig. 30 shows a comparative evaluation of SNAILS, together with ssEPI with and without parallel imaging, demonstrating the potential superiority of multishot scans for DWIBS.

The use of multishot scans often makes the scan duration of DWIBS prohibitively long, especially in abdominal scans when breath-holds are warranted to limit motion artifacts. Although free breathing is typically tolerable in the pelvis, respiratory motion in the abdomen is too severe to allow free breathing. Alternatively, respiratory gating can be used but, again, leads to a considerable prolongation of the entire DWIBS examination. A possible alternative is the recently introduced tracking-only navigator (TRON) technique.[112] This technique does not use the navigator for gating image acquisition but for the tracking of movement. The tracking data are then retrospectively used to correct for displacement of structures, such as, for example, that caused by breathing motion. The technique only corrects for linear displacement of subdiaphragmatic tissues. For relatively small structures, such as lymph nodes, this is probably fine. For larger structures, such as the liver, which not only translate but deform during respiratory motion, this remains to be investigated. Nevertheless, the first data indicate that TRON may improve image quality of DWIBS, with minimal prolongation of acquisition time.

Aside from being sensitive to lymph nodes, DWIBS reveals nerve fibers and paraspinal ganglions well. However, DWIBS is nothing else other than a regular DWI sequence, and thus it is sensitive to anisotropic diffusion (Fig. 31). The ability to perform neurographic imaging outside the CNS has been demonstrated with DTI for the median nerve before; however, recently, DWIBS was also used to examine the brachial[113] and lumbosacral[114] plexus. The main advantage of using DWIBS, again, is in the suppression of background detail. This is especially beneficial to neurography, because DWI can suppress the signal from blood vessels, which often course alongside nerves in neurovascular bundles. Suppression of background also allows MIP visualization of the often complex anatomy of a nerve plexus and aids in, for example, the discrimination of primary neuronal diseases, such as tumors, from extraneuronal pathologic conditions compressing or infiltrating the plexus.

SUMMARY

Fifteen years ago DWI was performed mostly on systems with special gradient hardware or insert gradients and with limited EPI upgrades, which resulted in only a few isolated institutions with access to DWI. Advances in MR scanner hardware over the past decade (eg, high-performance gradient coils, better magnet homogeneity, multichannel coils that facilitate parallel imaging) made EPI and DWI much more accessible to a broader user base. Nowadays, diffusion-weighted EPI belongs to the key sequences of a clinical MR system and DTI has been used in hundreds of research studies.

This article has described the major salient problems that still remain with DWI and potential solutions for solving these problems. After many years of struggling with mediocre image resolution and distortions, some of the solutions presented here offer possibilities to achieve DWI with image quality comparable to conventional structural imaging, which was probably unthinkable 10 years ago. This article has also provided the radiologist with an overview about the strengths and weaknesses of current DWI methods.

ACKNOWLEDGMENTS

The first author (RB) is grateful to his hosts during his sabbatical, when most of this manuscript was written: Prof. Joachim Hornegger (University of Erlangen) and Profs. Linda Chang, Thomas Ernst, and Andrew Stenger (University of Hawaii).

REFERENCES

1. Moseley ME, Cohen Y, Mintorovitch J, et al. Early detection of regional cerebral ischemia in cats: comparison of diffusion- and T2-weighted MRI and spectroscopy. Magn Reson Med 1990;14: 330–46.
2. Albers GW, Lansberg MG, O'Brien MW, et al. Evolution of cerebral infarct volume assessed by diffusion-weighted MRI: implications for acute stroke trials. Neurology 1999;52:A453.
3. Callaghan PT, Coy A, MacGowan D, et al. Diffraction-like effects in NMR diffusion studies of fluids in porous solids. Nature 1991;351:467–9.
4. Basser PJ, Mattiello J, LeBihan D. Estimation of the effective self-diffusion tensor from the NMR spin-echo. J Magn Reson B 1994;103:247–54.
5. Takahara T, Imai Y, Yamashita T, et al. Diffusion weighted whole body imaging with background body signal suppression (DWIBS): technical improvement using free breathing, stir and high resolution 3D display. Radiat Med 2004;22:275–82.
6. Torrey HC. Bloch equations with diffusion terms. Physiol Rev 1956;104:563–5.
7. Stejskal EO, Tanner JE. Spin diffusion measurements: spin-echoes in the presence of a time-dependent field gradient. J Chem Phys 1965;42: 288–92.
8. Basser PJ. Inferring microstructural features and the physiological state of tissues from diffusion-weighted images. NMR Biomed 1995;8:333–44.
9. Jones DK, Horsfield MA, Simmons A. Optimal strategies for measuring diffusion in anisotropic systems by magnetic resonance imaging. Magn Reson Med 1999;42:515–25.
10. Fliege J, Maier U. The distribution of points on the sphere and corresponding cubature formulae. IMA J Numer Anal 1999;19:317–34.
11. Skare S, Hedehus M, Moseley ME, et al. Condition number as a measure of noise performance of diffusion tensor data acquisition schemes with MRI. J Magn Reson 2000;147:340–52.
12. Basser PJ, Pajevic S, Pierpaoli C, et al. In vivo fiber tractography using DT-MRI data. Magn Reson Med 2000;44:625–32.
13. Mori S, Crain BJ, Chacko VP, et al. Three-dimensional tracking of axonal projections in the brain by magnetic resonance imaging. Ann Neurol 1999;45:265–9.
14. Frank LR. Anisotropy in high angular resolution diffusion-weighted MRI. Magn Reson Med 2001;45:935–9.
15. Frank LR. Characterization of anisotropy in high angular resolution diffusion-weighted MRI. Magn Reson Med 2002;47:1083–99.
16. Callaghan PT. Principles of nuclear magnetic resonance microscopy. Oxford (UK): Clarendon Press; 1993.
17. Assaf Y, Cohen Y. Structural information in neuronal tissue as revealed by q-space diffusion NMR spectroscopy of metabolites in bovine optic nerve. NMR Biomed 1999;12:335–44.
18. Assaf Y, Ben-Bashat D, Chapman J, et al. High b-value q-space analyzed diffusion-weighted MRI: application to multiple sclerosis. Magn Reson Med 2002;47:115–26.
19. Wedeen VJ, Wang RP, Schmahmann JD, et al. Diffusion spectrum magnetic resonance imaging (DSI) tractography of crossing fibers. Neuroimage 2008;41:1267–77.
20. Wedeen VJ, Hagmann P, Tseng WY, et al. Mapping complex tissue architecture with diffusion spectrum magnetic resonance imaging. Magn Reson Med 2005;54:1377–86.
21. Tuch DS. Q-ball imaging. Magn Reson Med 2004; 52:1358–72.
22. Liu C, Bammer R, Acar B, et al. Characterizing non-Gaussian diffusion by using generalized diffusion tensors. Magn Reson Med 2004;51(5):924–37.
23. Skare S, Andersson JL. On the effects of gating in diffusion imaging of the brain using single shot EPI. Magn Reson Imaging 2001;19:1125–8.
24. Poncelet BP, Wedeen VJ, Weisskoff RM, et al. Brain parenchyma motion: measurement with cine echo-planar MR imaging. Radiology 1992; 185:645–51.
25. Chow LC, Bammer R, Moseley ME, et al. Single breath-hold diffusion-weighted imaging of the abdomen. J Magn Reson Imaging 2003;18:377–82.
26. Chow LC, Chang R, Bammer R. Diffusion weighted imaging in the assessment of renal dysfunction. 12th Annual Meeting of the ISMRM. Kyoto (Japan), May 15–21, 2004.
27. Anderson AW, Gore JC. Analysis and correction of motion artifacts in diffusion weighted imaging. Magn Reson Med 1994;32:379–87.
28. Butts K, de Crespigny A, Pauly JM, et al. Diffusion-weighted interleaved echo-planar imaging with a pair of orthogonal navigator echoes. Magn Reson Med 1996;35:763–70.

29. Meiboom S, Gill D. Modified spin-echo method for measuring nuclear relaxation times. Rev Sci Instrum 1958;29:688–91.

30. Poon CS, Henkelman RM. Practical $t2$ quantitation for clinical applications. J Magn Reson Imaging 1992;2:541–53.

31. Le Roux P. Non-CPMG fast spin-echo with full signal. J Magn Reson 2002;155:278–92.

32. Mansfield P. Multi-planar image formation using NMR spin-echoes. J Phys Chem 1977;10:L55–8.

33. Glover GH. Basic and advanced concepts of spiral imaging. Presented at the ISMRM Fast MRI Workshop: Methodological Perspectives and Advances in Cardiac, Neuro, Angiography and Abdominal Imaging. Asilomar, CA, October 27–28, 1997.

34. Li TQ, Takahashi AM, Hindmarsh T, et al. ADC mapping by means of a single-shot spiral MRI technique with application in acute cerebral ischemia. Magn Reson Med 1999;41:143–7.

35. Liu C, Bammer R, Kim DH, et al. Self-navigated interleaved spiral (SNAILS): application to high-resolution diffusion tensor imaging. Magn Reson Med 2004;52(6):1388–96.

36. Bammer R, Glover GH, Moseley ME. Diffusion tensor spiral imaging. 10th Annual Meeting of the International Society of Magnetic Resonance in Medicine. Honolulu, HI, May 18–24, 2002.

37. Liu C, Bammer R, Acar B, et al. Generalized diffusion tensor imaging (GDTI) using higher order tensor (HOT) statistics. Magn Reson Med 2004;51:924–37.

38. Ozarslan E, Mareci TH. Generalized diffusion tensor imaging and analytical relationships between diffusion tensor imaging and high angular resolution diffusion imaging. Magn Reson Med 2003;50:955–65.

39. Ozarslan E, Shepherd TM, Vemuri BC, et al. Fast orientation mapping from HARDI. Med Image Comput Comput Assist Interv Int Conf Med Image Comput Comput Assist Interv 2005;8:156–63.

40. Tuch DS, Reese TG, Wiegell MR, et al. High angular resolution diffusion imaging reveals intra-voxel white matter fiber heterogeneity. Magn Reson Med 2002;48(4):577–82.

41. Farzaneh F, Riederer SJ, Pelc NJ. Analysis of T2 limitations and off-resonance effects on spatial resolution and artifacts in echo-planar imaging. Magn Reson Med 1990;14:123–39.

42. Chang H, Fitzpatrick JM. A technique for accurate magnetic resonance imaging in the presence of field inhomogeneities. IEEE Trans Med Imaging 1992;11:319–29.

43. Andersson JL, Skare S, Ashburner J. How to correct susceptibility distortions in spin-echo echo-planar images: application to diffusion tensor imaging. Neuroimage 2003;20(2):870–88.

44. Reese TG, Heid O, Weisskoff RM, et al. Reduction of eddy-current-induced distortion in diffusion MRI using a twice-refocused spin-echo. Magn Reson Med 2003;49:177–82.

45. Bammer R, Auer M. Correction of eddy-current induced image warping in diffusion-weighted single-shot EPI using constrained non-rigid mutual information image registration. Presented at the 9th Annual Meeting of ISMRM. Glasgow (Scotland), April 21–27, 2001.

46. Andersson JL, Skare S. A model-based method for retrospective correction of geometric distortions in diffusion-weighted EPI. Neuroimage 2002;16:177–99.

47. Haselgrove JC, Moore JR. Correction for distortion of echo-planar images used to calculate the apparent diffusion coefficient. Magn Reson Med 1996;36:960–4.

48. Pruessmann KP, Weiger M, Scheidegger MB, et al. SENSE: sensitivity encoding for fast MRI. Magn Reson Med 1999;42:952–62.

49. Griswold MA, Jakob PM, Heidemann RM, et al. Generalized autocalibrating partially parallel acquisitions (GRAPPA). Magn Reson Med 2002;47(6):1202–10.

50. Brau AC, Beatty PJ, Skare S, et al. Comparison of reconstruction accuracy and efficiency among autocalibrating data-driven parallel imaging methods. Magn Reson Med 2008;59:382–95.

51. Bammer R, Auer M, Keeling SL, et al. Diffusion tensor imaging using single-shot SENSE-EPI. Magn Reson Med 2002;48:128–36.

52. Bammer R, Keeling SL, Augustin M, et al. Improved diffusion-weighted single-shot echo-planar imaging (EPI) in stroke using sensitivity encoding (SENSE). Magn Reson Med 2001;46:548–54.

53. Jaermann T, Crelier G, Pruessmann KP, et al. SENSE-DTI at 3 T. Magn Reson Med 2004;51:230–6.

54. Skare S, Bammer R. Spatial modeling of the GRAPPA weights. 13th Annual Meeting of the ISMRM. Miami Beach, FL, May 7–13, 2005.

55. Brau ACS, Beatty PJ, Skare S, et al. Efficient computation of autocalibrating parallel imaging reconstruction. 14th Annual Meeting of the ISMRM. Seattle, WA, May 6–12, 2006.

56. Skare S, Newbould RD, Clayton DB, et al. Clinical multishot DW-EPI through parallel imaging with considerations of susceptibility, motion, and noise. Magn Reson Med 2007;57:881–90.

57. Newbould RD, Skare ST, Jochimsen TH, et al. Perfusion mapping with multiecho multishot parallel imaging EPI. Magn Reson Med 2007;58:70–81.

58. Pipe JG. Motion correction with PROPELLER MRI: application to head motion and free-breathing cardiac imaging. Magn Reson Med 1999;42:963–9.

59. Pipe JG, Farthing VG, Forbes KP. Multishot diffusion-weighted FSE using PROPELLER MRI. Magn Reson Med 2002;47:42–52.

60. Skare S, Newbould R, Clayton DB, et al. PROPELLER EPI in the other direction. Magn Reson Med 2006;55(6):1298–307.

61. de Crespigny AJ, Marks MP, Enzmann DR, et al. Navigated diffusion imaging of normal and ischemic human brain. Magn Reson Med 1995; 33:720–8.

62. Bammer R, Stollberger R, Augustin M, et al. Diffusion-weighted imaging with navigated interleaved echo-planar imaging and a conventional gradient system. Radiology 1999;211:799–806.

63. Butts K, Pauly J, de Crespigny A, et al. Isotropic diffusion-weighted and spiral-navigated interleaved EPI for routine imaging of acute stroke. Magn Reson Med 1997;38:741–9.

64. Storey P, Frigo FJ, Hinks RS, et al. Partial k-space reconstruction in single-shot diffusion-weighted echo-planar imaging. Magn Reson Med 2007;57: 614–9.

65. Miller KL, Pauly JM. Nonlinear navigated motion correction for diffusion imaging. Presented at the 10th Annual Meeting of ISMRM. Honolulu, HI, May 18–24, 2002.

66. Liu C, Moseley ME, Bammer Roland. Simultaneous phase correction and SENSE reconstruction for navigated multi-shot DWI with non-Cartesian k-space sampling. Magn Reson Med 2005;54: 1412–22.

67. Liu C, Moseley ME, Bammer R. Simultaneous off-resonance and phase correction for multi-shot DWI. 13th Annual Meeting of the ISMRM. 2005:5.

68. Aksoy M, Liu C, Moseley ME, et al. Single-step nonlinear diffusion tensor estimation in the presence of microscopic and macroscopic motion. Presented at the 16th Annual Meeting of ISMRM. Toronto, Canada, May 3–9, 2008.

69. Atkinson D, Porter DA, Hill DL, et al. Sampling and reconstruction effects due to motion in diffusion-weighted interleaved echo planar imaging. Magn Reson Med 2000;44:101–9.

70. Arfanakis K, Tamhane AA, Pipe JG, et al. K-space undersampling in PROPELLER imaging. Magn Reson Med 2005;53(3):675–83.

71. Pipe JG, Zwart N. TurboPROP: improved PROPELLER imaging. Magn Reson Med 2006;55: 380–5.

72. Oshio K, Feinberg DA. GRASE (gradient- and spin-echo) imaging: a novel fast MRI technique. Magn Reson Med 1991;20:344–9.

73. Arfanakis K, Gui M, Lazar M. White matter tractography by means of turboPROP diffusion tensor imaging. Ann N Y Acad Sci 2005;1064: 78–87.

74. Chuang TC, Huang TY, Lin FH, et al. PROPELLER-EPI with parallel imaging using a circularly symmetric phased-array RF coil at 3.0 T: application to high-resolution diffusion tensor imaging. Magn Reson Med 2006;56: 1352–8.

75. Wang FN, Huang TY, Lin FH, et al. PROPELLER EPI: an MRI technique suitable for diffusion tensor imaging at high field strength with reduced geometric distortions. Magn Reson Med 2005;54: 1232–40.

76. Deng J, Omary RA, Larson AC. Multishot diffusion-weighted splice PROPELLER MRI of the abdomen. Magn Reson Med 2008;59:947–53.

77. Deng J, Virmani S, Young J, et al. Diffusion-weighted PROPELLER MRI for quantitative assessment of liver tumor necrotic fraction and viable tumor volume in vx2 rabbits. J Magn Reson Imaging 2008;27:1069–76.

78. Deng J, Miller FH, Salem R, et al. Multishot diffusion-weighted PROPELLER magnetic resonance imaging of the abdomen. Invest Radiol 2006;41: 769–75.

79. Robson MD, Anderson AW, Gore JC. Diffusion-weighted multiple shot echo planar imaging of humans without navigation. Magn Reson Med 1997;38:82–8.

80. Porter DA, Mueller E. Multi-shot diffusion-weighted EPI with readout mosaic segmentation and 2D navigator correction. 11th Annual Meeting of the ISMRM. 2004:442.

81. Holdsworth SJ, Skare S, Newbould RD, et al. Readout-segmented EPI for rapid high resolution diffusion imaging at 3T. Eur J Radiol 2008;65(1): 36–46.

82. Holdsworth S, Skare S, Newbould R, et al. GRAPPA-accelerated readout-segmented EPI for high resolution diffusion imaging. Presented at the 16th Annual Meeting of ISMRM. Toronto, Canada, May 3–9, 2008.

83. Holdsworth S, Skare S, Newbould R, et al. Practical considerations for GRAPPA-accelerated readout-segmented EPI in diffusion-weighted imaging. Presented at the 16th Annual Meeting of ISMRM. Toronto, Canada, May 3–9, 2008.

84. Holdsworth S, Skare S, Newbould R, et al. Comparison of short-readout trajectories for diffusion-weighted imaging. Presented at the 16th Annual Meeting of ISMRM. Toronto, Canada, May 3–9, 2008.

85. Kim DH, Chung S, Vigneron DB, et al. Diffusion-weighted imaging of the fetal brain in vivo. Magn Reson Med 2008;59:216–20.

86. Glover GH, Lai S. Self-navigated spiral fMRI: interleaved versus single-shot. Magn Reson Med 1998; 39:361–8.

87. Glover GH, Law CS. Spiral-in/out BOLD fMRI for increased SNR and reduced susceptibility artifacts. Magn Reson Med 2001;46(3): 515–22.

88. Kim DH, Adalsteinsson E, Spielman DM. Simple analytic variable density spiral design. Magn Reson Med 2003;50:214–9.

89. Kim DH, Adalsteinsson E, Spielman DM. Spiral readout gradients for the reduction of motion artifacts in chemical shift imaging. Magn Reson Med 2004;51:458–63.

90. Kim DH, Spielman DM. Reducing gradient imperfections for spiral magnetic resonance spectroscopic imaging. Magn Reson Med 2006;56:198–203.

91. Spielman DM, Pauly JM, Meyer CH. Magnetic resonance fluoroscopy using spirals with variable sampling densities. Magn Reson Med 1995;34:388–94.

92. Miller KL, Pauly JM. Nonlinear phase correction for navigated diffusion imaging. Magn Reson Med 2003;50:343–53.

93. Maudsley AA. Carr-Purcell-Meiboom-Gill sequence for NMR Fourier imaging applications. J Magn Reson 1997;38:527–33.

94. Murdoch JB. An "effective" method for generating spin-echo intensity expression. Annual Meeting of the SMR. 1994:1145.

95. Shaka AJ, Rucker SP, Pines A. Iterative Carr-Purcell trains. J Magn Reson 1988;77:606–11.

96. Conolly SM, Nishimura DG, Macovski A. Variable-rate selective excitation. J Magn Reson 1988;78:440–58.

97. Norris DG, Bornert P, Reese T, et al. On the application of ultra-fast RARE experiments. Magn Reson Med 1992;27:142–64.

98. Norris DG. Selective parity rare imaging. Magn Reson Med 2007;58:643–9.

99. Alsop DC. Phase insensitive preparation of single-shot RARE: application to diffusion imaging in humans. Magn Reson Med 1997;38:527–33.

100. Buxton RB. The diffusion sensitivity of fast steady-state free precession imaging. Magn Reson Med 1993;29:235–43.

101. Miller KL, Hargreaves BA, Gold GE, et al. Steady-state diffusion-weighted imaging of in vivo knee cartilage. Magn Reson Med 2004;51:394–8.

102. Baur A, Stabler A, Bruning R, et al. Diffusion-weighted MR imaging of bone marrow: differentiation of benign versus pathologic compression fractures. Radiology 1998;207:349–56.

103. Le Bihan D, Turner R, MacFall JR. Effects of intravoxel incoherent motions (IVIM) in steady-state free precession (SSFP) imaging: application to molecular diffusion imaging. Magn Reson Med 1989;10:324–37.

104. Hennig J. Echoes—how to generate, recognize, use or avoid them in MR-imaging sequences: part 1. Concepts Magn Reson 1991;3:125–43.

105. Hennig J. Echoes—how to generate, recognize, use or avoid them in MR-imaging sequences: part 2. Concepts Magn Reson 1991;3:179–92.

106. McNab JA, Miller KL. Sensitivity of diffusion weighted steady state free precession to anisotropic diffusion. Magn Reson Med 2008;60:405–13.

107. Low RN, Gurney J. Diffusion-weighted MRI (DWI) in the oncology patient: value of breathhold DWI compared to unenhanced and gadolinium-enhanced MRI. J Magn Reson Imaging 2007;25:848–58.

108. Kwee TC, Takahara T, Ochiai R, et al. Diffusion-weighted whole-body imaging with background body signal suppression (DWIBS): features and potential applications in oncology. Eur Radiol 2008;18:1937–52.

109. Lauenstein TC, Goehde SC, Herborn CU, et al. Whole-body MR imaging: evaluation of patients for metastases. Radiology 2004;233:139–48.

110. Squillaci E, Manenti G, Mancino S, et al. Staging of colon cancer: whole-body MRI vs. whole-body PET-CT—initial clinical experience. Abdom Imaging 2008;33:676–88.

111. Schmidt GP, Schoenberg SO, Schmid R, et al. Screening for bone metastases: whole-body MRI using a 32-channel system versus dual-modality PET-CT. Eur Radiol 2007;17:939–49.

112. Takahara T, Ogino T, Okuaki T, et al. Respiratory gated body diffusion weighted imaging avoiding prolongation of scan time: tracking only navigator echo (TRON) technique. Presented at the 15th Annual Meeting of ISMRM. Berlin (Germany), May 19–25, 2007.

113. Takahara T, Hendrikse J, Yamashita T, et al. Diffusion-weighted MR neurography of the brachial plexus: feasibility study. Radiology 2008;249:653–60.

114. Zhang ZW, Song LJ, Meng QF, et al. High-resolution diffusion-weighted MR imaging of the human lumbosacral plexus and its branches based on a steady-state free precession imaging technique at 3T. AJNR Am J Neuroradiol 2008;29:1092–4.

Diffusion MR Tractography As a Tool for Surgical Planning

Jeffrey Berman, PhD

KEYWORDS

- MR imaging • Diffusion tensor imaging
- Tractography • Surgical planning • Brain
- Motor tract

Diffusion MR tractography has rapidly become an important clinical tool that can delineate functionally important white matter tracts for surgical planning. One of the goals of brain surgery is to avoid damage to eloquent cortex and subcortical white matter. Diffusion tractography remains the only noninvasive method capable of segmenting the subcortical course of a white matter tract. This article reviews the technical and clinical issues surrounding presurgical diffusion tractography, including traditional diffusion tensor imaging (DTI) methods and more advanced high angular resolution diffusion imaging (HARDI) approaches, such as q-ball imaging. An overview of the presurgical DTI and q-ball tractography protocols used at our institution is also provided.

Tractography based on diffusion MR exploits the correlation between water diffusion and brain structure to delineate the course of white matter pathways.[1–5] The brain's white matter is highly organized into fasciculi comprised of densely packed axons. Axonal membranes, myelin, and other structures affect the pattern of Brownian motion of water within white matter.[6] Tractography follows a white matter tract from voxel to voxel in three dimensions by assuming that the direction of least restricted diffusion corresponds with the orientation of axons.

The quantitative assessments of tissue microstructure central to the scientific applications of diffusion MR are not directly used for presurgical tractography. Instead, the goal of presurgical tractography is simply to identify the position of eloquent pathways, such as the motor, sensory, and language tracts. The shortcomings of DTI fiber tracking have driven the development of advanced HARDI techniques to provide more accurate presurgical tractography. This article includes a description of the most recent applications of q-ball tractography, one of these HARDI methods, to surgical planning. As DTI and HARDI tractography become more widely used for patient diagnosis and treatment, it is critical for users to understand the capabilities and limitations of these techniques.

SPECTRUM OF BRAIN MAPPING TECHNIQUES

Tractography complements the information available from an array of brain mapping techniques available for surgical planning. Brain mapping techniques are differentiated by invasiveness, accuracy, and their physiologic basis. Diffusion MR is inherently noninvasive and does not, in most applications, directly detect brain function. Instead, tractography uses the diffusion of water to observe the microstructure of brain tissue, construct the gross anatomy of major white matter pathways, and then infer the trajectory of the delineated tract. Other noninvasive functional mapping techniques, such as functional MR imaging,[7–10] magnetoencephalography,[11–13] and electrocorticography,[14] observe physiologic changes associated with brain function. However, these techniques are restricted to localizing activity in the gray matter.

Cortical and subcortical electrical stimulation directly determines the function of neurons and remains the gold standard for functional mapping during neurosurgery.[15,16] Stimulation is highly invasive, however, and subcortical stimulation

Department of Radiology and Biomedical Imaging, University of California, San Francisco, 185 Berry Street, Suite 350, San Francisco, CA 94107, USA
E-mail address: jberman@radiology.ucsf.edu

Magn Reson Imaging Clin N Am 17 (2009) 205–214
doi:10.1016/j.mric.2009.02.002
1064-9689/09/$ – see front matter

cannot be performed until the resection cavity is close to the target pathway.[17] Localization with stimulation also is subject to inaccuracies from the penetration of electrical current into surrounding tissues and variations in excitation thresholds.[18,19] In the clinical setting, it is advantageous to use more than one brain mapping technique. Independent aspects of physiology are observed with each mapping technique, and their combined results can be used to validate each other and improve the confidence of surgical planning decisions.

ROUTINE PRESURGICAL DIFFUSION TENSOR IMAGING TRACTOGRAPHY PROTOCOL

Translating DTI tractography into a useful clinical tool requires efficient integration of the technique into presurgical protocols. This section describes the presurgical DTI fiber-tracking protocol developed and routinely performed at University of California San Francisco. DTI tractography of the motor tract is prescribed for any brain tumor case with a lesion near the motor tract that involves awake or asleep intraoperative cortical stimulation mapping. The protocol involves image acquisition, post processing, quality assurance, and integration with a surgical navigation system.

DTI acquisition sequences are readily available on all commercial MR scanner platforms. The following discussion provides several general guidelines for acquiring diffusion MR data suitable for tractography; more detailed specifications can be found in a recent review.[20,21] A minimum of six diffusion gradient directions is required to calculate the diffusion tensor; however, significant improvements in data quality can be obtained by increasing the number of directions.[22] For tractography, the slices must be contiguous and should not be thicker than 3 mm. At our institution, a typical acquisition at 1.5 T on a GE scanner has TR/TE = 11 s/78 ms, 3-mm thick slices, matrix = 128 × 128, field of view = 260 × 260 mm, ASSET factor = 2, and 15 diffusion directions with two averaged acquisitions at b = 1000 s/mm^2. Total diffusion imaging time is less than 8 minutes. In addition to diffusion MR, high-resolution three-dimensional T1- and T2-weighted anatomic images are acquired for use with the surgical navigation system. The postcontrast three-dimensional T1-weighted spoiled gradient recalled and the three-dimensional T2-weighted fast spin echo volumes have voxel resolution of 1 × 1 × 1.5 mm.

DTI tractography is performed with multiple regions of interest using an algorithm based on the deterministic fiber assignment by continuous tracking method.[4] Fiber tracks are first generated from a region drawn in the cerebral peduncle with the aid of the b = 0 s/mm^2 echo planar images from the DTI sequence (Fig. 1A) and the postprocessed DTI anisotropy map. The starting region encompasses the entire cerebral peduncle, although the motor tract only occupies a fraction of this region. An overly large starting region reduces the potential for user-introduced error. Tractography algorithms such as the fiber assignment by continuous tracking method require a minimum anisotropy threshold to be specified for propagation of the "streamline" outlining the fiber trajectory. If the fiber track encounters a voxel with anisotropy below the threshold, which is usually caused by the presence of gray matter or cerebrospinal fluid, the streamline is terminated at that location. A relatively low fractional anisotropy threshold of 0.1 is used for presurgical tractography to assist in following white matter tracts through regions of edema or tumor infiltration, which exhibit low diffusion anisotropy.[23] Each voxel in the starting region is densely seeded with 27 starting points evenly arranged in a 3 × 3 × 3 grid to improve fiber tracking performance.[2]

Extraneous fiber tracks are removed through the use of multiple target regions of interest (Fig. 1). The fiber tracks are first targeted to a region drawn in the posterior limb of the internal capsule. Then a second target region is drawn around fiber track bundles anterior to the central sulcus within the precentral gyrus. Fiber tracks passing through all three regions are retained as the delineated pyramidal tract (See Fig. 1).

The echo planar images are unsuitable for surgical navigation because of poor image contrast and geometric warping artifacts that compromise anatomic fidelity, so the DTI tractography must be co-registered to the high-resolution anatomic images. The b = 0 s/mm^2 echo planar images are first aligned to the anatomic images using automated image registration.[24,25] A three-dimensional affine 12-parameter model with a maximum of 50 iterations is used for registration. The registration's performance is checked by comparing the position of sulci, ventricles, and cortex. The transformation matrix is applied to the DTI fiber track mask, and the registered mask is fused to the high-resolution anatomic images. Voxels that contain fiber tracks are given intensities 1.5 times higher than the brightest anatomic feature in the image (Fig. 1C, D). This "hot white" intensity ensures that fiber tracks can be distinguished easily from T2-hyperintense lesions and cerebrospinal fluid.

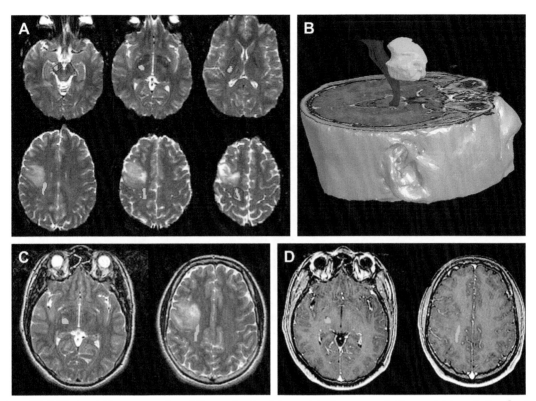

Fig. 1. (A) Diffusion MR tractography of the motor tract (*green*) is shown overlaid on axial b = 0 s/mm² echo planar images. Starting and target regions of interest (*red outlines*) are shown in the cerebral peduncle, posterior limb of the internal capsule, and precentral gyrus. (B) The resultant fiber tracks (*red*) are shown adjacent to the lesion (*green*) in three dimensions. (C) Tractography (*green*) is registered to the T2-weighted fast spin echo anatomic volume and (D) T1-weighted spoiled gradient recalled volume.

Black and white anatomic images fused with the DTI tractography easily can be made Digital Imaging and Communications in Medicine (DICOM) compliant and recognized by multiple systems, including PACS and surgical navigation systems (Fig. 2). The DICOM standard and newer surgical navigation systems allow tractography to be viewed as a color overlay. The advantage of color overlays is that they can be removed easily if the surgeon desires to view the anatomic images beneath the tractography. Multiple white matter pathways can be represented by different colors and simultaneously viewed. Diffusion MR fiber tracks also can be viewed in relation to the tumor and skull as three-dimensional streamlines, streamtubes, glyphs, and solid volumes.[26]

TRACTOGRAPHY OF PATHWAYS OTHER THAN THE MOTOR TRACT

Most presurgical tractography studies have focused on the motor tract because it is important for patient quality of life and is easy to track. However, tractography of functional pathways other than the cerebral corticospinal tract have

been integrated with a surgical navigation system or studied before surgery. A brainstem cavernous angioma was safely removed with the aid of sensory and motor pathway tractography.[27] The optic radiation is a challenging pathway to delineate with tractography because it is a thin ribbon of white matter and turns at a sharp angle through Meyer's loop (Fig. 3). Studies have shown the feasibility of using tractography to plan radiation therapy and guide surgical resection of arteriovenous malformations.[28,29]

The anatomy and operation of the language pathways are still under investigation. Tractography has been launched from mouth motor, speech arrest, and anomia stimulation sites on the frontal cortex.[30,31] The subcortical language network was observed to include connections to the supplementary motor area, cerebral peduncle, and thalamus. Language tracts including the arcuate fasciculus and the uncinate fasciculus have been delineated with tractography and their position confirmed with stimulation.[32,33] In patients undergoing anterior temporal lobectomy in the language dominant hemisphere, preoperative tractography has been used to predict language deficits.[34]

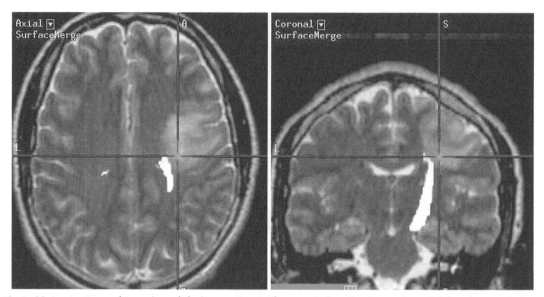

Fig. 2. Motor tractography as viewed during surgery with a surgical navigation system. Axial and coronal views are shown of the T2-weighted anatomic volume fused with the tractography. Voxels through which the fiber tracks pass are assigned bright white intensities. The red crosshairs indicate the location of a mouth motor subcortical stimulation site.

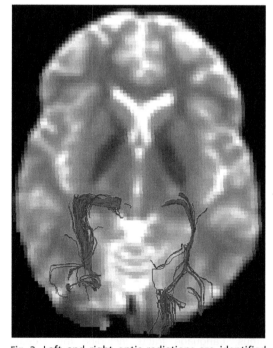

Fig. 3. Left and right optic radiations are identified with DTI tractography in an epileptic patient before surgery. Fiber tracks in three dimensions (*purple*) are projected on a b = 0 s/mm² axial echo planar slice. The anterior extent of Meyer's loop is not fully delineated with DTI tractography because of the tract's tight turn and thin dimensions.

OTHER MAPPING TECHNIQUES USED WITH TRACTOGRAPHY

Diffusion MR should never be solely relied on to guide a resection. Because diffusion MR measures a structural property of the brain's tissue, functional information always must be added to infer the location of eloquent pathways. In most presurgical cases, our knowledge of brain anatomy enables us to draw starting and target regions in the cerebral peduncle and the precentral gyrus. In some brain tumor cases, however, the tumor has shifted or infiltrated the surrounding white matter, changing the geometry of the brain's anatomy.[35,36] These situations necessitate additional functional mapping to guide the placement of tractography starting and target regions. Motor functional MR imaging has been used to locate the motor and language cortex in patients who have brain tumor and define the starting region for diffusion tractography.[37–39] The use of functional MR imaging allows detailed functional specificity to be assigned to the generated tractography.[40] The subsection of the motor tract or language pathways specific to a particular muscle group or language function can be delineated. There is a disjoint between the functional MR imaging–activated volume in the gray matter and brain tissue with diffusion anisotropy in the white matter, however. The tractography starting region can be drawn manually in the white matter of the gyrus adjacent to the functional MR imaging activation.

Validation of DTI tractography is necessary if the technique is to be trusted for surgical planning. Electrical stimulation of cortical and subcortical brain tissue has aided in the preservation of functional brain tissue for many decades.[16] Comparison to electrical stimulation has been a necessary step to validate tractography's use during surgery. Electrical stimulation studies test tractography and its integration with the surgical navigation system in a real clinical situation. **Fig. 4** demonstrates the combination of DTI tractography and cortical stimulation to delineate the portion of the motor tract that controls jaw motions.

Diffusion tractography launched from stimulation sites on the primary motor cortex has been observed to follow the expected anatomic course and maintain somatotopic organization through the internal capsule.[30] An initial study observed a gap between tractography and subcortical motor stimulation.[41] The diffusion tractography was capable of revealing the relative position of

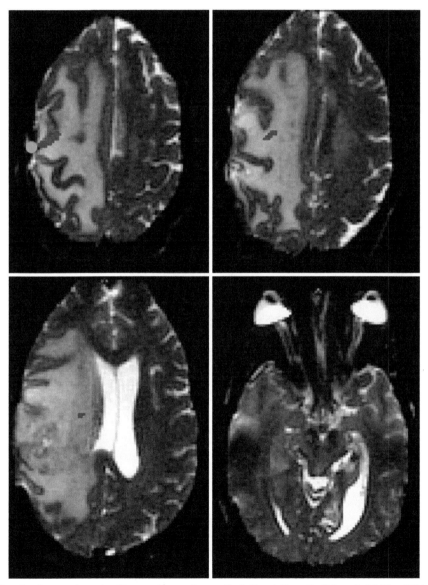

Fig. 4. DTI fiber tracks were launched from a jaw motor cortical stimulation site (*blue circle*). The DTI tractography (*red*) represents only the portion of the motor pathway descending from the cortical stimulation site. This case demonstrated the feasibility of using DTI fiber tracking to follow white matter tracts through some T2-hyperintense lesions.

the tumor and corticospinal tract; however, the borders of the tract were underestimated. Additional subcortical motor stimulation studies have repeatedly observed an approximately 1-cm gap between the electrode tip and tractography.[42–44]

The gap between DTI tractography and bipolar stimulation represents the cumulative errors from diffusion tensor uncertainty, registration inaccuracies, and brain shift during surgery. Noise in the diffusion MR signal results in uncertainty in the orientation of the diffusion tensor and the position of fiber tracks.[45,46] Geometric distortions are common on the echo planar images used to acquire diffusion MR. Care must be taken when registering echo planar images to the high-resolution anatomic volumes. Numerous studies have examined the effect of brain shift during surgery.[47–51] It is possible for the brain to shift either inward or outward, altering the position of tractography as perceived on the surgical navigation system. Bipolar stimulation currents can penetrate several millimeters into surrounding brain tissue.[18] Stimulation of neurons distant from the tip of the bipolar electrode always contributes to the approximately 1-cm discrepancy between the stimulation coordinates reported by the navigation system and the tractography.

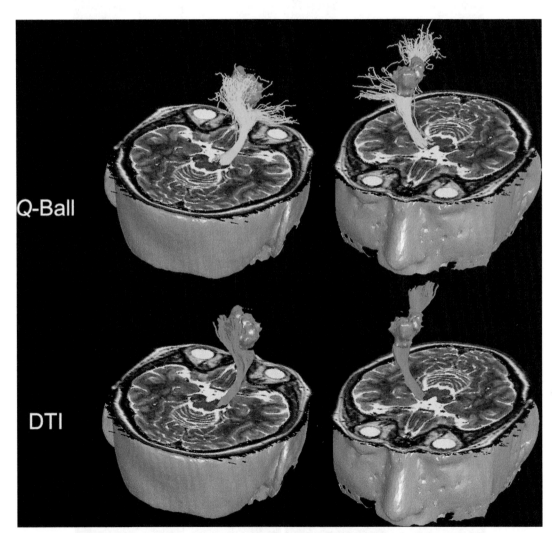

Fig. 5. Q-ball fiber tracks (*green, top row*) are compared with DTI fiber tracks (*blue, bottom row*). The tumor is in orange. The DTI fiber tracks are restricted to the portion of the motor tract originating in the superior-medial aspect of the motor cortex controlling lower extremity functions. The q-ball fiber tracks delineate a larger portion of the motor tract than the DTI fiber tracks. The q-ball fiber tracks show connectivity to the lateral portion of the motor cortex controlling facial motor functions.

HIGH ANGULAR RESOLUTION DIFFUSION IMAGING FOR FIBER TRACKING

The diffusion tensor model is limited to a single fiber population per voxel, and DTI fiber tracking fails in regions with crossing white matter fibers or intravoxel partial volume averaging of adjacent tracts with different fiber orientations. This shortcoming of DTI can be overcome by sampling many more diffusion-weighted directions than the minimum of six required for DTI and acquiring the images with stronger diffusion weighting than the clinical standard of b = 1000 s/mm^2 for DTI. This technique is known as HARDI, and many different mathematical approaches have been devised recently to reconstruct fiber pathways based on HARDI information. One of the most popular of these is known as q-ball imaging.[3,5] The q-ball reconstruction of HARDI data can distinguish distinct fiber populations in regions of complex white matter fiber architecture.[3,5] Tractography based on these advanced diffusion MR methods has been shown to traverse

white matter regions with crossing fibers and reveal a greater portion of tracts.[52–54]

The major limitation of HARDI's clinical application is the lengthy scan time required for acquiring many diffusion gradient directions. With only 55 gradient directions and parallel imaging at 3 T, however, scan time can be reduced to approximately 13 minutes or less.[3,55] A typical acquisition at our institution on a 3 T GE Signa EXCITE scanner has parallel imaging reduction factor of 2, TR/TE = 12.4 s/73 ms, 2.2 × 2.2 × 2.2 isotropic voxels, field of view = 280 × 280 mm, and a 128 × 128 matrix zero-filled to a 256 × 256 matrix. The 55 diffusion gradient directions are acquired with b = 2000 s/mm^2. Although 13 minutes still may be a bit lengthy for many clinical situations, it can be anticipated that the required scan time will decrease with hardware and HARDI methodologic improvements. Our institution has begun using q-ball tractography for a limited number of patients who have brain tumors.[55]

As seen in **Fig. 5**, q-ball fiber tracking is able to delineate the motor tract from the midbrain to the

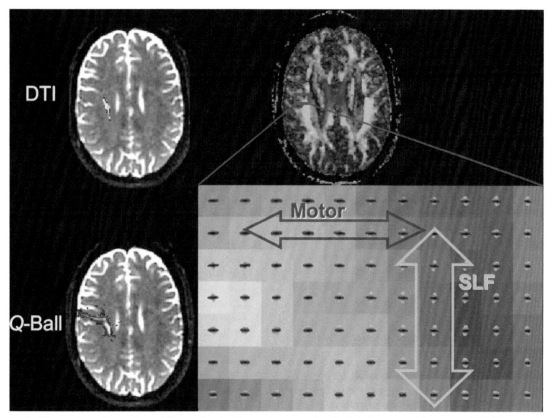

Fig. 6. The region of complex white matter in the centrum semiovale (*pink rectangle*) prevents DTI fiber tracks from traversing laterally to the motor cortex. The q-ball orientation density function distinguishes the motor pathway from the superior longitudinal fasciculus (SLF) and enables fiber tracks to course laterally through the centrum semiovale to the motor cortex.

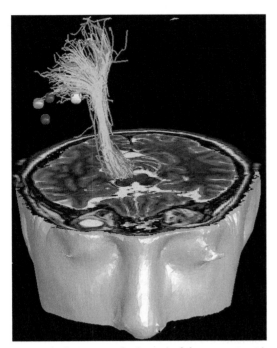

Fig. 7. Q-ball tractography (*green*) of the motor tract is shown in three dimensions in a patient who has a brain tumor. Cortical tongue motor (*purple spheres*) and subcortical mouth motor (*orange sphere*) stimulation sites are indicated. A cortical tongue sensory site (*blue sphere*) is also visible. The q-ball tractography generated presurgically showed connectivity from one cortical motor site, through the subcortical motor site, to the cerebral peduncle.

superior-medial and lateral portions of the motor cortex in our patients. The lateral sections of the motor tract control facial movements and are necessary for language functions. DTI fiber tracking revealed connectivity from the midbrain to only the medial-superior aspect of the motor cortex. The centrum semiovale is a region that contains multiple crossing white matter pathways, and DTI fails to accurately characterize this complex structure (**Fig. 6**). Initial studies have shown cortical and subcortical stimulations to be in good agreement with the course of the motor tract predicted by q-ball tractography (**Fig. 7**).[55]

IMPACT ON PATIENT CARE AND FUTURE DIRECTIONS

Many studies have been conducted to improve tractography techniques and assess the accuracy of diffusion tractography. Recently a few studies were conducted to assess the technique's impact on patient care. Mikuni examined postoperative motor function after tractography-guided surgery in patients who had brain tumors.[56,57] Subcortical

motor evoked potentials were combined with tractography to preserve motor function. This clinical outcome study and other subcortical stimulation validation studies suggested that stimulation be continually applied when resections are within 1 cm of motor tractography. Tractography can speed up radical resections by indicating which borders of a resection cavity deserve extensive stimulation.

Future improvements in MR hardware and HARDI methods will further enable tractography's clinical use for surgical planning. Protecting subcortical pathways and functional cortices is important during surgery. It is important to understand and account for the limitations of tractography and include multiple mapping techniques when planning surgeries.

ACKNOWLEDGMENTS

I am grateful to Roland Henry, PhD, for his guidance on analyzing the data for many of the figures, and to Pratik Mukherjee, MD, PhD, for his help preparing this article.

REFERENCES

1. Basser PJ, Mattiello J, LeBihan D. Estimation of the effective self-diffusion tensor from the NMR spin echo. J Magn Reson B 1994;103(3):247–54.
2. Conturo TE, Lori NF, Cull TS, et al. Tracking neuronal fiber pathways in the living human brain. Proc Natl Acad Sci USA 1999;96(18):10422–7.
3. Hess CP, Mukherjee P, Han ET, et al. Q-ball reconstruction of multimodal fiber orientations using the spherical harmonic basis. Magn Reson Med 2006; 56(1):104–17.
4. Mori S, Crain BJ, Chacko VP, et al. Three-dimensional tracking of axonal projections in the brain by magnetic resonance imaging. Ann Neurol 1999; 45(2):265–9.
5. Tuch DS. Q-ball imaging. Magn Reson Med 2004; 52(6):1358–72.
6. Beaulieu C. The basis of anisotropic water diffusion in the nervous system – a technical review. NMR Biomed 2002;15(7–8):435–55.
7. Guye M, Parker GJ, Symms M, et al. Combined functional MRI and tractography to demonstrate the connectivity of the human primary motor cortex in vivo. Neuroimage 2003;19(4):1349–60.
8. Krishnan R, Raabe A, Hattingen E, et al. Functional magnetic resonance imaging-integrated neuronavigation: correlation between lesion-to-motor cortex distance and outcome. Neurosurgery 2004;55(4): 904–14 [discusssion 914–5].
9. Ruff IM, Petrovich Brennan NM, Peck KK, et al. Assessment of the language laterality index in

patients with brain tumor using functional MR imaging: effects of thresholding, task selection, and prior surgery. AJNR Am J Neuroradiol 2008; 29(3):528–35.

10. Schulder M, Maldjian JA, Liu WC, et al. Functional image-guided surgery of intracranial tumors located in or near the sensorimotor cortex. J Neurosurg 1998;89(3):412–8.

11. Ganslandt O, Buchfelder M, Hastreiter P, et al. Magnetic source imaging supports clinical decision making in glioma patients. Clinical Neurology and Neurosurgery 2004;107(1):20–6.

12. Nagarajan S, Kirsch H, Lin P, et al. Preoperative localization of hand motor cortex by adaptive spatial filtering of magnetoencephalography data. J Neurosurg 2008;109(2):228–37.

13. Schiffbauer H, Berger MS, Ferrari P, et al. Preoperative magnetic source imaging for brain tumor surgery: a quantitative comparison with intraoperative sensory and motor mapping. J Neurosurg 2002;97(6):1333–42.

14. Engel AK, Moll CK, Fried I, et al. Invasive recordings from the human brain: clinical insights and beyond. Nat Rev Neurosci 2005;6(1):35–47.

15. Ojemann G. Brain organization for language from the perspective of electical stimulation mapping. The Behavioral and Brain Sciences 1983;6:189–230.

16. Penfield W, Rasmussen T. The cerebral cortex of man: a clinical study of localization of function. New York: Macmillan; 1950. xv, 248.

17. Keles GE, Lundin DA, Lamborn KR, et al. Intraoperative subcortical stimulation mapping for hemispherical perirolandic gliomas located within or adjacent to the descending motor pathways: evaluation of morbidity and assessment of functional outcome in 294 patients. J Neurosurg 2004;100(3):369–75.

18. Haglund MM, Ojemann GA, Blasdel GG. Optical imaging of bipolar cortical stimulation. J Neurosurg 1993;78(5):785–93.

19. Pouratian N, Cannestra AF, Bookheimer SY, et al. Variability of intraoperative electrocortical stimulation mapping parameters across and within individuals. J Neurosurg 2004;101(3):458–66.

20. Mukherjee P, Berman JI, Chung SW, et al. Diffusion tensor MR imaging and fiber tractography: theoretic underpinnings. AJNR Am J Neuroradiol 2008;29(4):632–41.

21. Mukherjee P, Chung SW, Berman JI, et al. Diffusion tensor MR imaging and fiber tractography: technical considerations. AJNR Am J Neuroradiol 2008;29(5):843–52.

22. Jones DK. The effect of gradient sampling schemes on measures derived from diffusion tensor MRI: a Monte Carlo study. Magn Reson Med 2004;51(4):807–15.

23. Stadlbauer A, Nimsky C, Buslei R, et al. Diffusion tensor imaging and optimized fiber tracking in glioma patients: Histopathologic evaluation of tumor-invaded white matter structures. Neuroimage 2007;34(3):949–56.

24. Woods RP, Grafton ST, Holmes CJ, et al. Automated image registration: I. General methods and intrasubject, intramodality validation. Journal of Computer Assisted Tomography 1998;22(1):139–52.

25. Woods RP, Grafton ST, Watson JDG, et al. Automated image registration: II. Intersubject validation of linear and nonlinear models. Journal of Computer Assisted Tomography 1998;22(1):153–65.

26. Nimsky C, Ganslandt O, Enders F, et al. Visualization Strategies for Major White Matter Tracts for Intraoperative Use. International Journal of Computer Assisted Radiology and Surgery 2006;1:13–22.

27. Chen X, Weigel D, Ganslandt O, et al. Diffusion tensor-based fiber tracking and intraoperative neuronavigation for the resection of a brainstem cavernous angioma. Surg Neurol 2007;68(3):285–91 [discussion 291].

28. Kikuta K, Takagi Y, Nozaki K, et al. Early experience with 3-T magnetic resonance tractography in the surgery of cerebral arteriovenous malformations in and around the visual pathway. Neurosurgery 2006;58(2):331–7 [discussion 331–7].

29. Maruyama K, Kamada K, Shin M, et al. Optic radiation tractography integrated into simulated treatment planning for Gamma Knife surgery. J Neurosurg 2007;107(4):721–6.

30. Berman JI, Berger MS, Mukherjee P, et al. Diffusion-tensor imaging-guided tracking of fibers of the pyramidal tract combined with intraoperative cortical stimulation mapping in patients with gliomas. J Neurosurg 2004;101(1):66–72.

31. Henry RG, Berman JI, Nagarajan SS, et al. Subcortical pathways serving cortical language sites: initial experience with diffusion tensor imaging fiber tracking combined with intraoperative language mapping. Neuroimage 2004;21(2):616–22.

32. Bello L, Gambini A, Castellano A, et al. Motor and language DTI Fiber Tracking combined with intraoperative subcortical mapping for surgical removal of gliomas. Neuroimage 2008;39(1):369–82.

33. Kamada K, Todo T, Masutani Y, et al. Visualization of the frontotemporal language fibers by tractography combined with functional magnetic resonance imaging and magnetoencephalography. J Neurosurg 2007;106(1):90–8.

34. Powell HW, Parker GJ, Alexander DC, et al. Imaging language pathways predicts postoperative naming deficits. J Neurol Neurosurg Psychiatry 2008;79(3):327–30.

35. Fernandez-Miranda JC, Rhoton AL Jr, Alvarez-Linera J, et al. Three-dimensional microsurgical and tractographic anatomy of the white matter of the human brain. Neurosurgery 2008;62(6 Suppl. 3):989–1026 [discussion 1026–8].

36. Wieshmann UC, Symms MR, Parker GJ, et al. Diffusion tensor imaging demonstrates deviation of fibres in normal appearing white matter adjacent to a brain tumour. J Neurol Neurosurg Psychiatry 2000;68(4): 501–3.

37. Hendler T, Pianka P, Sigal M, et al. Delineating gray and white matter involvement in brain lesions: three-dimensional alignment of functional magnetic resonance and diffusion-tensor imaging. J Neurosurg 2003;99(6):1018–27.

38. Holodny AI, Ollenschleger MD, Liu WC, et al. Identification of the corticospinal tracts achieved using blood-oxygen-level-dependent and diffusion functional MR imaging in patients with brain tumors. AJNR Am J Neuroradiol 2001;22(1):83–8.

39. Schonberg T, Pianka P, Hendler T, et al. Characterization of displaced white matter by brain tumors using combined DTI and fMRI. Neuroimage 2006; 30(4):1100–11.

40. Smits M, Vernooij MW, Wielopolski PA, et al. Incorporating functional MR imaging into diffusion tensor tractography in the preoperative assessment of the corticospinal tract in patients with brain tumors. AJNR Am J Neuroradiol 2007;28(7):1354–61.

41. Kinoshita M, Yamada K, Hashimoto N, et al. Fiber-tracking does not accurately estimate size of fiber bundle in pathological condition: initial neurosurgical experience using neuronavigation and subcortical white matter stimulation. Neuroimage 2005; 25(2):424–9.

42. Berman JI, Berger MS, Chung SW, et al. Accuracy of diffusion tensor magnetic resonance imaging tractography assessed using intraoperative subcortical stimulation mapping and magnetic source imaging. J Neurosurg 2007;107(3):488–94.

43. Kamada K, Todo T, Masutani Y, et al. Combined use of tractography-integrated functional neuronavigation and direct fiber stimulation. J Neurosurg 2005; 102(4):664–72.

44. Mikuni N, Okada T, Nishida N, et al. Comparison between motor evoked potential recording and fiber tracking for estimating pyramidal tracts near brain tumors. J Neurosurg 2007;106(1):128–33.

45. Anderson AW. Theoretical analysis of the effects of noise on diffusion tensor imaging. Magn Reson Med 2001;46(6):1174–88.

46. Lazar M, Alexander AL. An error analysis of white matter tractography methods: synthetic diffusion tensor field simulations. Neuroimage 2003;20(2): 1140–53.

47. Coenen VA, Krings T, Weidemann J, et al. Sequential visualization of brain and fiber tract deformation during intracranial surgery with three-dimensional ultrasound: an approach to evaluate the effect of brain shift. Neurosurgery 2005;56(1 Suppl):133–41 [discussion 133–41].

48. Keles GE, Lamborn KR, Berger MS. Coregistration accuracy and detection of brain shift using intraoperative sononavigation during resection of hemispheric tumors. Neurosurgery 2003;53(3):556–62 [discussion 562–4].

49. Nimsky C, Ganslandt O, Hastreiter P, et al. Preoperative and intraoperative diffusion tensor imaging-based fiber tracking in glioma surgery. Neurosurgery 2005;56(1):130–7.

50. Reinges MHT, Nguyen HH, Krings T, et al. Course of brain shift during microsurgical resection of supratentorial cerebral lesions: limits of conventional neuronavigation. Acta Neurochirurgica 2004;146(4): 369–77.

51. Roberts DW, Hartov A, Kennedy FE, et al. Intraoperative brain shift and deformation: a quantitative analysis of cortical displacement in 28 cases. Neurosurgery 1998;43(4):749–58 [discussion 758–60].

52. Berman JI, Chung S, Mukherjee P, et al. Probabilistic streamline Q-Ball tractography using the residual bootstrap. Neuroimage 2008;39:215–22.

53. Campbell JS, Siddiqi K, Rymar VV, et al. Flow-based fiber tracking with diffusion tensor and q-ball data: validation and comparison to principal diffusion direction techniques. Neuroimage 2005;27(4): 725–36.

54. Wedeen VJ, Wang RP, Schmahmann JD, et al. Diffusion spectrum magnetic resonance imaging (DSI) tractography of crossing fibers. Neuroimage 2008; 41(4):1267–77.

55. Berman JI, Clark DJ, Berger MS, et al. Improved Diffusion MR Fiber Tracking for Neurosurgical Application. ISMRM 2008; Toronto.

56. Mikuni N, Okada T, Enatsu R, et al. Clinical impact of integrated functional neuronavigation and subcortical electrical stimulation to preserve motor function during resection of brain tumors. J Neurosurg 2007; 106(4):593–8.

57. Mikuni N, Okada T, Enatsu R, et al. Clinical significance of preoperative fibre-tracking to preserve the affected pyramidal tracts during resection of brain tumours in patients with preoperative motor weakness. J Neurol Neurosurg Psychiatry 2007; 78(7):716–21.

Update on Diffusion Tensor Imaging in Alzheimer's Disease

Christopher P. Hess, MD, PhD

KEYWORDS
- Alzheimer's disease • Diffusion imaging
- DTI • Mild cognitive impairment • Tractography

Millions of Americans now have Alzheimer's disease (AD), and the prevalence of the disease is accelerating rapidly as the population ages. It is now estimated that someone develops AD every 71 seconds (Alzheimer's Association), making it the most common cause for dementia in the United States. Beyond the significant individual and societal burden of the disease, the economic impact of AD is staggering, with estimated direct and indirect costs to the United States of over $100 billion per year. Unfortunately, the diagnosis of AD can be made with high accuracy only in its late stages, at a time when there is little hope for therapeutic intervention. There is an urgent need for development of accurate AD biomarkers to define individual prognosis, to understand the underlying pathophysiology of the disease, and to monitor the effects of the disease-modifying therapies that are currently under development. Among several putative biomarkers that include genetic testing, spinal fluid and plasma analysis, and neuropsychological evaluation, neuroimaging is poised to take a primary role in the evaluation of patients who have cognitive complaints. Widespread availability in the medical community and its current use in clinical practice make MR imaging particularly well suited to further development.

Mild cognitive impairment (MCI) has been described as a transitional period from healthy aging to clinically probable AD, when patients experience problems with memory, language, or other mental functions that are severe enough to be noticed by other people, but not serious enough to interfere with daily life. The population of patients who have MCI is very heterogeneous, containing a larger group who will remain at a stable cognitive function for life and a smaller subset who go on to develop clinically definite AD. Patients who have amnestic MCI, suffering from symptoms that relate primarily to memory loss, are at the greatest risk of ultimately developing AD, and as a group convert to clinically probable AD over time at a rate of 10%–15% per year. This group is the primary target of several pharmacologic and vaccine treatments that are aimed at slowing or possibly halting the progression of AD pathology.

The number of MR imaging biomarkers for MCI and Alzheimer's mirrors the breadth of information that can be derived using pulse sequences available on modern scanners; high-resolution structural T1, perfusion, magnetization transfer, diffusion imaging, and functional MR imaging have all been proposed as potential biomarkers. Some of these sequences are currently available only in the research setting, but most are now available on commercial scanners. This article surveys the current state of research on the application of diffusion imaging for the evaluation of patients who have MCI and AD.

There is now sufficient data to indicate that measurement of water diffusion in some brain regions, such as the hippocampus, can serve as a useful adjunct to conventional high-resolution T1-weighted imaging in support of a clinical impression of probable AD. However, much work remains to determine whether diffusion may also

Department of Radiology and Biomedical Imaging, University of California, San Francisco, 505 Parnassus Avenue, Room L-358, San Francisco, CA 94143-0628, USA
E-mail address: chess@radiology.ucsf.edu

Magn Reson Imaging Clin N Am 17 (2009) 215–224
doi:10.1016/j.mric.2009.02.003
1064-9689/09/$ – see front matter © 2009 Elsevier Inc. All rights reserved.

be useful to distinguish between healthy elders and patients who have early symptoms of MCI and AD, whether altered diffusion within specific tracts correlates with deficits in individual cognitive domains on a patient-by-patient basis, and whether longitudinal changes in diffusion predict the course of disease progression.

CURRENT STATE OF STRUCTURAL MR IMAGING IN DEMENTIA

The current role for MR imaging evaluation of patients who have cognitive complaints is to exclude a potentially reversible structural abnormality. According to DSM-IV criteria, clinical diagnosis of AD requires that symptoms of progressive decline in memory and cognition reflect a primary process that is not due to other central nervous system conditions.[1] Most practice guidelines for the evaluation of patients who have dementia thus include some type of structural neuroimaging.[2,3] CT and MR imaging are notoriously unrewarding in this role, however, as a brain tumor, subdural hematoma, hydrocephalus, or other potentially reversible abnormality is found in at most 5% of patients, depending on the referral population.[4] Despite its low yield in this regard, imaging is routinely used to guide the management of patients, and not infrequently alters initial diagnostic impressions. MR imaging is particularly helpful in the differential diagnosis of dementia and in the characterization of comorbid disease, because it may suggest other pathologies such as significant vascular disease, infectious diseases such as progressive multifocal leukoencephalopathy or HIV, prion disease, or cerebrovascular amyloidosis.

Most memory and aging experts now use morphologic changes on MR imaging examinations as supplementary evidence for certain types of dementia (Fig. 1). For example, selective medial temporal lobe atrophy distinguishes AD from healthy aging and from certain types of frontotemporal dementia with relatively high accuracy. There is moderately strong evidence that visual hippocampal atrophy can accurately distinguish between patients who have AD and cognitively normal elders.[5] Qualitative assessment of hippocampal atrophy, as manifest by increased width of the temporal horn, decreased height of the hippocampus, and increased width of the choroidal fissure, has relatively low interobserver variability. Frontotemporal dementia is a clinically heterogeneous disease, but in late stages is typified by volume loss within the temporal and frontal lobes that is amenable to visual analysis.[6] Global atrophy is a feature of dementia with Lewy bodies, although there is relative sparing of the temporal lobes in comparison with AD.[7] While MR imaging features like these may aid in differential diagnosis, there are no specific patterns of regional atrophy that reliably distinguish different types of dementia in the preclinical stages, before the onset of overt cognitive or behavioral symptoms.

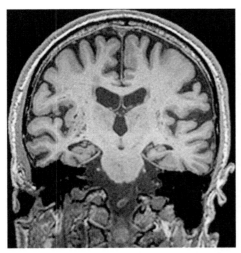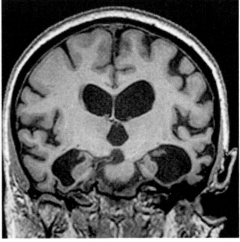

Fig. 1. Structural changes within the temporal lobes on high-resolution T1-weighted volumetric MR imaging. Hippocampal atrophy in a patient carrying a diagnosis of AD (*left*), showing enlargement of the temporal horns, decrease in hippocampal height and enlargement of the choroidal fissure that are more prominent on the left. Hippocampal atrophy is also present in a patient with semantic frontotemporal dementia (*right*), though much more striking atrophy is evident within the medial temporal lobes outside of the hippocampi. Memory and aging specialists routinely use different patterns of atrophy to confirm a clinical diagnosis of different types of dementia.

ALZHEIMER'S EFFECTS ON WHITE MATTER: RATIONALE FOR USING DIFFUSION MR IMAGING

As first described by Alois Alzheimer in 1907, the hallmark neuropathological changes in AD consist of extracellular, insoluble amyloid beta peptide (Aβ) and intracytoplasmic tau-associated neurofibrillary tangles (NFTs). According to the amyloid hypothesis of AD, it is the abnormal processing of amyloid precursor protein and consequent cumulative deposition of Aβ that ultimately leads to the development of symptoms. This theory is based on ex vivo examination of brain specimens from demented and nondemented subjects. Little is known about the intermediate steps that result in Aβ and NFT accumulation. However, there is sufficient evidence to suggest that there exists a programmed sequence of biochemical and structural changes that begins on a cellular and synaptic level and ultimately culminates in the loss of specific bundles of vulnerable neurons.[8] Initially, this process involves a decline in synaptic function and decreased structural integrity of the neuron. This is followed by internal redistribution of intracellular organelles and cytoskeletal elements from the neuronal periphery to the soma. Degeneration of the dendritic processes, axonal loss, and a progressive decline in neuronal function then ensue. When the neuronal death becomes sufficiently widespread to significantly decrease neuronal density, the result is regional atrophy in predictable areas of the brain that can be identified macroscopically.

Autopsy studies indicate that AD pathology precedes the development of cognitive symptoms by many years, and that some patients accrue Aβ plaques and NFTs but do not develop AD. Entorhinal pre-alpha cells, which give rise to axons within the perforant pathway in the medial temporal lobe, are reduced in number early in AD and may be among the earliest sites of disease in patients who do develop clinical symptoms.[9,10] During the early onset of symptoms, the loss of neurons that initially began in the medial temporal lobes spreads locally to neighboring neurons within the allocortex.[11] Involvement of the neocortex is a later phenomenon, with accumulation of neuritic plaques outside of the mesial temporal lobes, predominantly in regions of the brain that give rise to the long corticocortical tracts that interconnect the associative cortices of the temporal, parietal, and frontal lobes.[10,12] Injury to these tracts may be secondary to gray matter injury, localizing to the soma and dendritic processes of susceptible neurons, although research on both autopsy specimens and transgenic mouse models[13] suggests that AD pathology may also directly injure white matter. Several histopathology studies indicate that changes in white matter in AD consist not only of axonal loss, which would be typical of a primary gray matter process, but also oligodendrogliocyte death and reactive astrocytosis, microscopic features that are more characteristic of primary white matter disease.[8,14,15]

Noninvasive imaging in living patients who have MCI and AD also lends support to the idea that white matter is directly involved in the pathogenesis of AD. There have been several studies using high-resolution structural MR imaging that document not only gray matter loss, but also global and regional atrophy of deep and subcortical white matter.[16–18] White matter disruption also helps to explain the observation of spatially disparate involvement of the medial temporal lobes on MR imaging and the metabolic and perfusion deficits in the posterior cingulate cortex on functional positron emission tomography and single photon emission computed tomography studies in subjects who have AD. Specifically, by reducing the number of efferent neurons that project outside of the limbic system, hippocampal atrophy may secondarily give rise to cerebral blood flow reductions in more posterior regions of the brain outside of the medial temporal lobe.[19] Further in support of this hypothesis, a strong correlation between medial temporal atrophy and gray matter hypometabolism and hypoperfusion has recently been shown.[20]

The recognition that white matter is affected in patients who have MCI and AD has motivated a number of research groups to try and use diffusion MR imaging to detect subtle changes in white matter that are otherwise occult on conventional T1- and T2-weighted imaging. The role of diffusion MR imaging in dementia research is reflected in the growing number of research papers that have been published on the subject (Fig. 2). As is the case for most applications of diffusion, apparent diffusion coefficient (ADC) and fractional anisotropy (FA) are the two parameters that have most commonly been used to characterize white matter injury in the majority of these studies. Regional increases in ADC within white matter are thought to reflect the net increase in extracellular volume that occurs with the loss of neurons, axons and dendrites.[21] In contrast, reductions in FA are associated with alterations in tissue cytoarchitecture, axonal demyelination and gliosis. Several recent studies of diffusion in dementia have also employed measurements of directional diffusivity.[22–24] These parameters, axial (DA) and radial (DR) diffusivity, quantify the magnitude of water diffusion parallel and perpendicular to the principal orientation of white matter. They may relate more closely to

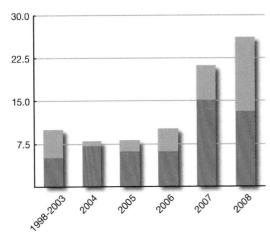

Fig. 2. Growth of research on the application of diffusion imaging to MCI and AD. Plot of published reports using diffusion MR imaging for the evaluation of patients with MCI (*green*) and AD (*blue*) through 2008, retrieved using PubMed with criteria "diffusion tensor imaging" and "mild cognitive impairment" and "diffusion tensor imaging" and "Alzheimer's," respectively.

underlying pathology, because decreases in DA have correlated with axonal loss in some studies, whereas increases in DR are most characteristic of demyelination. Wallerian degeneration, for example, results in reduced DA;

whereas chronic ischemia increases both DR and DA.

REGIONAL CHANGES IN WATER DIFFUSION

The majority of studies applying diffusion imaging in MCI and AD employ region-of-interest (ROI) techniques, which rely upon expert measurement of ADC, FA, or other diffusion parameters in specific brain regions. ROIs may be drawn on b = 0 diffusion-weighted images, on anisotropy maps, or on T1-weighted images that have been spatially coregistered with diffusion data. Typical ROIs used for hypothesis testing in research on MCI and AD are illustrated in **Fig. 3**. More recent work by several authors[24–26] has employed whole-brain analysis methods, in which voxel-by-voxel statistical testing is performed after transforming calculated diffusion parameters for each subject into a standard measurement space. This approach avoids measurement bias through automated identification of regions of involved white matter, but introduces uncertainty during the spatial transformation step that may limit sensitivity to subtle changes.

Initial work on diffusion in subjects who have MCI[27,28] and AD[27,29,30] used diffusion-weighted imaging to characterize localized changes in mean diffusivity and anisotropy in the medial temporal lobes, especially within the hippocampal

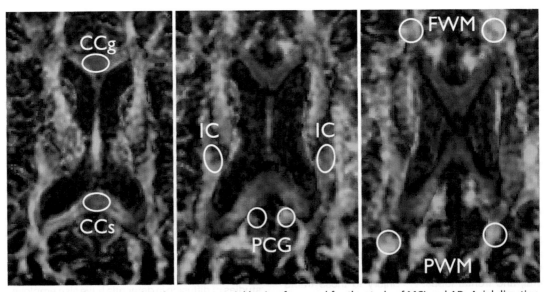

Fig. 3. Regions of interest within the supratentorial brain often used for the study of MCI and AD. Axial directionally encoded colormaps of fractional anisotropy within the brain of a patient with Alzheimer's disease (*green = anterior–posterior, blue = craniocaudal, red = left–right*). Manually drawn regions of interest have been placed within the genu (CCg) and splenium (CCs) of the corpus callosum, internal capsules (IC), posterior cingulate gyrus (PCG), frontal white matter (FWM) and parietal white matter (PWM). These tracts are relatively well defined on FA maps, but ROIs drawn on maps of ADC may be subject to partial volume averaging between tracts.

formation. Technical constraints at the time limited acquisition to relatively large voxel sizes of 5 × 5 × 5 mm or more and only three directional diffusion measurements, such that reliable calculation of the diffusion tensor was not feasible. Subject to these limitations, initial published reports of increased values of ADC within one or both hippocampi in subjects who have MCI have been subsequently reproduced in later work on modern scanners. In the earliest work on the subject, Kantarci and colleagues[27] observed that among multiple ROIs within the anterior and posterior lobar white matter, the thalami and cingulate gyri, only the hippocampus exhibited ADC values that differed significantly between normal control subjects and subjects who have MCI. However, while hippocampal ADC was up to 80% sensitive in separating healthy elders from subjects who have AD, it showed a disappointing 47% sensitivity in distinguishing between healthy elders and patients who have MCI. Asymmetry in the magnitude of ADC changes between the right and left hippocampus remains a point of debate, with some studies suggesting greater involvement on the left[31,32] and others indicating no significant asymmetry across the midline.[29,33,34] At least some increase in ADC is likely a diagnostic feature of AD and possibly MCI, but it should be noted that the reliability of the ADC measurements obtained in much of the work supporting this finding is uncertain because partial volume averaging with cerebrospinal fluid may have spuriously increased measurements of ADC in cases of significant hippocampal atrophy.

A growing body of literature also provides evidence for changes in water diffusion outside of the hippocampal complex in the lobar white matter. Among the most consistent findings are a significant increase in ADC and/or reduction in FA within the extralimbic temporal lobe.[23,25,26,29,33,35–38] Elevated ADC in the parietal lobe without accompanying changes in FA has been described by several groups in subjects who have both MCI[37,39] and AD.[31,33,38] Reduced FA has also been reported in the parietal lobes in AD subjects,[23,26,35,40] though it has not been cited as consistently as increased ADC. Reports of altered diffusion within the frontal lobes are considerably more variable in the literature,[22,35,41] confounded by the observation in many studies of age-related decreases in FA in the frontal white matter of cognitively normal elderly subjects.[41–43]

EVIDENCE FOR INVOLVEMENT OF SPECIFIC WHITE MATTER TRACTS

Variability in ROI placement presents a significant obstacle to consensus identification of white matter regions involved in AD. In any part of the brain, an ROI may encompass several white matter pathways that may or may not be individually affected by AD pathology. As diffusion pulse sequences with higher spatial resolution and less distortion by eddy-current and susceptibility artifacts have become more widely available, it is becoming increasingly evident that MCI and AD preferentially involve specific white matter pathways. Using field strengths of 3T and higher with modern gradient coils, voxel sizes of 4 × 4 × 4 mm or less are now routinely attained. Moreover, using a larger number of diffusion-encoding directions, fiber tractography can now more reliably parcellate the white matter tracts that have been implicated in the development of symptoms related to MCI and AD (**Fig. 4**).

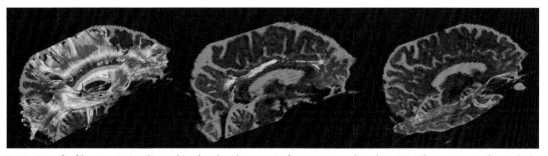

Fig. 4. Specific fiber tracts implicated in the development of symptoms related to AD. Fibers passing through the corpus callosum (*left*) represent the primary route of interhemispheric transfer of information. Axons within the cingulum bundle (*center*) interconnect the frontal cortex, cingulate cortex, retrosplenial cortex, and ventral temporal lobe, serving as a major conduit for emotional response and memory consolidation. The uncinate fasciculus (*right*), a much smaller tract that links the frontal and temporal lobes through the insular white matter, also plays a role in the storage and retrieval of long-term memory.

Corpus Callosum

The corpus callosum is comprised of axons with varying diameters that arise from pyramidal neurons in cortical layers 3 and 5, a group of neurons known to be involved in AD by neuropathology.[44,45] These fibers exhibit a consistent topographic organization, with an anterior-to-posterior arrangement from rostrum to splenium to interconnect homologous cortical regions across the hemispheres. Axons passing through the posterior aspect of the callosum to link the temporal, parietal, and occipital lobes tend to have larger diameters and faster conduction velocities, thereby facilitating the rapid interhemispheric exchange of visual and somatosensory information. In contrast, the tracts that pass through the anterior aspect of the callosum to interconnect the frontal lobes are comprised largely of smaller diameter, slower-conducting axons. There are also a smaller number of the slow-conducting fibers that pass through the posterior callosum, to connect the higher-order processing areas of the temporal and parietal lobes that are characteristically involved in AD. Involvement of these axons may explain the poor performance that has been observed in subjects who have AD on motor, somatosensory and visual tests of interhemispheric transfer.[46]

Mirroring neuropathology evidence that points to the later involvement of the neocortex, it appears that the changes within the corpus callosum that are evident on diffusion imaging are a feature of more advanced disease. A number of studies have described reduced anisotropy and increased ADC and/or reduced FA within the posterior corpus callosum in subjects who have AD.[22,31,33,35–37,40,41,47–49] While similar reports of changes in MCI have also been described,[28,50] this is an inconsistent finding. The anterior callosum appears to be relatively spared in this process, although there have been some reports showing changes of a smaller magnitude within the genu and rostrum of the callosum.[41,50,51] Notably, the detection of any anterior callosum involvement in AD is confounded by the loss of frontal lobe neurons that occurs with normal aging, because there have now been multiple studies confirming increased ADC or reduced FA within the genu and anterior body of the callosum in healthy elders. The degree to which altered diffusion within the corpus callosum in subjects who have AD reflects secondary neuronal loss versus primary white matter injury remains to be determined, but recent work by Sydykova and colleagues[52] suggests that Wallerian degeneration plays a significant role. In this study, a significant regional correlation was observed between FA within the corpus callosum and gray matter thickness in the lobes these fibers connect.

Uncinate Fasciculus

The uncinate fascicle (UF) is a monosynaptic association pathway that couples the frontal and temporal lobes via white matter tracts coursing through the insular region. Within the temporal lobe, neurons arising from the amygdala, hippocampus, temporal pole, and superior temporal gyri contribute to this tract, which passes underneath the putamen and claustrum within the limen insulae to terminate within the ipsilateral orbitofrontal cortex. Disruption of this tract, which consists primarily of cholinergic fibers, may result in memory deficits after traumatic brain injury[53] and is associated with neuropsychological deficits after neurosurgical resection.[54] While ROI measurements of diffusion in the temporal lobe may have included segments of the UF in early studies, there are very few studies that specifically assess the integrity of the UF. In one study by Taoka and colleagues,[55] both a reduction in FA and an increase in mean diffusivity were observed within the UF bilaterally in AD subjects relative to healthy controls, while in another study by Yasmin and colleagues,[56] FA was reduced but mean diffusivity was preserved. Interestingly, a correlation between FA in the left UF in subjects who have amnestic MCI and performance on tests of episodic memory and emotional recognition has also been described.[57]

Superior Longitudinal Fasciculus

The superior longitudinal fasciculus (SLF) is a massive bidirectional tract that connects different regions of the cortex within the same hemisphere. Using DTI, the tract has been divided by Makris and colleagues[58] into four primary components, each serving a different function: SLF I-III and an arcuate fascicle. The tract has been implicated in the pathology of AD through several studies using diffusion imaging.[34,36,40,47,49] Xie and colleagues[26] have suggested that there is predominant involvement within the SLF II component of the tract, a bundle of fibers that connects the inferior parietal lobe to the prefrontal cortex and serves as the major route for the conscious perception of visual space. This segment of the SLF plays a role in the modulation of spatial attention, and its disruption results in disorders of spatial working memory. Involvement of SLF II may contribute to deficits in spatial short-term memory experienced by some patients who have AD.

Cingulum Bundle and Parahippocampal Gyrus

The cingulum bundle is composed primarily of bidirectional association fibers that interconnect cingulate cortex, retrospenial cortex, frontal cortex and the ventral temporal lobe.[59] As part of the hippocampal/mammillothalamic circuit of Papez, this tract is important for the control of emotion and the long-term consolidation of memories. ROI measurements of diffusion have shown both elevated ADC and reduced FA within the cingulum bundle of subjects who have AD.[35,36,48,49,60,61] Measurements of FA using tractography methods to specifically define the margins of this structure suggest that there is a reduction in anisotropy along the entire length of the tract.[62] The magnitude of these changes relative to healthy controls varies across studies, confounded by differences in ROI placement or clinical heterogeneity in the cohorts of subjects evaluated. It is notable that among several ROIs evaluated by Zhang and colleagues,[48] the region with the largest effect size in discerning between healthy controls and MCI or AD was the posterior cingulate, at the apex of the posterior curve of the tract. In this study, medial temporal lobe volume was only 63% accurate for distinguishing between healthy subjects and subjects who have MCI, but accuracy increased to 78% with the additional consideration of left posterior cingulate FA. Similarly, the accuracy of separating healthy subjects from subjects who have AD increased from 78% to 91% when left posterior cingulate FA was included. Several authors have also described reduction in FA within the more rostral and ventral continuation of this tract, within the white matter of the parahippocampal gyrus.[24,25,47] In a study of 20 subjects who have probable AD, Salat and colleagues[24] observed that reduced FA in parahippocampal white matter exhibited an anterior-to-posterior gradient.

Perforant Pathway

The perforant pathway (PP) represents the major route of input to the hippocampus, with axons that originate within the entorhinal cortex and project to the dentate gyrus, Ammon's horn and subiculum. The tract serves as a node within a much larger network, transmitting information from several neocortical association areas through the entorhinal cortex and hippocampus to ultimately distribute information throughout the limbic system. The PP is particularly important to the pathology of AD, because its disruption results in the functional disconnection of higher-level sensory input to the hippocampus. Early involvement of these neurons has been documented through autopsy specimens,[9,12] making it a prime region of the brain for evaluation using diffusion MR imaging. Unfortunately, the pathway is difficult to identify with accuracy using diffusion imaging due to its relatively small volume, proximity to other neighboring tracts, and frequent geometric distortion from susceptibility artifacts. In a relatively small study of 10 subjects who have MCI by Kalus and colleagues,[63] reduced anisotropy within the PP was the solitary parameter that distinguished this group from healthy controls. In this study, decreases in anisotropy further correlated with MMSE score.

FUTURE WORK

The role for diffusion imaging in the evaluation of patients who have MCI and AD remains to be determined. To date, the strongest evidence from the literature supports the idea that early changes in white matter can be detected using diffusion in the hippocampus, the temporal stem, and the posterior corpus callosum in subjects who have AD. Results are considerably more variable in subjects who have MCI, in part reflecting the clinical heterogeneity of this population. Paralleling the early allocortical involvement on neuropathology, the earliest changes in water diffusion are found in the temporal lobes. In contrast, changes outside of this region, in structures such as the corpus callosum and parietal lobes, appear to arise later in the course of disease, during the period of the disease in which there is pathologic involvement of the neocortex. More work is clearly necessary to define the temporal and spatial course of changes in white matter diffusion in subjects who have MCI and AD, and to determine the degree to which these changes correlate with cognitive function on an individual basis.

Despite considerable progress in research in this area, there remain several challenges that must be overcome before diffusion imaging can become a reliable tool for dementia evaluation. As noted above, most studies to date have been undertaken in relatively small cohorts of 20 or fewer subjects, making it difficult to generalize the results of any one study with confidence. There has been a lack of consistent inclusion criteria for enrolling patients who have both MCI and AD among imaging studies. Well-defined study populations are especially important for MCI, because many patients who carry this diagnosis do not ultimately progress to Alzheimer's. Significant variations in imaging technique, including differences in voxel size, the number of diffusion-encoding directions and field strength, may account for some of the variability in observed outcomes between studies. Finally, there have been substantial differences in the methods used for data analysis, with most studies using ROI-based techniques that may suffer from interobserver variability and a smaller number of studies using whole-brain analysis techniques that may lower overall sensitivity.

Several recent technical advances in diffusion imaging promise to improve future work on patients who have dementia. Images obtained with the long echo times typically used for single-shot echo planar diffusion imaging are subject to significant geometric distortion. This is particularly problematic in evaluation of the medial temporal lobes, because their proximity to the pneumatized central skull base renders them vulnerable to artifacts from magnetic susceptibility. To overcome this problem, several postprocessing algorithms for correcting geometric distortion in echo planar imaging data have been developed. Perhaps more importantly, shorter echo parallel imaging techniques, which are less sensitive to susceptibility effects,[64] are now more widely available on scanners in both the research and clinical setting. Finally, a number of methods for improving characterization of diffusion in more complex white matter have started to be applied clinically. Techniques such as diffusion spectrum imaging and high angular resolution diffusion imaging, which permit more accurate fiber tracking within brain regions where white matter tracts cross, converge, or pass through one another, will become especially important for accurate evaluation of the long association tracts that are the primary site of involvement in later-stage AD.[65,66]

As research up to this point illustrates, the idea that diffusion MR imaging will identify subtle changes in white matter in a single brain region or tract before macroscopic gray matter loss is apparent is attractive. However, it is more likely that several functionally coupled tracts must become involved before the overt symptoms of the disease become apparent. Disruption in the flow of information between the larger-scale, corticocortical networks that link different areas of the brain is a likely culprit for the development of deficits that span several cognitive domains. While AD pathology may be present for many years, the disease may become evident only after a sufficient number of efferent and afferent connections between the hippocampal complex and the remainder of the brain have been interrupted.[67] Tools for noninvasive brain network analysis using diffusion MR imaging have recently been proposed,[68,69] making possible for the first time integrated analysis of changes in large-scale connectivity between different brain regions and suggesting the next step in the evolution of diffusion MR imaging as a powerful biomarker for Alzheimer's disease.

REFERENCES

1. American Psychiatric Association. Diagnostic and statistical manual of mental disorders: DSM-IV. 4th edition. Washington,DC: American Psychiatric Association; 1994.
2. Knopman DS, DeKosky ST, Cummings JL, et al. Practice parameter: diagnosis of dementia (an evidence-based review). Report of the quality standards subcommittee of the American Academy of Neurology. Neurology 2001;56:1143–53.
3. Petersen RC, Stevens JC, Ganguli M, et al. Practice parameter: early detection of dementia: mild cognitive impairment (an evidence-based review). Report of the quality standards subcommittee of the American Academy of Neurology. Neurology 2001;56:1133–42.
4. Kantarci K, Jack CR. Neuroimaging in Alzheimer disease: an evidence-based review. Neuroimaging Clin N Am 2003;13:197–209.
5. Wahlund LO, Almkvist O, Blennow K, et al. Evidence-based evaluation of magnetic resonance imaging as a diagnostic tool in dementia workup. Top Magn Reson Imaging 2005;16:427–37.
6. Kipps CM, Davies RR, Mitchell J, et al. Clinical significance of lobar atrophy in frontotemporal dementia: application of an MRI visual rating scale. Dement Geriatr Cogn Disord 2007;23:334–42.
7. Barber R, Ballard C, McKeith IG, et al. MRI volumetric study of dementia with Lewy bodies: a comparison with AD and vascular dementia. Neurology 2000;54:1304–9.
8. Brun A, Englund E. A white matter disorder in dementia of the Alzheimer type: a pathoanatomical study. Ann Neurol 1986;19:253–62.
9. Hyman BT, Van Hoesen GW, Damasio AR, et al. Alzheimer's disease: cell-specific pathology isolates the hippocampal formation. Science 1984;225:1168–70.
10. Gómez-Isla T, Price JL, McKeel DW, et al. Profound loss of layer II entorhinal cortex neurons occurs in very mild Alzheimer's disease. J Neurosci 1996;16:4491–500.
11. Braak H, Braak E. Neuropathological staging of Alzheimer-related changes. Acta Neuropathol 1991;82:239–59.
12. Braak H, Braak E. On areas of transition between allocortex and temporal isocortex in human brain. Normal morphology and lamina-specific pathology in Alzheimer's disease. Acta Neuropathol 1985;68:325–32.
13. Song SK, Kim JH, Lin SJ, et al. Diffusion tensor imaging detects age-dependent white matter

changes in a transgenic mouse model with amyloid deposition. Neurobiol Dis 2004;15:640–7.

14. Englund E. Neuropathology of white matter changes in Alzheimer's disease and vascular dementia. Dement Geriatr Cogn Disord 1998;9:6–12.

15. Bronge L, Bogdanovic N, Wahalund LO. Postmortem MRI and histopathology of white matter changes in Alzheimer brains: a quantitative, comparative study. Dement Geriatr Cogn Disord 2002;13:205–12.

16. Stout JC, Jernigan TL, Archibald SL, et al. Association of dementia severity with cortical gray matter and abnormal white matter volumes in dementia of the Alzheimer type. Arch Neurol 1996;53:742–9.

17. Salat DH, Kaye JA, Janowsky JS, et al. Prefrontal gray and white matter volumes in healthy aging and Alzheimer disease. Arch Neurol 1999;56:338–44.

18. Stoub TR, de Toledo-Morrell L, Stebbins GT, et al. Hippocampal disconnection contributes to memory dysfunction in individuals at risk for Alzheimer's disease. Proc Natl Acad Sci U S A 2006;26:10041–5.

19. Jobst KA, Smith AD, Barker CS, et al. Association of atrophy of the medial temporal lobe with reduced blood flow in the posterior parietotemporal cortex in patients with a clinical and pathological diagnosis of Alzheimer's disease. J Neurol Neurosurg Psychiatr 1992;55:190–4.

20. Villain N, Desgranges B, Viader F, et al. Relationships between hippocampal atrophy, white matter disruption, and gray matter hypometabolism in Alzheimer's disease. J Neurosci 2008;28:6174–81.

21. Beaulieu C. The basis of anisotropic water diffusion in the nervous system - a technical review. NMR Biomed 2002;15:435–55.

22. Choi SJ, Lim KO, Moteiro I, et al. Diffusion tensor imaging of frontal white matter microstructure in early Alzheimer's disease: a preliminary study. J Geriatr Psychiatry Neurol 2005;18:12–9.

23. Huang J, Friedland RP, Auchus AP, et al. Diffusion tensor imaging of normal-appearing white matter in mild cognitive impairment and early Alzheimer disease: preliminary evidence of axonal degeneration in the temporal lobe. AJNR Am J Neuroradiol 2007;28:1943–8.

24. Salat DH, Tuch DS, Van der Kouwe AJW, et al. White matter pathology isolates the hippocampal formation in Alzheimer's disease. Neurobiol Aging 2008 [Epub ahead of print].

25. Teipel SJ, Stahl R, Dietrich O, et al. Multivariate network analysis of fiber tract integrity in Alzheimer's disease. Neuroimage 2007;34:985–95.

26. Xie S, Xiao JX, Gong GL, et al. Voxel-based detection of white matter abnormalities in mild Alzheimer disease. Neurology 2006;66:1845–9.

27. Kantarci K, Jack CR Jr, Xu YC, et al. Mild cognitive impairment and Alzheimer disease: regional diffusivity of water. Radiology 2001;219:101–7.

28. Wang H, Su MY. Regional pattern of increased water diffusivity in hippocampus and corpus callosum in mild cognitive impairment. Dement Geriatr Cogn Disord 2006;22:223–9.

29. Hanyu H, Sakurai H, Iwamoto T, et al. Diffusion-weighted MR imaging of the hippocampus and temporal white matter in Alzheimer's disease. J Neurol Sci 1998;156:195–200.

30. Sandson TA, Felician O, Edelman RR, et al. Diffusion-weighted magnetic resonance imaging in Alzheimer's disease. Dement Geriatr Cogn Disord 1999;10:166–71.

31. Fellgiebel A, Wille P, Müller MJ, et al. Ultrastructural hippocampal and white matter alterations in mild cognitive impairment: a diffusion tensor imaging study. Dement Geriatr Cogn Disord 2004;18:101–8.

32. Müller MJ, Greverus D, Dellani PR, et al. Functional implications of hippocampal volume and diffusivity in mild cognitive impairment. Neuroimage 2005;28:1033–42.

33. Naggara O, Oppenheim C, Rieu D, et al. Diffusion tensor imaging in early Alzheimer's disease. Psychiatry Res 2006;146:243–9.

34. Ray KM, Wang H, Chu Y, et al. Mild cognitive impairment: apparent diffusion coefficient in regional gray matter and white matter structures. Radiology 2006;241:197–205.

35. Bozzali M, Falini A, Franceschi M, et al. White matter damage in Alzheimer's disease assessed in vivo using diffusion tensor magnetic resonance imaging. J Neurol Neurosurg Psychiatr 2002;72:742–6.

36. Takahashi S, Yonezawa H, Takahashi J, et al. Selective reduction of diffusion anisotropy in white matter of Alzheimer disease brains measured by 3.0 Tesla magnetic resonance imaging. Neurosci Lett 2002;332:45–8.

37. Stahl R, Dietrich O, Teipel SJ, et al. White matter damage in Alzheimer disease and mild cognitive impairment: assessment with diffusion-tensor MR imaging and parallel imaging techniques. Radiology 2007;243:483–92.

38. Rose SE, Janke AL, Chalk JB. Gray and white matter changes in Alzheimer's disease: a diffusion tensor imaging study. J Magn Reson Imaging 2008;27:20–6.

39. Rose SE, McMahon KL, Janke AL, et al. Diffusion indices on magnetic resonance imaging and neuropsychological performance in mild cognitive impairment. J Neurol Neurosurg Psychiatr 2006;77:1122–8.

40. Medina D, Detoledo-Morell L, Urresta F, et al. White matter changes in mild cognitive impairment and AD: a diffusion tensor imaging study. Neurobiol Aging 2006;27:663–72.

41. Head D, Buckner RL, Shimony JS, et al. Differential vulnerability of anterior white matter in nondemented aging with minimal acceleration in dementia of the

Alzheimer type: evidence from diffusion tensor imaging. Cereb Cortex 2004;14:410–23.

42. Salat DH, Tuch DS, Hevelone ND, et al. Age-related changes in prefrontal white matter measured by diffusion tensor imaging. Ann N Y Acad Sci 2005; 1064:37–49.

43. Grieve SM, Williams LM, Paul RH, et al. Cognitive aging, executive function, and fractional anisotropy: a diffusion tensor MR imaging study. AJNR Am J Neuroradiol 2007;28:226–35.

44. Giannakopoulos P, Hof PR, Michel JP, et al. Cerebral cortex pathology in aging and Alzheimer's disease: a quantitative survey of large hospital-based geriatric and psychiatric cohorts. Brain Res Brain Res Rev 1997;25:217–45.

45. Doron KW, Gazzaniga MS. Neuroimaging techniques offer new perspectives on callosal transfer and interhemispheric communication. Cortex 2008; 44:1023–9.

46. Lakmache Y, Lassonde N, Gauthier S, et al. Interhemispheric disconnection syndrome in Alzheimer's disease. Proc Natl Acad Sci U S A 1998;95:9042–6.

47. Rose SE, Chen F, Chalk JB, et al. Loss of connectivity in Alzheimer's disease: an evaluation of white matter tract integrity with colour coded MR diffusion tensor imaging. J Neurol Neurosurg Psychiatr 2000; 69:528–30.

48. Zhang Y, Schuff N, Jahng GH, et al. Diffusion tensor imaging of cingulum fibers in mild cognitive impairment and Alzheimer disease. Neurology 2007;68: 13–9.

49. Parente DB, Gasparetto EL, da Cruz LC Jr, et al. Potential role of diffusion tensor MRI in the differential diagnosis of mild cognitive impairment and Alzheimer's disease. AJR Am J Roentgenol 2008;190: 1369–74.

50. Hanyu H, Asano T, Sakurai H, et al. Diffusion-weighted and magnetization transfer imaging of the corpus callosum in Alzheimer's disease. J Neurol Sci 1999;67:37–44.

51. Ukmar M, Makuc E, Onor ML, et al. Evaluation of white matter damage in patients with Alzheimer's disease and patients with mild cognitive impairment by using diffusion tensor imaging. Radiol Med 2008; 113:915–22.

52. Sydykova D, Stahl R, Dietrich O, et al. Fiber connections between the cerebral cortex and the corpus callosum in Alzheimer's disease: a diffusion tensor imaging and voxel-based morphometry study. Cereb Cortex 2007;17:2276–82.

53. Niogi SN, Mukherjee P, Ghajar J, et al. Structural dissociation of attentional control and memory in adults with and without mild traumatic brain injury. Brain 2008;131:3209–21.

54. Ebeling U, von Cramon D. Topography of the uncinate fascicle and adjacent temporal fiber tracts. Acta Neurochir 1992;115:143–8.

55. Taoka T, Iwasaki S, Sakamoto M, et al. Diffusion anisotropy and diffusivity of white matter tracts within the temporal stem in Alzheimer disease: evaluation of the "tract of interest" by diffusion tensor tractography. AJNR Am J Neuroradiol 2006;29: 1329–34.

56. Yasmin H, Nakata Y, Aoki S, et al. Diffusion abnormalities of the uncinate fasciculus in Alzheimer's disease: diffusion tensor tract-specific analysis using a new method to measure the core of the tract. Neuroradiology 2008;50:293–9.

57. Fujie S, Namiki C, Nishi N, et al. The role of the uncinate fasciculus in memory and emotional recognition in amnestic mild cognitive impairment. Dement Geriatr Cogn Disord 2008;26:432–9.

58. Makris N, Kennedy DN, McInerney S, et al. Segmentation of subcomponents within the superior longitudinal fascicle in humans: a quantitative, in vivo, DT-MRI study. Cereb Cortex 2005;15:854–69.

59. Schmahmann J, Pandya D. Fiber pathways of the brain. Oxford: Oxford University Press; 2006.

60. Fellgeibel A, Müller MJ, Wille P, et al. Color-coded diffusion-tensor imaging of posterior cingulate fiber tracts in mild cognitive impairment. Neurobiol Aging 2005;26:1193–8.

61. Yoshiura T, Mihara F, Ogomori K, et al. Diffusion tensor in posterior cingulate gyrus: correlation with cognitive decline in Alzheimer's disease. Neuroreport 2002;13:2299–302.

62. Xie S, Xiao JX, Wang YH, et al. Evaluation of bilateral cingulum with tractography in patients with Alzheimer's disease. Neuroreport 2005;16: 1275–8.

63. Kalus P, Slotboom J, Gallinat J, et al. Examining the gateway to the limbic system with diffusion tensor imaging: the perforant pathway in dementia. Neuroimage 2006;30:713–20.

64. Jaermann T, Crelier G, Pruessmann KP, et al. SENSE-DTI at 3T. Magn Reson Med 2004;51: 230–6.

65. Hess CP, Mukherjee P. Visualizing white matter pathways in the living human brain: diffusion tensor imaging and beyond. Neuroimaging Clin N Am 2007;17:407–26.

66. Wedeen VJ, Wang RP, Schmahmann JD, et al. Diffusion spectrum imaging (DSI) tractography of crossing fibers. Neuroimage 2008;41:1267–77.

67. Delbeuck X, Van der Linden M, Collette F. Alzheimer's disease as a disconnection syndrome? Neuropsychol Rev 2003;13:79–92.

68. Hagmann P, Cammoun L, Gigandet X, et al. Mapping the structural core of the human cerebral cortex. PLoS Biol 2008;6:e159.

69. Iturria-Medina Y, Sotero RC, Canales-Rodríguez EJ, et al. Studying the human brain anatomical network via diffusion-weighted MRI and graph theory. Neuroimage 2008;40:1064–76.

Diffusion-Weighted Imaging, Diffusion-Tensor Imaging, and Fiber Tractography of the Spinal Cord

Majda M. Thurnher, MD[a], Meng Law, MD, FRACR[b,c],*

KEYWORDS

• Diffusion tensor • Fiber tractography • Spinal cord

In the brain, diffusion-weighted imaging (DWI) is an established and reliable method for the characterization of neurologic lesions. Although the diagnostic value of DWI in the early detection of ischemia has not diminished with time, many new clinical applications of DWI have also emerged, including differentiation of pyogenic abscess from necrotic tumor, metabolic disorders, epilepsy, tumor characterization, posttherapeutic change, and monitoring of chemoradiation therapy.

Diffusion-tensor imaging (DTI) and fiber tractography (FT) have more recently been developed and optimized, allowing quantification of the magnitude and direction of diffusion along three principal eigenvectors. The information provided by DTI acquisition allows measurement of various metrics, and generation of three-dimensional white matter FT. These metrics provide unique information about central nervous system tissue microstructure. DTI and FT is proving useful in clinical neuroradiology practice, with application to several categories of disease and a powerful research tool.

This article describes some of the applications of DWI and DTI in the evaluation of the diseases of the spinal cord listed below (this is a short subset of a long list of potential applications):

• Normal anatomy (ultra–high field imaging in vivo and ex vivo imaging)
• Multiple sclerosis
• Spinal cord tumors and arteriovenous malformations
• Degenerative myelopathy–cord compression and canal stenosis
• HIV-associated spinal cord abnormalities
• Transverse myelitis
• Traumatic spinal cord injury
• Spinal cord ischemia

To appreciate the clinical application of DWI, DTI, and FT requires an understanding of basic underlying principles and potential imaging pitfalls that are pertinent particularly to imaging the spinal cord, a small structure that has physiologic motion surrounded by very inhomogeneous structures.

[a] Department of Radiology, Medical University of Vienna, Vienna, Austria
[b] Department of Radiology, University of Southern California Imaging Center, University of Southern California Keck School of Medicine, Health Science Campus, University of Southern California, 1520 San Pablo Street, Lower Level, Suite 1600, Los Angeles, CA 90033, USA
[c] Department of Neurosurgery, University of Southern California Imaging Center, University of Southern California Keck School of Medicine, Health Science Campus, University of Southern California, 1520 San Pablo Street, Lower Level, Suite 1600, Los Angeles, CA 90033, USA
* Corresponding author. Departments of Radiology and Neurosurgery, University of Southern California Imaging Center, Health Science Campus, University of Southern California, 1520 San Pablo Street, Lower Level, Suite 1600, Los Angeles, CA 90033, USA.
E-mail address: meng.law@gmail.com (M. Law).

Magn Reson Imaging Clin N Am 17 (2009) 225–244
doi:10.1016/j.mric.2009.02.004

PRINCIPLES OF DIFFUSION-TENSOR IMAGING
Diffusion, Apparent Diffusion, and Anisotropy

Water molecules undergo random diffusion over time according to Fick's law. Diffusion in a given volume of tissue may be quantified as the diffusion coefficient, D, which is normalized for observation time according to the Einstein equation, and expressed in millimeter squared per second. Diffusion of water molecules may also occur in response to differences in pressure or temperature, caused by ion-ion interactions, or in response to other factors. In DWI, the apparent diffusion of water molecule protons is detected as a combination of true diffusion and these other mechanisms, and quantified as the apparent diffusion coefficient (ADC). Although diffusion is a random process, directional preference may result from local barriers; for example, barriers to diffusion in white matter tracts include axonal proteins and myelin. Diffusion is considered isotropic if it shows no directional dependence (eg, in gray matter) or anisotropic if directional dependence is present (eg, in white matter).

Diffusion-Weighted Imaging

A DWI sequence may be generated by application of paired diffusion-weighted gradient pulses before and after the 180-degree refocusing pulse of a T2-weighted spin echo sequence. Using this sequence, signal loss occurs compared with a baseline T2-weighted (non-DWI) image, according to

$$SI = SI_0 \exp(-b \times ADC)$$

where SI_0 represents the baseline signal intensity and b represents the diffusion sensitivity factor, which depends on the gyromagnetic ratio, magnitude and width of the diffusion-weighted gradient pulses, and time between the two diffusion-weighted gradient pulses. If anisotropic diffusion is present, the degree of signal loss is dependent on the direction of the diffusion-weighted gradient pulses; to negate this effect, three DWIs with diffusion-weighted gradient pulses in orthogonal directions may be obtained and ADC calculated as an average. **Fig. 1** demonstrates sagittal and axial ADC maps of a normal spinal cord acquired using a multishot echo planar imaging sequence at 3 T.

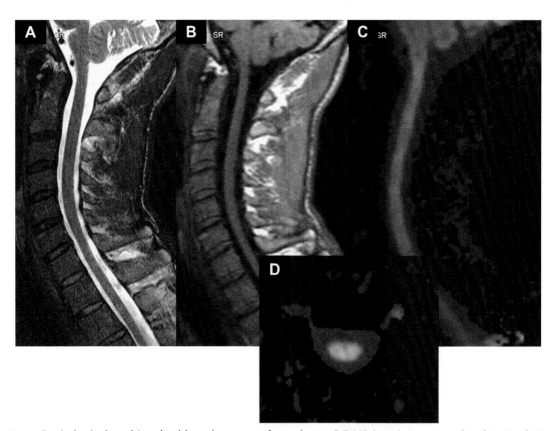

Fig. 1. Cervical spinal cord in a healthy volunteer performed on a 3-T MR imaging scanner. (*A, B*) Sagittal T2-weighted and T1-FLAIR MR images of the cervical spine. Sagittal (*C*) and axial (*D*) DWI of the cervical spinal cord performed using a multishot echo planar imaging DWI technique.

DIFFUSION-TENSOR IMAGING
Obtaining the Diffusion Tensor

Anisotropic diffusion may be described in terms of an ellipsoid tensor. The tensor consists of three vectors, a major eigenvector (or principle eigenvector) and two minor eigenvectors, with magnitudes being the major eigenvalue and minor eigenvalues, respectively. Because the eigenvectors are by definition orthogonal to each other, the diffusion tensor has six degrees of freedom and may be expressed in terms of a symmetric 3×3 matrix:

$$\mathbf{ADC} = \begin{bmatrix} ADC_{xx} & ADC_{xy} & ADC_{xz} \\ ADC_{yx} & ADC_{yy} & ADC_{yz} \\ ADC_{zx} & ADC_{zy} & ADC_{zz} \end{bmatrix} \qquad (1)$$

where $ADC_{xy} = ADC_{yx}$, $ADC_{xz} = ADC_{zx}$, and $ADC_{yz} = ADC_{zy}$. In DTI, the scalar elements of this diffusion tensor matrix may be calculated on a voxel-by-voxel basis from data obtained by performing multiple DWI sequences, applying the diffusion-weighted gradient along six or more noncollinear directions, with an additional, non–diffusion weighted ($b = 0$) sequence. The elements along the diagonal of the diffusion tensor matrix correspond to the directional ADC along the x, y, and z axes, respectively, referenced to the scanner; the off-diagonal elements provide information as to the correlation of the directional ADCs from pairs of axes.

Using the eigen decomposition theorem, the diffusion tensor matrix may be expressed as

$$\mathbf{ADC} = \mathbf{E} \begin{bmatrix} \lambda_1 & 0 & 0 \\ 0 & \lambda_2 & 0 \\ 0 & 0 & \lambda_3 \end{bmatrix} \mathbf{E}^{-1} \qquad (2)$$

where λ_1 is the major eigenvalue, and λ_2 and λ_3 are the minor eigenvalues; by definition, $\lambda_1 \geq \lambda_2 \geq \lambda_3$. The 3×3 matrix $\mathbf{E}$ contains the three eigenvectors.

Diffusion-Tensor Imaging Metrics

From the diffusion tensor matrix, several scalar metrics may be calculated. These commonly include fractional anisotropy (FA) and mean diffusivity (MD). FA is a measure of the degree of anisotropy, calculated as

$$FA = \frac{1}{\sqrt{2}} \sqrt{\frac{(\lambda_1 - \lambda_2)^2 + (\lambda_2 - \lambda_3)^2 + (\lambda_1 - \lambda_3)^2}{\lambda_1^2 + \lambda_2^2 + \lambda_3^2}} \qquad (3)$$

FA varies from 0 to 1, with FA = 0 representing isotropic diffusion ($\lambda_1 = \lambda_2 = \lambda_3$) and FA = 1 ($\lambda_1, \lambda_2 = \lambda_3 = 0$) representing 100% directional

preference along the major eigenvector. Relative anisotropy, a similar measure, is less commonly used.

MD is the trace of the diffusion tensor matrix, and may be calculated as

$$MD = (\lambda_1 + \lambda_2 + \lambda_3)/3 \qquad (4)$$

MD is analogous to the scalar ADC used in routine DWI.

DISPLAY OF THE DIFFUSION-TENSOR IMAGING DATA
Tensor Maps and Maps of Metrics

All the major MR imaging vendors now provide users with robust DTI postprocessing software that allows for depiction of color FA, MD maps, FT, and even quantitation of individual eigenvalues. This is sufficient for most clinical and even some research applications. A search of the literature provides a number of "freeware" software that can be downloaded to handle DTI data. An example of this is the "DTI studio" software available from http://lbam.med.jhmi.edu/DTIuser/DTIuser.asp.

Several methods are used to visualize the large amount of data obtained at DTI. Diffusion tensor maps may be generated using a workstation with three-dimensional display capability. In addition, the metrics FA, relative anisotropy, or MD may be calculated on a voxel-by-voxel basis and displayed as two-dimensional color or gray-scale images; the major and minor eigenvalues may also be displayed in this fashion. From these images, the average metric values within user-defined regions of interest (ROIs) may be calculated. In addition, the maps may be interrogated using such methods as histogram analysis.

Three-Dimensional Fiber Tractography

In white matter, the direction of the major eigenvector tends to be parallel with the orientation of axonal fibers. Using this observation, algorithms have been developed that may generate three-dimensional representations of axonal fibers, or three-dimensional FT. These algorithms "string together" adjacent voxels based on similarity in the direction of their major eigenvectors. Fiber tracking is typically performed using a line propagation technique based on continuous number fields called "fiber assignment using continuous tracking."[1] Tracking is launched from a seed voxel from which a line is propagated in both retrograde and antegrade directions according to the principal eigenvector at each voxel. Tracking propagates on the basis of the orientation of the eigenvector that is associated with the largest eigenvalue. Tracking is terminated when it reaches a voxel with FA lower than a threshold of 0.25 to 0.35 and when the angle between the two principal eigenvectors is greater than 35 to 40 degrees. These threshold values are generally applicable in the brain and spinal cord, although few validation studies have been performed to determine the most optimal FA and angle thresholds for spinal cord FT.

Although useful in tract visualization, white matter FT represents a more postprocessed representation of DTI data compared with visualization of tensor maps and maps of metrics, and is prone to the addition of error. In voxels that contain crossing fiber tracts from two or more directions, the association between the diffusion tensor measurement and the axonal fiber direction is less direct; algorithms have been developed to mitigate this problem, which arises commonly in central nervous system structures, such as the brainstem, and in areas with complex crossing association fibers. Various data smoothing and interpolation techniques have also been used to minimize the propagation of noise error. In addition, FT algorithms require user-defined ROIs and threshold values, which affect the number of fibers tracked and degree of noise effects. All of these

differences potentially limit reproducibility and may limit the comparison of various investigations. **Figs. 2** and **3** demonstrate FA maps and FT.

FT algorithms may be grouped into single-ROI and multiple-ROI techniques. Single-ROI techniques trace all fibers that pass through the user-defined ROI. Multiple ROI techniques trace the fibers that pass through all of the user-defined ROIs, ignoring any tracking patterns that track to other locations. The multiple ROI method allows discrete visualization of known anatomic tracts that pass through high-branching areas, such as the corticospinal tract as it passes through the brainstem, at the expense of nonvisualization of any associated branching tracts.

TECHNIQUES AND SEQUENCES FOR ACQUISITION OF DIFFUSION-TENSOR IMAGING DATA

Obtaining spinal cord DWI and DTI has a number of challenges because of its inherent technical difficulty. The spinal cord's small size requires the use of small voxel sizes (higher matrix) for spatial resolution that decreases the signal-to-noise ratio.[2] Images may be degraded because of macroscopic motion related to physiologic cerebrospinal fluid pulsations, breathing, and

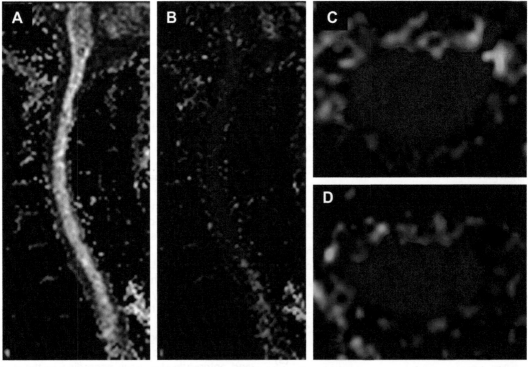

Fig. 2. Sagittal (*gray scale and color*) (*A, B*) and axial (*C, D*) fractional anisotropy maps from a normal volunteer obtained at 3 T. Note on the axial acquisitions the ability to resolve the gray and white matter. The gray matter has lower FA compared with the white matter. The axial acquisition allows for quantitation of DTI metrics, such as FA and ADC.

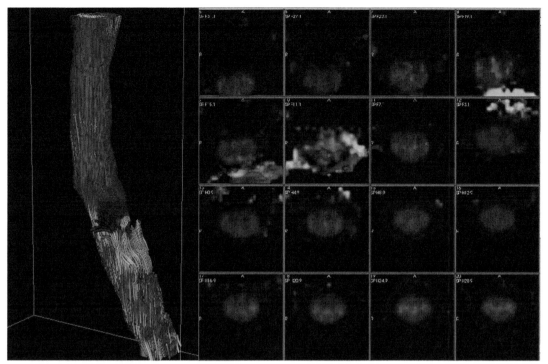

Fig. 3. FT from a DTI acquisition at 3 T. Fiber tracking is performed with "fiber assignment using continuous tracking."[1] Tracking is terminated when it reaches a voxel with FA lower than a threshold of 0.25–0.35 and when the angle between the two principal eigenvectors is greater than 35–40 degrees. These threshold values are currently arbitrary and have not been validated in the brain or spinal cord.

swallowing.[3] In addition, local field inhomogeneities prevent efficient rephasing of proton spins, thereby further reducing the image resolution. The use of routine echo-planar sequences typically used for brain DWI and DTI further increases susceptibility. Because of these technical challenges, limited data exist regarding not only pathologic processes, but also normal parameters. This difficulty leads to a relative paucity of information regarding normal cervical spinal cord gray and white matter regional DTI metrics (FA, MD), and minor and major eigenvectors in the axial plane. With faster alternative techniques being developed for acquiring DTI datasets, such as multishot echo planar imaging, diffusion weighted PROPELLER, spin echo navigator spiral DTI, and parallel imaging methods, such as sensitivity encoding, acquisition times have been reduced to allow data to be acquired from structures like the human spinal cord.[4,5] The spinal cord has intrinsic cord motion and cerebrospinal fluid pulsation, which makes for acquisition of DTI metrics difficult unless faster sequences are used. Most of the vendor provided sequences use parallel imaging techniques, which helps to reduce susceptibility and speed up the acquisition to negate some of the effects of physiology motion, such as cerebrospinal pulsation, swallowing, and

respiration. Parallel imaging techniques, such as sensitivity encoding, array spatial sensitivity encoding technique, and generalized autocalibrating partially parallel acquisition, can all be used to shorten the echo-train length of echo planar imaging. Experimentation with cardiac-pulse gating can be useful, although typically with cardiac gating the acquisition of the DTI data during the resting "R-R" interval further lengthens the acquisition time thereby increasing the likelihood of swallowing and respiratory artifact. Line scan diffusion imaging is a spin echo technique that relies on the sequential single-shot acquisition of columns. Line scan diffusion imaging is relatively insensitive to magnetic field inhomogeneities, eddy currents, and bulk motion, and can provide rectangular images, diffusion-weighted along six encoding axes in as little as 25 seconds per section.[2] A summary of the possible sequences and techniques used and proposed with their advantages and disadvantages is presented in Table 1. The typical parameters used for brain DTI can be applied to the spinal cord using clinical b-values in the range of 0 to 1000 s/mm.[2] Using these parameters but reducing the field of view in the axial plane is most optimal, although the acquisition could also be applied in the sagittal plane.

Table 1
Various techniques and sequences with advantages and disadvantages for spinal cord diffusion-tensor imaging

Technique and Sequence	Advantages	Disadvantages
Navigated pulsed-gradient spin echo	Motion correction	30-min scan, cardiac/respiratory gating needed
Spin echo single-shot echo-planar imaging	Fast, easy (1–2 min), good SNR	Nyquist ghosting, chemical shift, magnetic field inhomogeneity, local susceptibility effects
Interleaved multishot echo planar	Reduces susceptibility, lower echo train	Not as fast as single-shot echo-planar imaging
Fast spin echo/turbo spin echo propeller DTI	Reduces susceptibility	Longer scan time, oversample center of k
Spin echo navigated DTI (spiral)	Overcome motion	Not readily available
Line scan spin echo DTI	25-s scan/section, relatively insensitive to inhomogeneity, eddy currents, motion	Scan rectangular field of view in sagittal plane
Parallel imaging/multishot echo-planar imaging DTI	Reduces susceptibility, fast scans	Increasing iPAT, generalized autocalibrating partially parallel acquisition, sensitivity encoding, array spatial sensitivity encoding technique reduces SNR

Abbreviations: DTI, diffusion-tensor imaging; SNR, signal to noise ratio.

APPLICATIONS OF DIFFUSION-TENSOR IMAGING IN SPINAL CORD DISEASES
Normal Spinal Cord

Regional differences in DTI metrics in normal volunteers were found, which can be explained by intrinsic differences in the white matter tracts, such as density, diameter, and myelination.[6,7] These regional differences in FA have been correlated with axonal density, axonal diameter, degree of myelination, and the integrity and density of cytoskeletal structures in the rat spinal cord.[8,9]

The changes in diffusion properties of the human spinal cord in subjects of different ages were studied and measured in a recently published study. DTI measurements of the cervical spinal cord were acquired on 42 healthy volunteers.[10] The FA, MD, and eigenvalues were compared for the ROI and DTI-based segmentation methods. The results of that and other studies suggest that, independent of the segmentation approach used, the diffusion characteristics are age-dependent. There are also regional differences in FA and MD in various tracts of the spinal cord (Fig. 4).

Because of cord motion and cerebrospinal fluid pulsation, DTI of the lower spinal cord is perhaps even more challenging than the cervical spinal cord. Tsuchiya and colleagues[11] used a single-shot echo-planar sequence in combination with parallel imaging for tractography of the lower spinal cord and assessed the feasibility of this technique at 1.5 T using a five-channel receiver coil. The scan time was 5 minutes, 15 seconds. The conus medullaris and cauda equina were able to be visualized, the cord was demonstrated as a bundle of tracts color-coded in the z-axis. Nerve roots were depicted showing color-coding in the x- and y-axes. DTI using parallel imaging is likely the most robust technique for routine tractography of the upper and lower spinal cord.

Diffusion-Tensor Imaging in Multiple Sclerosis of the Spinal Cord

Multiple sclerosis (MS) is primarily an inflammatory demyelinating disorder of the brain and spinal cord.[12] In recent years, MR imaging has been established as an important tool for the assessment of clinical diagnosis, natural history, and treatment effects in MS. MS lesions in the brain are pathologically heterogeneous and demonstrate different imaging patterns on MR imaging, with variable sizes and appearance; some

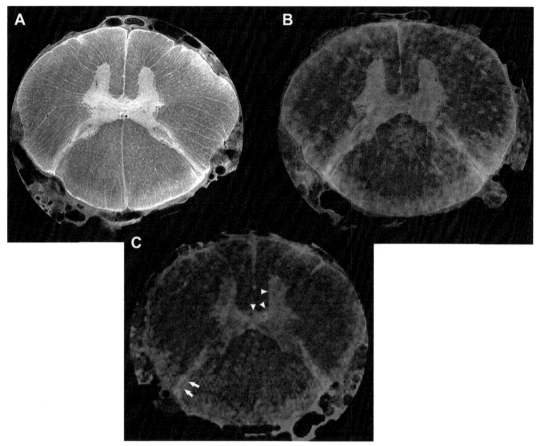

Fig. 4. (A) Anatomic image through the upper thoracic cord of a formalin-fixed specimen at 9.4 T. Distinction between gray and white matter is easily made. Even internal laminations of the central gray are resolved. (B, C) Ex vivo MR microscopic diffusion tensor color map through the upper thoracic cord at 9.4 T. Because most of the tracts run craniocaudal, much of the white matter is homogeneously blue. Prominent areas of transverse white matter include the ventral commissure (*arrowheads*) where one can trace, from anterolateral to the midline, green (*anteroposterior*) through yellow (*oblique*) through red (*transverse*). This same pattern is seen in curved tracts elsewhere in the central nervous system, such as the forceps of the callosum. Areas of gray matter that have prominent entry tracts, such as the dorsolateral horns (*arrows*), may also demonstrate enough anisotropy to resolve a dominant tract orientation (*green = anteroposterior*). (*Courtesy of* Bradley Delman and Thomas Naidich, New York, NY.)

undergo acute inflammatory changes, whereas others may show extensive tissue destruction.

The spinal cord is frequently involved in MS, with cord lesions found in up to 99% of autopsy cases.[13,14] Three main types of MS lesions in the cord have been described: (1) focal high signal intensity lesions, (2) diffuse abnormalities, and (3) spinal cord atrophy and axonal loss. Focal MS lesions have wedge shape if they are located in the lateral portions of the cross-sectional area and round shape if they are not in contact with the surface of the cord. Cord swelling may be present and it is usually found in the relapsing-remitting form of MS.

Clark and colleagues[15] have used a conventional, cardiac-gated, navigated diffusion-sensitized spin echo sequence for in vivo DWI of the spinal cord in MS patients. Increased rates of diffusivity have

been found in focal MS lesions, with a significantly higher isotropic diffusion coefficient compared with healthy controls. The decrease in anisotropy was explained by several factors: loss of myelin from white matter fiber tracts, expansion of the extracellular space fraction, and perilesional inflammatory edema. The large standard deviation in the lesion values observed in that study was explained by lesion heterogeneity. MD and FA histograms were acquired from the cervical cords obtained from 44 MS patients and 17 healthy controls in another study.[16] The measurements have clearly shown that the average cervical cord FA was significantly lower in MS patients compared with controls. Good correlation was found between the average FA and average MD and the degree of disability. In subsequent study, axial DTI was performed in 24 patients with relapsing-remitting MS and 24 age- and sex-matched control subjects.[7] FA and MD were calculated in the anterior, lateral, and posterior spinal cord, bilaterally, and the central spinal cord, at the C2-C3 level. Significantly lower FA values were found in the lateral, dorsal, and central parts of the normal-appearing white matter in MS patients. The results of this and subsequent studies show that significant changes in DTI metrics are present in the cervical spinal cord of MS patients, in the absence of spinal cord signal abnormality at conventional MR examination.[7] By means of FA measurements in 21 MS patients and controls, Ohgiya and colleagues[17] were able to distinguish between areas with T2 abnormalities versus normal-appearing white matter, and between normal-appearing white matter of MS patients versus white matter of neurologically healthy controls. FA was significantly lower in all regions of the spinal cord in MS patients than in control subjects.

The measurement of DTI metrics in the cervical spinal cord in MS patients may prove useful in aiding the diagnosis of MS (because secondary causes of demyelination are more likely to have normal DTI in normal-appearing spinal cord); in correlating with clinical disability; and in

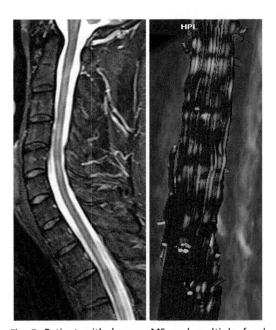

Fig. 5. Patient with known MS and multiple focal lesions in the cervical spinal cord. The lesions are typically short-segment lesions involving the dorsolateral columns of the cord on T2-weighted imaging typical for MS. FT demonstrates, on the whole, the fiber tracts to be intact. Enhancing acute demyelinating lesions may, however, sometimes cause fiber tracts to stop if the FA falls below the threshold selected for FT (see Fig. 6).

monitoring disease progression and therapeutic effect (Figs. 5 and 6).

Diffusion-Tensor Imaging in Spinal Cord Tumors and Arteriovenous Malformations

The most common spinal cord tumors are astrocytomas and ependymomas. Ependymomas arise from the ependymal cells lining the central canal and grow concentrically outward, whereas astrocytomas are typically infiltrating and arise from the astrocytic cells, typically from an eccentric location. Based on imaging characteristics on conventional MR imaging sequences, it is difficult to distinguish an ependymoma from an astrocytoma. Promising results in the characterization of tissues have been shown using DWI and DTI in brain tumors. Highly cellular tumors demonstrate low ADC values, whereas low cellular tumors and necrotic neoplasms have high ADC. Studies using DWI and DTI in spinal cord tumors have been somewhat limited. In one published study using DTI in characterization of spinal cord lesions, FA values measured were similar for astrocytomas, ependymomas, and metastases but different for hemangioblastomas.[18] The lowest FA values were measured in metastases and the highest in hemangioblastomas. The authors suggested that FA maps may be useful in distinguishing surrounding edema from tumor. FT was also used in that study showing displacement of the fibers in ependymomas and infiltration of fibers in astrocytoma. Ducreux and colleagues[18] described DTI findings in five cases of spinal cord astrocytoma. The data suggest that FT can be used for visualization of warped and destroyed fibers in cases of solid astrocytomas, but showed some limitations in cystic astrocytomas (Figs. 7–13).

In spinal cord arteriovenous malformations, DTI with FA measurements may help to understand better the pathophysiology of arteriovenous malformations. Interestingly, FA values may improve after embolization and correlate with improved patient outcome. FT shows that at the level of the arteriovenous malformation nidus, the tracts can be displaced, shifted without spreading, interrupted, or normal. FT shows no fibers running through the nidus, an observation that may become important if surgical resection is considered. Away from the nidus, congestive edema or a "cavitation" pattern may be found. In congestive edema, FT shows spreading of the fiber tracts.[19]

Diffusion-Tensor Imaging in Cervical Degenerative Disease

Cervical spondylotic myelopathy is the most frequent cause of spinal cord dysfunction in

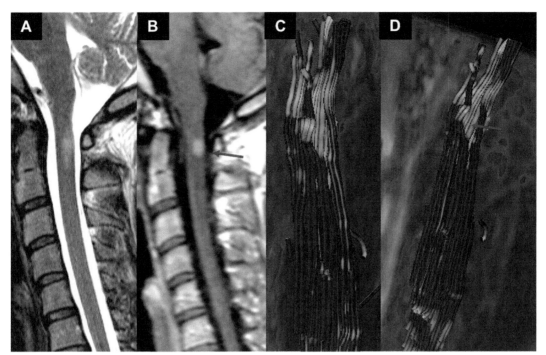

Fig. 6. (A, B) Patient with known MS demonstrates a lesion at the C2 level in the dorsal aspect of the cord. Following contrast administration there is contrast enhancement suggesting an acutely demyelinating lesion (*arrow*). (C, D) Enhancing acute demyelinating lesions may, however, sometimes cause fiber tracts to stop if the FA falls below the threshold selected for fiber tracking (*arrow*).

elderly patients.[20–22] By age 60, 70% of women and 85% of men show changes consistent with cervical spondylosis. As a result of narrowing of the spinal canal because of spondylosis, spinal cord ischemia occurs because of the impaired microcirculation resulting from compression. Initial symptoms of degenerative compression myelopathy consist of mild motor and sensory impairment

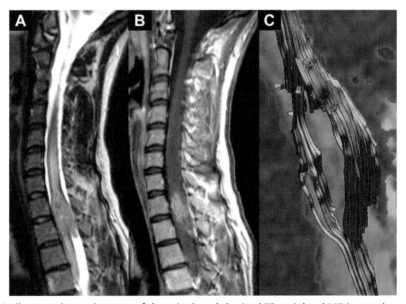

Fig. 7. Histologically proved ependymoma of the spinal cord. Sagittal T2-weighted MR image demonstrates bulky mass expanding the spinal cord detected at the level of T1-T3 with edema (A) and patchy enhancement on the postcontrast study (B). FT clearly shows displacement of the fiber tracts concentrically outward at the level of the tumor (C) suggesting an ependymoma arising from the ependymal cells of the central canal.

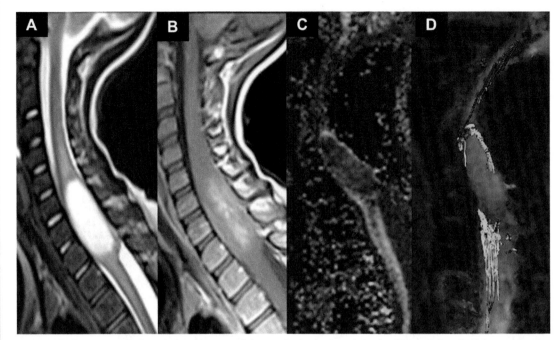

Fig. 8. Pathology proved pilocytic astrocytoma of the cervical spinal cord. Sagittal T2-weighted MR image demonstrates a primarily cystic expanding the spinal cord detected at the level of C7-T1 with a small amount of edema (A) and patchy enhancement on the postcontrast study (B). (C, D) FA and FT clearly show displacement of the fiber tracts concentrically outward at the level of the tumor in keeping with a cystic tumor.

that, if left untreated, may progress to quadriplegia. The time course of neurologic deterioration is variable and there is controversy regarding the most appropriate timing of surgical decompression of the spinal cord.[23] Currently, MR imaging is the most commonly used tool for delineating the extent of the spondylotic changes in the spine. MR imaging findings in cervical

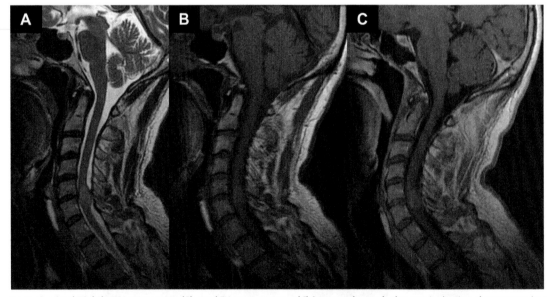

Fig. 9. Sagittal T2 (A), T1 precontrast (B), and T1 postcontrast (C) images through the cervical spine demonstrating a well-circumscribed lesion at the C5-6 level expanding the cervical spinal cord. The well-circumscribed nature and lack of significant edema tends to favor an ependymoma; however, the lack of blood products in A and enhancement in C tends to favor an astrocytoma. The DTI and FT in Figs. 10 and 11 help in the differentiation and in planning the surgical approach.

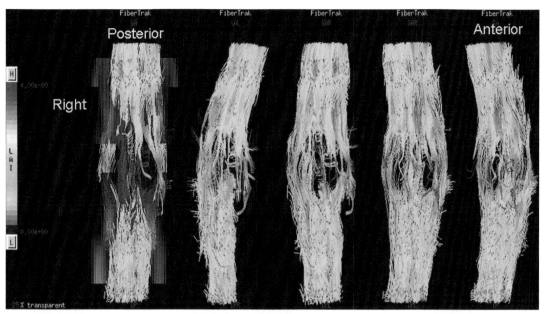

Fig. 10. Rotating figures from posterior to anterior of FT of the lesion in Fig. 9 acquired in the axial plane demonstrate the lesion to displace the fiber tracts rather than to infiltrate the fiber tracts, suggestive of a well-circumscribed ependymoma, which pathologically has a plane of resection between the lesion and the normal spinal cord allowing for a surgical resection compared with a diffusely infiltrating astrocytoma.

spondylotic myelopathy include the degree of narrowing of spinal canal (measured with compression ratio) and focal increased T2 signal within the spinal cord, secondary to edema, ischemia, myelomalacia, or gliotic changes, and spondylotic and disk degenerative changes.[24-26] Findings on conventional MR imaging are not only nonspecific, but also unable to discriminate potentially reversible edema and ischemia from irreversible myelomalacia and gliosis. More importantly, such conventional tools are inadequate for predicting the surgical benefit and identifying the subset of candidates who benefit from decompressive surgery because of the low sensitivity in detecting cord dysfunction.[27]

The pathologic changes in the cord related to cervical spondylotic myelopathy progress over time, beginning with normal-appearing cord on conventional MR imaging techniques progressing to focal increased T2-signal changes related to edema and later to chronic myelomalacia and gliotic changes, eventually leading to cavitation or syrinx formation, and atrophy of the cord.[28]

Using DWI, six healthy volunteers and 12 patients with cervical myelomalacia caused by chronic cord compression were imaged. The spinal cord was well seen in all subjects without the distortion associated with echo-planar DWI. In the patients, lesions appeared as areas of low or isointense signal on DWI. Calculated ADC of the lesions ($3.30 \pm 0.38 \times 10^{-3}$ mm^2/s) was

significantly higher than that of normal volunteers ($2.26 \pm 0.08 \times 10^{-3}$ mm^2/s). Increased diffusion in areas of cervical myelomalacia, suggesting irreversible damage, seem to be able to be detected using DWI.[29]

There is only preliminary evidence in the medical literature suggesting increased sensitivity of DTI for detection of early myelopathic changes in the setting of cervical spondylotic myelopathy.[28,30,31]

The changes found on DTI typically consist of decreased FA and increased MD. These changes in FA and MD may not be sufficient to differentiate between potentially reversible edema and irreversible gliosis in patients with spondylosis. The evaluation of major (E1) and minor (E2, E3) eigenvalues, from which FA is calculated, however, may assist in identifying subgroups of patients who may benefit from surgery. Diffusion tensor metrics in the white matter tracts of the cervical spinal cord in patients with severe multilevel spondylosis with normal volunteers, evaluating changes in FA and MD and the major and minor eigenvalues were measured in a recent study.[32] Increased minor eigenvalues in the setting of chronic spondylosis, with preservation of the major eigenvalue, were found. In the spinal cord, the minor eigenvalues typically correspond to transverse diffusion, perpendicular to the longitudinal axis of the spinal cord. Animal studies have suggested that increases in the minor eigenvalues occur in the setting of demyelination, increased axonal

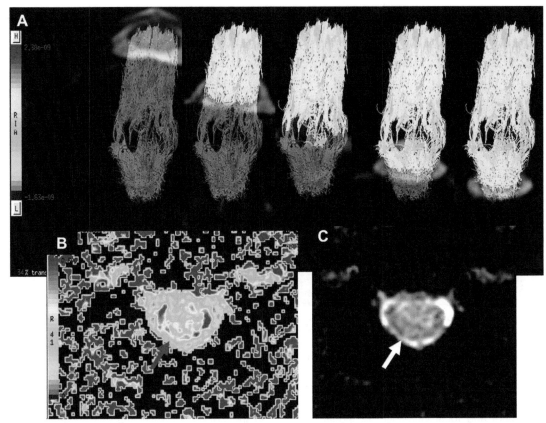

Fig. 11. FT (*A*) and axial color-coded and gray scale FA maps (*B, C*) demonstrating a paucity of fiber tracts on the right dorsal aspect of the spinal cord (*arrow*) in this patient with an ependymoma (see Fig. 9). This paucity of tracts suggested a possible surgical approach for the neurosurgeon to the ependymoma without compromising functional tracts. This can be confirmed with intraoperative electrophysiologic testing to validate the presence or absence of these fiber tracts. This has important clinical implications not only in the diagnosis of these lesions but also in the surgical approach and the postoperative recovery of these patients.

diameter, and additional factors including protein integrity.[8] The increased transverse diffusion seen in the normal-appearing spinal cord of patients with cervical spondylosis suggests possible microscopic demyelination and edema. By the same token, a decrease in the longitudinal diffusion may herald irreversible axonal damage and neurologic impairment. Most of this is conjecture and has not been adequately validated.

HIV-Associated Spinal Cord Abnormalities

A large number of conditions affect the central nervous system in patients with HIV infection. Involvement of the brain has been studied extensively, but involvement of the spinal cord is less well understood. The frequency of spinal cord involvement varies in different published clinical series.[33–35] In a neuropathologic study of 138 unselected autopsies, the spinal cord was involved in 40%. Petito and colleagues[33] first

described neuropathologic findings in a previously uncharacterized progressive myelopathy in AIDS patients. Pathologically, vacuolar myelopathy is characterized by vacuolization in the lateral and posterior columns of the thoracic spinal cord, resembling changes seen in vitamin B_{12} deficiency. Vacuoles are the result of edematous swelling within myelin, with splitting of the lamellae. The axons are usually normal until severe vacuolation occurs and secondary wallerian degeneration and axonal disruption occurs.[34–37] The vacuolization is not, however, confined to specific white matter tracts. Twenty percent to 55% of patients with AIDS have evidence of spinal cord disease consistent with vacuolar myelopathy. The exact cause of vacuolar myelopathy remains unclear. Published reports support an indirect relation between HIV and the pathogenesis of vacuolar myelopathy, peripheral neuropathy, and dementia. Because of the overlap between these syndromes, it is not completely clear whether

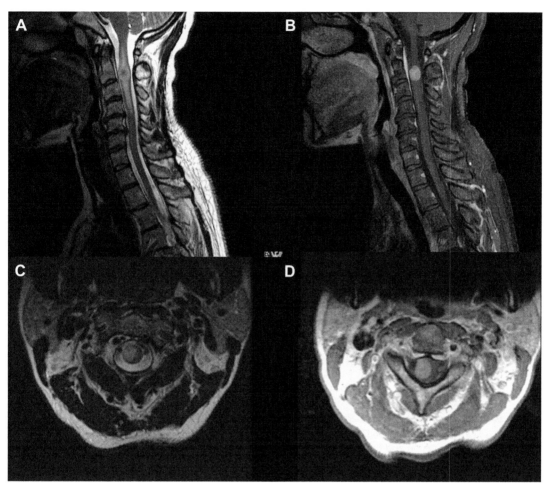

Fig. 12. Patient with a challenging lesion in the cervical spinal cord at C2-3, which seems to be fairly well circumscribed on both sagittal and axial imaging. (*A, B*) The presence of low signal on T2-weighted imaging suggests some blood products typically seen in ependymomas. (*C, D*) The degree of edema and the eccentric location seen best on axial imaging, however, suggests an astrocytoma. Clinically, this is an important question, which determines whether or not this lesion is resectable. DTI and FT is demonstrated in Fig. 13.

these are dealing with disease entities or parts of a spectrum of tissue damage.[38] The diagnosis is based on the clinical course and exclusion of other causes of myelopathy. MR imaging findings include bilaterally symmetric increased signal intensity on T2-weighted MR images, predominantly located in the lateral and dorsal parts of the cord.[39,40] In one study, symmetric, triangular, high-signal lesions were found within the gracile tract over several spinal segments, which correlated well with histopathologic findings.[40] Because the inflammatory component is missing in vacuolar myelopathy, the blood-brain barrier is not damaged, and no enhancement is present on postcontrast images. Vacuolar myelopathy may have been below the limits of resolution-detection of 1- to 1.5-T MR imaging units. With a high-field unit using optimized high-resolution imaging

acquisitions, the number and extent of intramedullary lesions detected on neuroimaging examinations will likely more closely approximate the actual number of cord lesions detected by the neuropathologist. A recently finished study performed at 3 T MR imaging using DTI in asymptomatic HIV-positive patients (Fig. 14) has shown that asymptomatic HIV-positive patients demonstrate changes in DTI metrics in cervical spinal cord compared with controls in the absence of abnormalities on conventional MR imaging.[41] A tendency toward decreased FA in lateral and posterior parts of the spinal cord was found. Predominance of changes in FA in lateral and posterior spinal cord may reflect the distribution pattern of vacuolar myelopathy. Inclusion of symptomatic HIV-positive patients with no abnormalities on conventional MR imaging, and correlation

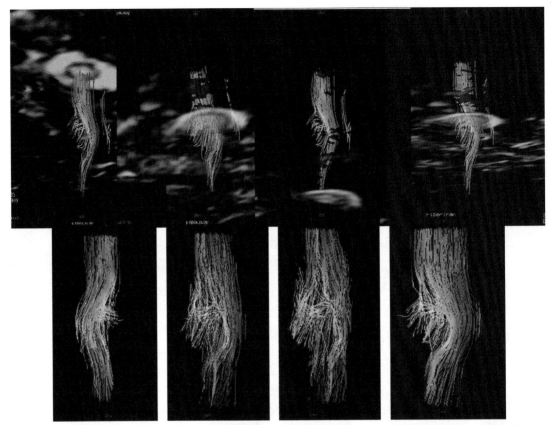

Fig. 13. DTI and FT demonstrates the lesion to displace rather than infiltrate the fiber tracts suggesting a plane of resection between the lesion and the normal-appearing spinal cord. This was resected and pathologically proved to be a spinal cord ependymoma.

of DTI metrics with CD4 count and virus load, is necessary before more solid conclusions can be made. Early identification of spinal cord abnormalities in asymptomatic HIV-positive patients identifies patients who benefit from antiretroviral therapy.

Diffusion-Tensor Imaging in Transverse Myelitis

Acute transverse myelitis is a clinical syndrome diagnosed when both halves of the cord are involved with an inflammatory process. The thoracic spine is the most commonly involved and middle-aged adults are usually affected. There are many etiologic associations with acute transverse myelitis, and despite extensive diagnostic work-ups, many cases of acute transverse myelitis are considered idiopathic. MR imaging findings include focal enlargement of the spinal cord and increased signal on T2-weighted MR images usually occupying more than two thirds of the cross-sectional area of the cord. Enhancement is usually absent, but when present two

patterns have been described: moderate patchy enhancement or diffusely abnormal enhancement.

Renoux and colleagues[42] found decreased FA values in areas of the spinal cord with abnormalities on T2-weighting in 15 patients with acute transverse myelitis. In a recently published study, sagittal DTI was performed in 10 patients with idiopathic acute transverse myelitis and 10 gender- and age-matched normal volunteers.[43] FA measurements were performed at the level of the T2-visible lesion, proximal normal-appearing spinal cord, and distal normal-appearing spinal cord. FA values in the lesion level and in distal normal-appearing spinal cord were significantly decreased in patients with idiopathic acute transverse myelitis. Severe decrease in FA values in the distal normal-appearing spinal cord was associated with poor clinical outcome.

Although the literature and the clinical experience with DTI in transverse myelitis are limited, the preliminary results suggest that DTI may be an additional tool for distinguishing myelitis from neoplasm of the spinal cord (**Fig. 15**).

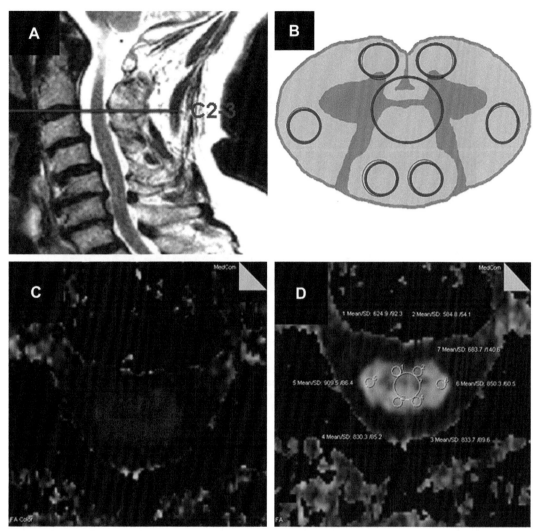

Fig. 14. Technique for DTI measurements in HIV-positive patient. Sagittal T2 (*A*) serves as a reference image for placing axial DTI to obtain diffusion tensor data, such as voxel-based anisotropy map (*B*). Measurements were done at the C2-3 levels. (*B–D*) On axial FA and ADC maps seven regions of interest were placed in the anterior, lateral, central, and posterior spinal cord. FA values, ADC values, and eigenvalues were compared with measurements done in healthy subjects.

Diffusion-Tensor Imaging in Spinal Cord Injury

Traumatic injury to the spinal cord occurs in 10% to 14% of spinal fractures and dislocations.[44] Injuries of the cervical spine are by far the most common cause of neurologic deficits, which occur in almost 40% of the cases.[45] Most injuries (85%) to the spinal cord occur at the time of trauma, and 5% to 10% are present in the immediate postinjury period.[46] MR imaging is the imaging modality of choice for assessing spinal cord injury.[47] The diagnosis of whiplash injury or whiplash-associated disorder is determined by the clinical history, by the mechanism of injury, and by the symptoms and the neurologic findings at examination. Whiplash injury is increasingly common and frequently caused by rear-end motor vehicle accidents with hyperextension and hyperflexion of the neck. Symptoms include neck pain, neck stiffness, paresthesias, upper extremity pain, jaw pain, and headache. Most imaging techniques in patients with suspected whiplash injury are inconclusive.[48] The role of imaging in the work-up of patients with whiplash injury remains controversial and has been suggested to be not cost-effective, at least not in the acute stage.[49–51] Most patients report recovery with resolution of symptoms. Some whiplash patients do develop chronic neck pain and in these patients with persistent symptoms,

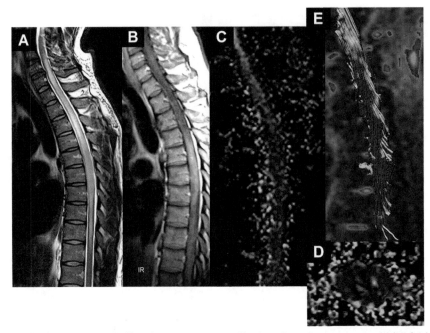

Fig. 15. Patient who has extensive infiltrating astrocytoma. The imaging appearance could be fairly similar for transverse myelitis and an infiltrating astrocytoma. A spinal cord ependymoma, however, demonstrates fiber tracts being displaced rather than infiltrated or separated as with transverse myelitis or astrocytoma. (*A, B*) Sagittal T2-weighted and postcontrast T1-weighted imaging demonstrate a typical long segment of increased signal within the cervicothoracic spinal cord with cord expansion and some patchy enhancement following the administration of contrast. (*C–E*) DTI, FA maps, and FT demonstrate a decrease in FA and a decrease in the number of fiber tracts demonstrated.

imaging might play a role.[52,53] The pathophysiology in spinal cord injuries has been described by McDonald and Sadowsky[54] and can be summarized as a primary injury caused by direct compression, disruption, or transection of neural elements by bony fracture fragments, epidural hematoma, gun bullets or weapons (penetrating trauma), and disk material, and by ligamentous injuries. Damage occurs to the blood vessels, there is disruption of axons, and microhemorrhages occur within minutes in the central gray matter and spread out within a few hours. The spinal cord swells within minutes after the injury, and when the cord swelling exceeds the venous pressure, secondary ischemia occurs. The ischemia and release of toxic chemicals from disrupted neural membranes trigger a second injury that results in spinal shock and kills neighboring cells.[54] The understanding of what happens secondarily is limited, but recent data suggest that cell death occurs days to weeks after the injury with apoptosis of the oligodendrocytes not only at the site of injury but also at several levels away from the injury site.[55]

The exact stage of spinal cord injury cannot be characterized by conventional MR imaging.

Furthermore, assessment of the functional integrity of the axons within the white matter tracts of the spinal cord cannot be accomplished with conventional MR imaging. Similarly, conventional MR imaging cannot detect possible therapeutic responses to neuroprotective drugs.

The use of DWI was evaluated first in rats with injured spinal cords.[56–58] Specifically, DWI was performed in injured rats treated with neuroprotective agents and compared with controls. The results showed a significant difference in anisotropy, with higher diffusion anisotropy in the spinal cords of the treated animals than in the untreated animals. In another animal study, diffusion MR imaging was used to demonstrate spontaneous regeneration in hemi-crushed rat spinal cords.[59] In this context, Sagiuchi and colleagues[60] reported recently a case of acute spinal cord injury with a type II odontoid fracture in a human, and described DWI findings. DWI, performed 2 hours after injury, showed intramedullary hyperintensity and decreased ADC values at the C1-C2 vertebral levels. Animal studies clearly demonstrate that DWI is more sensitive in the evaluation of spinal cord injury and the outcome and regeneration after neuroprotection than conventional MR imaging sequences. The results of animal research encourage further development of DWI as a useful method for detecting and visualizing spinal cord injury.

Investigators have used DWI with single-shot fast spin echo sequence in acute human cervical cord injury and evaluated the usefulness of this method for predicting the prognosis. A study of 14 patients examined 2 hours to 3 days after injury showed DWI hyperintensity in 10 patients, and no abnormal signal was noted in the remaining 4 patients. The ADC maps showed restricted diffusion in all patients with hyperintensity on DWI. Repeated MR imaging examinations obtained in 6 of the 10 patients showed either myelomalacia or exacerbation. Seven (70%) of the 10 patients required assistance and the other three were independent. DWI in acute cervical cord injury often reveals restricted diffusion. This finding seems to be able to predict an unfavorable functional prognosis.[61]

Diffusion-Tensor Imaging in Spinal Cordially, Ischemia

Acute spinal cord ischemia is a severe condition with a poor prognosis, associated with neuronal death, functional neurologic loss, and paraplegia in up to 33% of the cases.[62] Aortic dissection (3%–5% risk) and aortic surgery (1%–10% risk) are the most common causes of acute spinal cord ischemia.[62] In up to 36% of cases, however, the cause of spinal cord ischemia remains undefined.

On MR imaging, high signal on T2-weighted images in the cord with cord enlargement are usually present. The appearance of "snake-eyes," with bilateral hyperintensities on axial T2-weighted MR images, suggests involvement of the anterior part of the gray matter, which is known to have the highest vulnerability to ischemia.[63] Contrast enhancement is usually present only in the subacute stage. MR imaging is the method of choice in detection of spinal cord ischemia. In one clinical study, however, only 45% of the patients with acute spinal cord ischemia had signal intensity changes on T2-weighted MR images.[63]

Gass and colleagues[64] reported hyperintensity on DWI in the central portion of the lumbar cord performed 30 hours after symptom onset. Soon after that first reported case, Stepper and Lovblad[65] published a case of spinal cord infarction, seen on DWI, in a patient after aortic grafting 12 hours after onset of symptoms. In this particular case, ADC was decreased 75% compared with the normal spinal cord. Multiple series varying from three to six patients describing DWI findings in spinal cord infarction have since followed in the literature.[66–73]

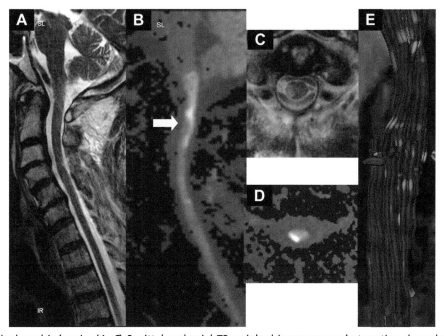

Fig. 16. Spinal cord ischemia. (A, C) Sagittal and axial T2-weighed image somewhat motion degraded demonstrates possible increase in signal in the cervical spinal cord at C2 and C3. (B, D) There is evidence of diffusion restriction on the sagittal acquired DWI in keeping with spinal cord ischemia (arrow). (E) FT demonstrates a decrease in the number of tracts at the level of ischemia.

The ADC measured in published series of spinal cord infarction ranged between 0.23 and 0.9 $\times$ 10^{-3} mm^2/s. The shortest time reported in the literature between the onset of clinical symptoms and abnormalities shown on DWI was 3 hours after onset of symptoms. Although the largest number of patients with described DWI findings does not exceed six patients, data and current experience suggest that DWI is a useful and feasible technique in early detection of the acute spinal infarction. Diffusion abnormality can be found after a few hours, but it may not last for longer than 1 week (**Fig. 16**).

SUMMARY

The ability of DWI, DTI, and FT in the measurement of microscopic water molecular diffusion and their interaction with cellular and extracellular structures provides a unique tool for characterizing and defining the extent of pathologic and microstructural alteration that occurs in diseases of the brain and spinal cord. This article reviews only a short list of potential applications in the human spinal cord that can potentially be investigated with DTI. DTI metrics and fiber tracking of different pathologies allow more accurate characterization of intrinsic integrity of tissues including cellular density and architecture. Careful studies to validate DTI and its metrics will allow it to become more applicable clinically and can affect therapeutic decision-making and eventually patient outcome. There are a number of limitations with the current techniques described in this article. Newer mathematic models, such as high angular resolution diffusion imaging[74–76] and diffusion spectrum imaging,[77] which promise to overcome the shortcomings of the diffusion tensor for representing complex white matter architecture, such as crossing fibers and intravoxel partial volume averaging, are on the horizon and should help to propel DWI and DTI into everyday clinical MR imaging practice.

REFERENCES

1. Melhem ER, Mori S, Mukundan G, et al. Diffusion tensor MR imaging of the brain and white matter tractography. AJR Am J Roentgenol 2002;178(1): 3–16.
2. Maier SE, Mamata H. Diffusion tensor imaging of the spinal cord. Ann N Y Acad Sci 2005;1064:50–60.
3. Mikulis DJ, Wood ML, Zerdoner OA, et al. Oscillatory motion of the normal cervical spinal cord. Radiology 1994;192(1):117–21.
4. Liu C, Bammer R, Kim DH, et al. Self-navigated interleaved spiral (SNAILS): application to high-resolution diffusion tensor imaging. Magn Reson Med 2004;52(6):1388–96.
5. von Mengershausen M, Norris DG, Driesel W. 3D diffusion tensor imaging with 2D navigated turbo spin echo. MAGMA 2005;18(4):206–16.
6. Hesseltine S, Law M, Lopez S, et al. Diffusion tensor imaging of the human spinal cord: determination of normal regional metrics. In: Proceedings of the ISMRM, 2006.
7. Hesseltine SM, Law M, Babb J, et al. Diffusion tensor imaging in multiple sclerosis: assessment of regional differences in the axial plane within normal-appearing cervical spinal cord. AJNR Am J Neuroradiol 2006;27(6):1189–93.
8. Schwartz ED, Cooper ET, Chin CL, et al. Ex vivo evaluation of ADC values within spinal cord white matter tracts. AJNR Am J Neuroradiol 2005;26(2):390–7.
9. Schwartz ED, Chin CL, Shumsky JS, et al. Apparent diffusion coefficients in spinal cord transplants and surrounding white matter correlate with degree of axonal dieback after injury in rats. AJNR Am J Neuroradiol 2005;26(1):7–18.
10. Van Hecke W, Leemans A, Sijbers J, et al. A tracking-based diffusion tensor imaging segmentation method for the detection of diffusion-related changes of the cervical spinal cord with aging. J Magn Reson Imaging 2008;27(5):978–91.
11. Tsuchiya K, Fujikawa A, Honya K, et al. Diffusion tensor tractography of the lower spinal cord. Neuroradiology 2008;50(3):221–5.
12. Compston A, Coles A. Multiple sclerosis. Lancet 2008;372(9648):1502–17.
13. Ikuta F, Zimmerman HM. Distribution of plaques in seventy autopsy cases of multiple sclerosis in the United States. Neurology 1976;26(6 Pt 2):26–8.
14. Toussaint D, Perier O, Verstappen A, et al. Clinico-pathological study of the visual pathways, eyes, and cerebral hemispheres in 32 cases of disseminated sclerosis. J Clin Neuroophthalmol 1983;3(3):211–20.
15. Clark CA, Werring DJ, Miller DH. Diffusion imaging of the spinal cord in vivo: estimation of the principal diffusivities and application to multiple sclerosis. Magn Reson Med 2000;43(1):133–8.
16. Valsasina P, Rocca MA, Agosta F, et al. Mean diffusivity and fractional anisotropy histogram analysis of the cervical cord in MS patients. Neuroimage 2005;26(3):822–8.
17. Ohgiya Y, Oka M, Hiwatashi A, et al. Diffusion tensor MR imaging of the cervical spinal cord in patients with multiple sclerosis. Eur Radiol 2007;17(10): 2499–504.
18. Ducreux D, Lepeintre JF, Fillard P, et al. MR diffusion tensor imaging and fiber tracking in 5 spinal cord astrocytomas. AJNR Am J Neuroradiol 2006;27(1): 214–6.
19. Ducreux D, Fillard P, Facon D, et al. Diffusion tensor magnetic resonance imaging and fiber tracking in

spinal cord lesions: current and future indications. Neuroimaging Clin N Am 2007;17(1):137–47.

20. Kadanka Z, Mares M, Bednanik J, et al. Approaches to spondylotic cervical myelopathy: conservative versus surgical results in a 3-year follow-up study. Spine 2002;27(20):2205–10 [discussion: 2210–1].

21. McCormick WE, Steinmetz MP, Benzel EC. Cervical spondylotic myelopathy: make the difficult diagnosis, then refer for surgery. Cleve Clin J Med 2003;70(10):899–904.

22. Healy JF, Healy BB, Wong WH, et al. Cervical and lumbar MRI in asymptomatic older male lifelong athletes: frequency of degenerative findings. J Comput Assist Tomogr 1996;20(1):107–12.

23. Hochman M. Cervical spondylotic myelopathy: a review. Proceedings of the Annual Meeting of the Radiological Society of North America; 2005.

24. Ohta K, Fujimura Y, Nakamura M, et al. Experimental study on MRI evaluation of the course of cervical spinal cord injury. Spinal Cord 1999;37(8):580–4.

25. Matsumoto M, Toyama Y, Ishikawa M, et al. Increased signal intensity of the spinal cord on magnetic resonance images in cervical compressive myelopathy. Does it predict the outcome of conservative treatment? Spine 2000;25(6):677–82.

26. Matsuda Y, Miyazaki K, Tada K, et al. Increased MR signal intensity due to cervical myelopathy: analysis of 29 surgical cases. J Neurosurg 1991;74(6):887–92.

27. Facon D, Ozanne A, Fillard P, et al. MR diffusion tensor imaging and fiber tracking in spinal cord compression. AJNR Am J Neuroradiol 2005;26(6):1587–94.

28. Fukuoka M, Matsui N, Otsuka T, et al. Magnetic resonance imaging of experimental subacute spinal cord compression. Spine 1998;23(14):1540–9.

29. Tsuchiya K, Katase S, Fujikawa A, et al. Diffusion-weighted MRI of the cervical spinal cord using a single-shot fast spin-echo technique: findings in normal subjects and in myelomalacia. Neuroradiology 2003;45(2):90–4.

30. Haughton V. Medical imaging of intervertebral disc degeneration: current status of imaging. Spine 2004;29(23):2751–6.

31. Kim P, Haisa T, Kawamoto T, et al. Delayed myelopathy induced by chronic compression in the rat spinal cord. Ann Neurol 2004;55(4):503–11.

32. Hesseltine S, Law M, Lopez S, et al. Evaluation of the spinal cord in spondylosis using diffusion tensor imaging: changes in regional minor Eigen values. In: Proceedings of the ISMRM, 2006.

33. Petito CK, Cho ES, Lemann W, et al. Neuropathology of acquired immunodeficiency syndrome (AIDS): an autopsy review. J Neuropathol Exp Neurol 1986;45(6):635–46.

34. Henin D, Smith TW, De Girolami U, et al. Neuropathology of the spinal cord in the acquired immunodeficiency syndrome. Hum Pathol 1992;23(10):1106–14.

35. Gray F, Geny C, Lionnet F, et al. [Neuropathologic study of 135 adult cases of acquired immunodeficiency syndrome (AIDS)]. Ann Pathol 1991;11(4):236–47.

36. Artigas J, Grosse G, Niedobitek F. Vacuolar myelopathy in AIDS: a morphological analysis. Pathol Res Pract 1990;186(2):228–37.

37. Dal Pan GJ, Glass JD, McArthur JC. Clinicopathologic correlations of HIV-1-associated vacuolar myelopathy: an autopsy-based case-control study. Neurology 1994;44(11):2159–64.

38. Bergmann M, Gullotta F, Kuchelmeister K, et al. AIDS-myelopathy: a neuropathological study. Pathol Res Pract 1993;189(1):58–65.

39. Thurnher MM, Post MJ, Jinkins JR. MRI of infections and neoplasms of the spine and spinal cord in 55 patients with AIDS. Neuroradiology 2000;42(8):551–63.

40. Sartoretti-Schefer S, Blattler T, Wichmann W. Spinal MRI in vacuolar myelopathy, and correlation with histopathological findings. Neuroradiology 1997;39(12):865–9.

41. Mueller-Mang C, Law M, Thurnher M. Diffusion tensor imaging of the cervical spinal cord in asymptomatic HIV-positive patients: preliminary results at 3.0 T. Proceedings of the Annual Meeting of the Radiological Society of North America; 2007.

42. Renoux J, Facon D, Fillard P, et al. MR diffusion tensor imaging and fiber tracking in inflammatory diseases of the spinal cord. AJNR Am J Neuroradiol 2006;27(9):1947–51.

43. Lee JW, Park KS, Kim JH, et al. Diffusion tensor imaging in idiopathic acute transverse myelitis. AJR Am J Roentgenol 2008;191(2):W52–7.

44. Riggins RS, Kraus JF. The risk of neurologic damage with fractures of the vertebrae. J Trauma 1977;17(2):126–33.

45. Castellano V, Bocconi FL. Injuries of the cervical spine with spinal cord involvement (myelic fractures): statistical considerations. Bull Hosp Joint Dis 1970;31(2):188–94.

46. Rogers WA. Fractures and dislocations of the cervical spine; an end-result study. J Bone Joint Surg Am 1957;39-A(2):341–76.

47. Flanders AE, Schaefer DM, Doan HT, et al. Acute cervical spine trauma: correlation of MR imaging findings with degree of neurologic deficit. Radiology 1990;177(1):25–33.

48. Spitzer WO, Skovron ML, Salmi LR, et al. Scientific monograph of the Quebec Task Force on whiplash-associated disorders: redefining whiplash and its management. Spine 1995;20(Suppl 8):1S–73S.

49. Ronnen HR, de Korte PJ, Brink PR, et al. Acute whiplash injury: is there a role for MR imaging? A prospective study of 100 patients. Radiology 1996;201(1):93–6.

50. Borchgrevink G, Smevik O, Haave I, et al. MRI of cerebrum and cervical columna within two days

after whiplash neck sprain injury. Injury 1997; 28(5–6):331–5.

51. Pettersson K, Hildingsson C, Toolanen G, et al. Disc pathology after whiplash injury: a prospective magnetic resonance imaging and clinical investigation. Spine 1997;22(3):283–7 [discussion: 288].

52. Rodriquez AA, Barr KP, Burns SP. Whiplash: pathophysiology, diagnosis, treatment, and prognosis. Muscle Nerve 2004;29(6):768–81.

53. Ovadia D, Steinberg EL, Nissan MN, et al. Whiplash injury: a retrospective study on patients seeking compensation. Injury 2002;33(7):569–73.

54. McDonald JW, Sadowsky C. Spinal-cord injury. Lancet 2002;359(9304):417–25.

55. Beattie MS, Farooqui AA, Bresnahan JC. Review of current evidence for apoptosis after spinal cord injury. J Neurotrauma 2000;17(10):915–25.

56. Nevo U, Hauben E, Yoles E, et al. Diffusion anisotropy MRI for quantitative assessment of recovery in injured rat spinal cord. Magn Reson Med 2001; 45(1):1–9.

57. Schwartz ED, Yezierski RP, Pattany PM, et al. Diffusion-weighted MR imaging in a rat model of syringomyelia after excitotoxic spinal cord injury. AJNR Am J Neuroradiol 1999;20(8):1422–8.

58. Ford JC, Hackney DB, Alsop DC, et al. MRI characterization of diffusion coefficients in a rat spinal cord injury model. Magn Reson Med 1994;31(5):488–94.

59. Nossin-Manor R, Duvdevani R, Cohen Y. q-Space high b value diffusion MRI of hemi-crush in rat spinal cord: evidence for spontaneous regeneration. Magn Reson Imaging 2002;20(3):231–41.

60. Sagiuchi T, Tachibana S, Endo M, et al. Diffusion-weighted MRI of the cervical cord in acute spinal cord injury with type II odontoid fracture. J Comput Assist Tomogr 2002;26(4):654–6.

61. Tsuchiya K, Fujikawa A, Honya K, et al. Value of diffusion-weighted MR imaging in acute cervical cord injury as a predictor of outcome. Neuroradiology 2006;48(11):803–8.

62. Nedeltchev K, Loher TJ, Stepper F, et al. Long-term outcome of acute spinal cord ischemia syndrome. Stroke 2004;35(2):560–5.

63. Hundsberger T, Thomke F, Hopf HC, et al. Symmetrical infarction of the cervical spinal cord due to spontaneous bilateral vertebral artery dissection. Stroke 1998;29(8):1742.

64. Gass A, Back T, Behrens S, et al. MRI of spinal cord infarction. Neurology 2000;54(11):2195.

65. Stepper F, Lovblad KO. Anterior spinal artery stroke demonstrated by echo-planar DWI. Eur Radiol 2001; 11(12):2607–10.

66. Loher TJ, Bassetti CL, Lovblad KO, et al. Diffusion-weighted MRI in acute spinal cord ischaemia. Neuroradiology 2003;45(8):557–61.

67. Kuker W, Weller M, Klose U, et al. Diffusion-weighted MRI of spinal cord infarction: high resolution imaging and time course of diffusion abnormality. J Neurol 2004;251(7):818–24.

68. Zhang JS, Huan Y, Sun LJ, et al. Temporal evolution of spinal cord infarction in an in vivo experimental study of canine models characterized by diffusion-weighted imaging. J Magn Reson Imaging 2007; 26(4):848–54.

69. Fujikawa A, Tsuchiya K, Takeuchi S, et al. Diffusion-weighted MR imaging in acute spinal cord ischemia. Eur Radiol 2004;14(11):2076–8.

70. Weidauer S, Nichtweiss M, Lanfermann H, et al. Spinal cord infarction: MR imaging and clinical features in 16 cases. Neuroradiology 2002;44(10): 851–7.

71. Weidauer S, Dettmann E, Krakow K, et al [Diffusion-weighted MRI of spinal cord infarction. Description of two cases and review of the literature]. Nervenarzt 2002;73(10):999–1003.

72. Sagiuchi T, Iida H, Tachibana S, et al. Case report: diffusion-weighted MRI in anterior spinal artery stroke of the cervical spinal cord. J Comput Assist Tomogr 2003;27(3):410–4.

73. Thurnher MM, Bammer R. Diffusion-weighted MR imaging (DWI) in spinal cord ischemia. Neuroradiology 2006;48(11):795–801.

74. Hess CP, Mukherjee P. Visualizing white matter pathways in the living human brain: diffusion tensor imaging and beyond. Neuroimaging Clin N Am 2007;17(4):407–26.

75. Mukherjee P, Berman JI, Chung SW, et al. Diffusion tensor MR imaging and fiber tractography: theoretic underpinnings. AJNR Am J Neuroradiol 2008;29(4): 632–41.

76. Mukherjee P, Chung SW, Berman JI, et al. Diffusion tensor MR imaging and fiber tractography: technical considerations. AJNR Am J Neuroradiol 2008;29(5): 843–52.

77. Wedeen VJ, Wang RP, Schmahmann JD, et al. Diffusion spectrum magnetic resonance imaging (DSI) tractography of crossing fibers. Neuroimage 2008; 41(4):1267–77.

Diffusion-Weighted MR Imaging for Whole Body Metastatic Disease and Lymphadenopathy

Russell N. Low, MD[a,b,*]

KEYWORDS

- Fast imaging • Echo planar imaging
- Diffusion-weighted imaging • MR imaging
- Diffusion-weighted whole-body imaging
  with background body signal suppression
- Whole body imaging

Diffusion is a physical property that describes the microscopic random movement of molecules in response to thermal energy. Also known as Brownian motion, diffusion may be affected by the biophysical properties of tissues such as cell organization and density, microstructure and microcirculation. Diffusion weighted (DW) imaging uses pulse sequences and techniques that are sensitive to very small-scale motion of water protons at the microscopic level. Single shot echo planar imaging (EPI) DW imaging is used to provide very rapid imaging sensitive to subtle small-scale alternations in diffusion. Areas of restricted water diffusion are displayed as areas of high signal intensity.[1–11]

The application of DW imaging for the evaluation of intracranial abnormalities, such as acute cerebral infarcts, is well established.[10] DW imaging often shows areas of altered diffusion in the abnormal brain long before any changes are manifested on conventional anatomic MR images. However, the challenges posed by DW imaging of the abdomen and pelvis initially limited its application for body MR imaging. With use of DW imaging, artifacts related to physiologic motion, susceptibility, and chemical shift are compounded by inherent limitations in signal-to-noise ratio and image resolution. The larger fields of view used for abdominal imaging accentuate many of the artifacts inherent in DW imaging and single shot EPI.[7,11]

Hardware and technical advances in MR imaging, including rapid echo planar imaging, larger amplitude gradient systems, multi channel coils, and parallel imaging techniques, have overcome many of these limitations and, as a result, DW imaging is feasible for abdominal and pelvic MR imaging. By allowing for more rapid imaging with shorter echo time, reduced echo train length, and more rapid k-space filling, many of the artifacts inherent to DW imaging can be reduced.[7,11,12]

Oncologic applications of DW imaging take advantage of restricted diffusion shown by most tumors.[4,7,9–11] The higher cellularity of solid tumors and their increase in cell membranes per unit volume results in restriction of water movement and corresponding high signal intensity on DW images (**Fig. 1**). Areas of tumor necrosis show a decrease in tumor cellularity with an associated increase in diffusion and loss of signal on DW images. Similarly, tumor edema or cystic components of a tumor will show an increase in water diffusion and loss of signal on DW images.[7]

The routine use of DW imaging for abdominal and pelvic oncologic MR imaging is being evaluated. Recent works have described the use of single shot EPI DW imaging for evaluation of lymphadenopathy,[11,13] liver tumors (**Fig. 2**),[14–23]

a Sharp and Children's MRI Center, 7901 Frost Street, San Diego, CA 92123, USA
b San Diego Imaging, Inc., 7901 Frost Street, San Diego, CA 92123, USA
* Sharp and Children's MRI Center, 7901 Frost Street, San Diego, CA 92123.
E-mail address: rlow52@yahoo.com

Magn Reson Imaging Clin N Am 17 (2009) 245–261
doi:10.1016/j.mric.2009.01.006
1064-9689/09/$ – see front matter © 2009 Published by Elsevier Inc.

mri.theclinics.com

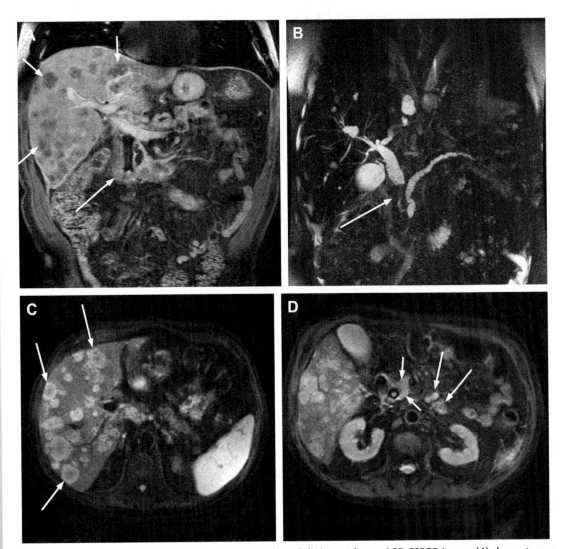

Fig. 1. 71-year-old man with pancreatic cancer. Coronal gadolinium-enhanced 3D FSPGR image (*A*) shows tumor (*long arrow*) encasing a biliary stent and liver metastases (*short arrows*). 3D MRCP (*B*) shows a double duct sign with obstruction of the common bile duct (*arrow*) and the pancreatic duct. Breath-hold DW image (*C*) b-value 400 s/mm² confirms multiple liver metastases (*arrows*) all showing restricted diffusion. Note the high contrast of the liver metastases and their sharp definition on this image obtained during suspended respiration. Breath-hold DW image (*D*) b-value 400 s/mm² at a lower level depicts tumor (*short arrows*) encasing the biliary stent and retroperitoneal nodal metastases (*long arrows*).

renal masses,[24–30] prostate cancer,[31,32] and colorectal cancer (see **Fig. 2**),[33,34] pancreatic cancer,[35] uterine cancer,[36–39] ovarian tumors,[39] peritoneal tumor,[40] and lung cancer.[41] Prior studies have documented the value of DW imaging for tumor detection in the abdomen and pelvis when added to routine unenhanced and gadolinium-enhanced MR imaging in the oncology patient.[4] The ability to generate qualitative and quantitative data using an entirely new contrast mechanism makes DW imaging an attractive tool for tumor assessment in the oncology patient.

TECHNICAL CONSIDERATIONS

Abdominal DW imaging can be performed on commercially available high field MR systems. Most vendors currently use a single shot spin–echo EPI pulse sequence for DW imaging. DW imaging can be performed as a breath-hold acquisition or as a breathing-averaged acquisition with multiple excitations.[1–4] The later may be acquired as a free breathing or respiratory triggered acquisition.[11] In the DW pulse sequence, paired diffusion sensitizing gradients are centered on either side

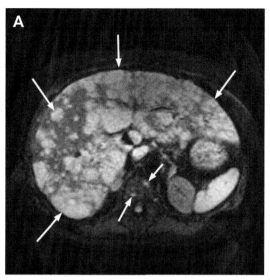
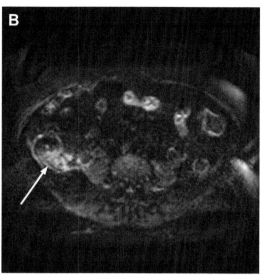

Fig. 2. 66-year-old man with colon cancer. Breath-hold DW image (*A*) b-value 400 s/mm² depicts innumerable liver metastases (*long arrows*) replacing most of the liver parenchyma. Osseous metastases (*short arrows*) are present in the thoracic spine vertebral bodies. Breath-hold DW image (*B*) b-value 400 s/mm² shows a mass in the right lower quadrant representing the patient's primary colon carcinoma.

of the 180 degree refocusing pulse. In the absence of motion, water molecules will acquire phase information from the first diffusion gradient that will be refocused by the second diffusion gradient with no net change in signal. However, with moving water molecules the situation is different. The water molecules will accumulate phase information from the first gradient that will not be completely refocused by the second diffusion gradient because of movement of the water molecule producing a loss of signal. The paired diffusion gradients will thus detect water motion as areas of signal loss.[1,7] Tumors with a higher cellular density possess more cell membranes per unit volume, which restricts mobility of water molecules and diffusion. These tumors will exhibit restricted diffusion and corresponding high signal on DW imaging.

The sensitivity of the DW imaging sequence to water motion can be varied by changing the b-value, which depends on the amplitude and the timing of the paired bipolar diffusion sensitizing gradients.[7] One typically acquires at least two b-values of 0 s/mm2, combined with a second intermediate to a high b-value of 400–1000 s/mm². Acquiring additional b-values will improve the accuracy of the quantitative data obtained from DW imaging. Higher b-values result in more diffusion weighting with better background suppression, at the expense of reduced signal and increasing artifacts.[7,11] At our institution, clinicians typically use b-value 0 s/mm² combined with intermediate b-values of 400–600 s/mm². For anatomic DW imaging, these intermediate

b-values achieve reasonable diffusion weighting while maintaining good image quality.

Diffusion experiments can be independently made in the phase, frequency, or slice directions by applying the diffusion gradient in the selected direction. One may also combine the diffusion signal from all three directions to create a summed image known as an index or magnitude diffusion image.[7] A summed diffusion image loses its directional information but will improve scanning efficiency, allowing for shorter breath hold scan times while maintaining signal–noise-ratio.

Fat suppression is implemented to improve the contrast to background ratio on the DW images. Fat suppression can be accomplished with a short inversion time inversion recovery prepulse (STIR) sequence for maximal background suppression.[7,11] This may be particularly advantageous for whole body diffusion where suppression of all background tissues is desirable when generating inverted maximum intensity projections (MIPs) of the DW dataset.[11] In our experience, for anatomic DW imaging, less complete suppression of background tissues is actually preferable to facilitate anatomic localization of tumors relative to adjacent anatomy. For anatomic DW imaging, fat suppression with spectral presaturation by inversion recovery (SPIR) prepulse or a frequency selective chemical shift selective (CHESS) prepulse achieves an optimal balance of partial background suppression to increase tumor conspicuity while maintaining anatomic landmarks for tumor localization.[7]

Phased array surface coils are used when performing anatomic DW imaging to improve signal-to-noise ratio and overall image quality. Surface coils also allow one to use parallel imaging, which reduces scan time. The read-out time is also decreased with SENSE, which reduces some of the artifacts that are inherent with DW imaging. Similarly, these artifacts may also be minimized by using a minimum echo time (TE) and decreasing the resolution in the frequency direction.[7,11]

The following is a typical protocol for breath-hold abdominal DW imaging used for anatomic imaging.

- Single Shot Spin-Echo EPI
- Phased array surface coil
- B-value 0, 500 s/mm^2
- Slice thickness 7 mm, 1 mm interslice gap
- FOV 320–400 cm
- TR 2700
- TE 58 (min)
- Matrix 115 x115
- SPIR fat suppression
- 24 slices
- 2–3 nex
- Direction of motion probing gradients: phase, frequency, slice
- Acceleration factor 2
- Time: 24 sec breath-hold

Whole-body DW imaging is performed with multiple stacks of axial DW acquisitions covering large anatomic areas that may include head, neck, chest, abdomen, pelvis and lower extremities.[11,42–47] The axial plane is chosen to minimize image distortion. A three- to five-station whole-body DW imaging protocol can be prescribed with overlap between the stations. Some MR systems allow for whole-body imaging with multiple surface coils. On other systems, whole-body DW imaging will require imaging with the integrated large body coil. After the multiple axial DW imaging stacks are prescribed and pre-scanned, automatic table movement between stations facilitates scanning and data acquisition.

Post-processing the whole-body DW imaging typically includes binding the multiple stacks of axial DW images into one large data set. The large whole-body DW data set can be further post processed by generating a 3D model using a MIP post-processing algorithm. The MIP can be inverted to create an image in which tumors are displayed as dark structures on a white background. Automation of post processing of the whole-body DW imaging dataset is available from some vendors.

Typical imaging parameters for whole-body DW imaging include:

- Single shot spin–echo EPI
- Body coil
- B-value 600–1000 s/mm^2
- 3 stations – axial
- 50 slices/station 6 mm thickness
- FOV 420 × 345
- TR 3560 TE 58 (min)
- Matrix 104 × 288 phase x frequency
- STIR fat suppression
- Covers 30 cm per stack
- NEX 4
- Direction of motion probing gradients: phase, frequency, slice
- Time: 1:39 per stack-free breathing

DIFFUSION-WEIGHTED IMAGE ANALYSIS AND DISPLAY

DW images can be evaluated qualitatively by observing changes in signal intensity from areas of the image with minimal restriction of water, such as liver parenchyma, to those with high restriction of water diffusion, such as tumors. In the author's experience, the DW images typically show excellent tumor conspicuity but relatively poor anatomic localization because of suppression of background tissues. For this reason, the DW images are often most useful when interpreted in conjunction with routine anatomic MR images. The DW images can be evaluated as a separate series side-by-side with the T1-, T2- and gadolinium-enhanced acquisitions. In the future, fusion of DW images with anatomic MR images may further improve image interpretation.

Simple visual inspection of magnitude DW images can lead to a potential pitfall and image misinterpretation because observed signal represents the combination of effects from water diffusion and T2 relaxation.[7,11,46] Tissues with prolonged T2 relaxation may appear bright on a DW image representing "T2 shine through." This effect is decreased with higher b-values. With an intermediate b-value, T2-shine through typically occurs with fluid-containing structures, such as gastrointestinal tract, gallbladder, urinary, bladder, and cerebrospinal fluid. Cystic lesions in the liver, kidney, and elsewhere may show similar high signal on DW images because of their prolonged T2 relaxation. Most of these fluid filled structures will show at least partial suppression on DW images obtained with an intermediate b-value. In practice, it is fairly simple to distinguish high signal on a DW image that is caused by T2 shine through from tumors with restricted diffusion. Tsushima and colleagues[8] confirmed the importance of comparing high b-value DW images with T2-weighted images or fused images for maximal accuracy in malignant tumor screening. By comparing the DW images with T2-weighted images or the B0 DW images, one can identify structures that are fluid-containing on the T2-weighted images or B0 images. A more rigorous elimination of high signal from T2 prolongation can be achieved using apparent diffusion coefficient (ADC) maps, which depict changes in signal intensity that are solely caused by water diffusion. On the ADC map, a tumor with restricted diffusion is displayed as an area with low signal intensity as opposed to the DW image in which the tumor is of high signal intensity.[7,42]

A qualitative display of DW images can also be performed following simple post-processing of the data set to generate thin section MIPs reformatted into the coronal or sagittal planes. A whole-volume MIP can also be generated creating a 3D model that can be rotated to display anatomic relationships of tumor to normal structures. This volumetric approach to displaying the DW imaging data requires maximal background suppression (see DWIBS below) and in our experience works best for lymphadenopathy.

Quantitative analysis of DW images can be performed if at least two b-values are obtained.[15,16,30,48–51] Obtaining additional b-values will increase the accuracy of measurements. This quantitative analysis can be performed easily on the MR scanner or workstation, generating ADC parametric maps that are independent of field strength and T2-shine through. By drawing regions of interest on the ADC map over tissues of interest, a numerical value known as the ADC is generated.[7] The ADC value can help to characterize tumors as benign or malignant and can assess interval change in a tumor in response to therapy. Areas of highly cellular tumor with restricted diffusion demonstrate low ADC values while tissues with free water diffusion demonstrate high ADC values. It has also been observed quantitatively that, following therapy, tumors show a significant increase in ADC values with a corresponding loss of signal on visual inspection of the DW image.[21,50–53]

TUMOR DETECTION

The addition of DW imaging to conventional abdominal and pelvic MR imaging improves the detection of many types of primary and metastatic tumor in oncology patients (**Fig. 3**).[4] This improved sensitivity for tumor is caused by the improved conspicuity of tumor on DW imaging compared with conventional T1-, T2-, and gadolinium-enhanced imaging. On DW imaging, background tissues are relatively suppressed while most forms of tumor show restricted water diffusion, which results in moderate to marked tumor conspicuity.

In a study of 169 oncology patients, the addition of breath-hold DW imaging to routine abdominal MR images resulted in detecting additional sites of tumor in 40% and 46% of patients for two observers[4] when compared with conventional MR imaging alone. An intermediate b-value 500 s/mm^2 was used. The additional sites of tumor detected on the DW imaging include 43 patients with lymphadenopathy, 15 with peritoneal metastases, 1 with a renal tumor, 12 with liver tumors, and 2 with osseous tumors. For observer two, the corresponding sites of addition tumor on DW images included 37 with lymphadenopathy, 12 with peritoneal tumors, 1 with renal tumors, 6 with liver tumor, 4 with osseous tumor, and 1 with a gastrointestinal

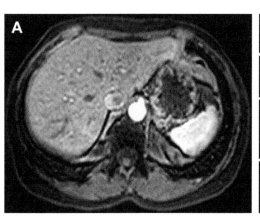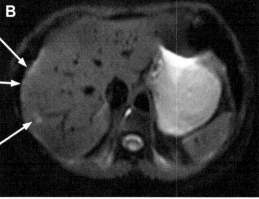

Fig. 3. 60-year-old woman with breast cancer. Arterial phase gadolinium-enhanced 3D FSPGR image (A) is unremarkable without evidence of liver metastasis. T1-weighted, T2-weighted, and portal venous phase gadolinium-enhanced images (not shown) were also normal. Breath-hold DW image (B) b-value 20 s/mm^2 shows small subcapsular and parenchymal liver metastases (*arrows*). Findings were confirmed by biopsy. This case demonstrates the sensitivity of DW imaging to small tumors. The "black blood" appearance of the DW image facilitates depiction of small perivascular tumors.

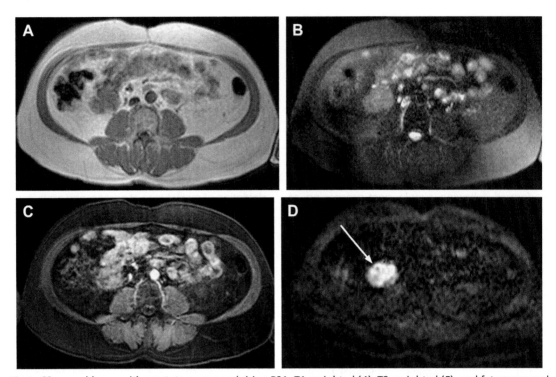

Fig. 4. 68-year-old man with prostate cancer and rising PSA. T1-weighted (*A*), T2-weighted (*B*), and fat suppressed gadolinium-enhanced SGE (*C*) images were interpreted as showing unopacified bowel but no evidence of tumor. Breath hold DWI (*D*) b-value 500 s/mm^2 shows a 3 cm right-sided retroperitoneal tumor (*arrow*).

tumor. The conventional MR examination was entirely normal while the DW images showed tumor in 6%–7% of patients (**Fig 4**).

Studies evaluating DW imaging for depicting liver metastases have found similar improvements in lesion detection compared with conventional unenhanced and contrast enhanced MR imaging (**Fig. 5**). Parikh and colleagues[23] compared DW imaging and breath-hold T2-weighted images for detection and characterization of liver metastases. Overall detection was significantly higher for DW imaging (87.7%) versus T2-weighted (70.1%) imaging, while lesion characterization was not significantly different. Nasu and colleagues[22] found that the addition of DW imaging to T1-weighted and T2-weighted MR imaging showed higher accuracy in the detection of hepatic metastases than did reading of SPIO-enhanced MR images. In a comparison, DW imaging performed before and after SPIO administration found a synergistic effect between iron oxides and DW imaging noting that post-SPIO DW imaging showed improved contrast-to-noise ratio between malignant lesions and liver.[54]

DW imaging can be useful to depict tumors in the nonsolid abdominal organs, such as the gastrointestinal tract and peritoneum (**Figs. 6** and **7**).[33,34,40] In evaluating patients with colorectal cancer, Nasu and colleagues[33] noted that tumors were hyperintense on DW images using a b-value 1000 s/mm^2 and were easily distinguished from the normal colon wall and feces, which was always hypointense. Primary and metastatic tumor in the chest, involving the lung parenchyma, mediastinum, pleura, and chest wall, are also well depicted on DW imaging (**Fig. 8**).[41]

DW imaging improves the depiction of a wide spectrum of primary and metastatic tumors in the abdomen and pelvis. When implemented as a breath-hold acquisition the DW imaging will add very little time to the examination and can be routinely performed in all patients.[4,7,11,42] It is important to note that areas of restricted diffusion on DW images are not specific for tumor. Normal lymph nodes show restricted diffusion and are displayed as hyperintense on DW images.[7,11,42] Similarly, infectious and inflammatory conditions will show restricted diffusion. For example, pancreatitis, cholecystitis, osteomyelitis, an abdominal abscess, and colitis will show restricted diffusion on DW imaging.[55–58] Therefore, interpretation of DW images requires consideration of the patient's clinical presentation and history, as well as an assessment of conventional MR images.

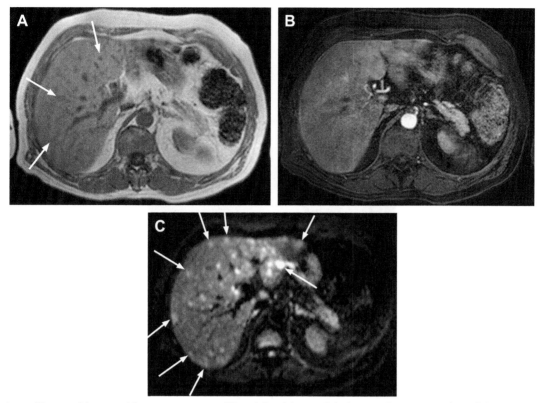

Fig. 5. 56-year-old man with prostate cancer. T1-weighted image (*A*) shows a few scattered small liver lesions (*arrows*). Arterial phase gadolinium-enhanced 3D FSPGR image (*B*) is unremarkable, as were the portal venous phase and equilibrium phase images (not shown). Breath-hold DW image (*C*) b-value 500 s/mm2 depicts many additional small liver metastases (*arrows*).

WHOLE-BODY DIFFUSION-WEIGHTED IMAGING

Diffusion-weighted whole-body imaging with background body signal suppression (DWIBS) was first described by Takahara and colleagues[11] in 2004 (Fig. 9). Using DW imaging with a short TI inversion recovery-echo planar imaging (STIR-EPI) sequence and free breathing scanning, the author generated

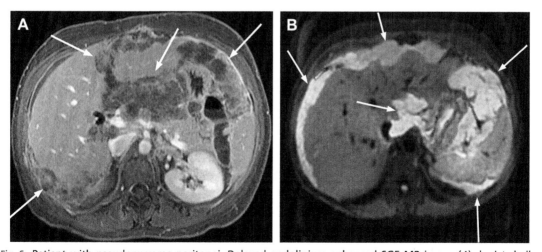

Fig. 6. Patient with pseudomyxoma peritonei. Delayed gadolinium enhanced SGE MR image (*A*) depicts bulky upper abdominal peritoneal tumors (*arrows*) encasing the liver, spleen, stomach, and pancreas. Breath hold DW image (*B*) b value 400 s/mm² depicts bulky upper abdominal peritoneal tumors (*arrows*) showing restricted diffusion. Ascites is low signal intensity on DW images while tumors are high signal intensity.

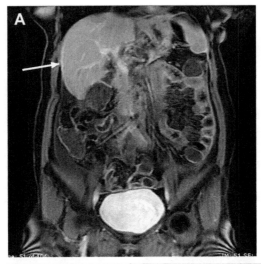

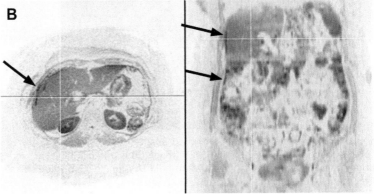

Fig. 7. Patient with treated ovarian cancer and rising serum CA-125 value. Coronal gadolinium enhanced 3D FSPGR image (A) depicts a thin rim of right subphrenic peritoneal tumor (arrow). Reformatted thin section axial and coronal DW images (B) b-value 400 s/mm² confirm a thin rim or right subphrenic peritoneal tumor adjacent to the right hepatic lobe. Thin section reformatted images are useful for anatomic localization of tumors in multiple planes.

whole-body DW images that depicted various tumors and lymphadenopathy, providing volumetric diffusion weighted images of the entire body. These projectional volumetric images provide a quick display of tumor in the chest, abdomen, and pelvis and can simplify display of complex cases facilitating comparison with follow-up MR examinations (Fig. 10).

Interpretation of DWIBS examinations should be performed by reviewing the source images (see Fig. 8). Projectional MIP images can be useful for displaying tumor relationships but can also mask a tumor or falsely create a pseudotumor.[11,42–47] The potential for false positive interpretations with whole-body diffusion may be because of incomplete background suppression, T2 shine-through, and susceptibility artifact. Because of the degree of background suppression, the DWIBS images often lack information for anatomic localization. For this reason, viewing the DWIBS images side-by-side with anatomic MR images is essential for accurate interpretation (Fig. 11). Fusion of the DW images and anatomic images may provide the most accurate means of image display.

Certainly, not all structures showing restricted diffusion on a whole-body DW imaging study are tumor. Some normal anatomic structures may show restricted diffusion and be displayed as hyperintense on DWIBS images. For example, normal lymph nodes are readily apparent on whole body DW images and probably cannot be distinguished from malignant nodes based solely upon their appearance on DW imaging.[7,42] Other normal structures including brain, salivary glands, tonsils, spleen, gallbladder, small intestine, colon, prostate, testes, endometrium, cerebrospinal fluid, and bladder may exhibit high signal intensity on DWIBS images.[42] Finally, just as with anatomic DW imaging, restricted diffusion can be seen in benign inflammatory and infectious diseases.[55–58]

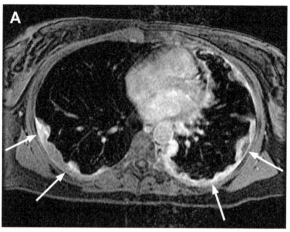
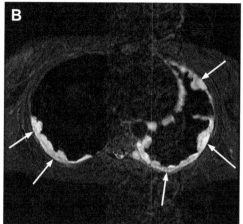

Fig. 8. Patient with appendiceal cancer. Gadolinium-enhanced SGE image (A) through the chest demonstrates bilateral enhancing pleural metastases (arrows). Breath hold DW image (B) b-value 500 s/mm² shows the bilateral pleural tumors. The marked tumor conspicuity facilitates depiction of the full extent of the pleural metastases.

Potential clinical applications for whole-body diffusion include staging of cancer because both the primary tumor and distant metastases demonstrate restricted diffusion.[7,42] Small metastases can be easily seen because of suppression of background tissues. Certain anatomic areas, including the diaphragms and heart, may be problematic because of artifacts from susceptibility or motion. Interpretation of whole-body DW images in conjunction with anatomic MR imaging will increase overall accuracy for tumor depiction and staging.[42]

Whole-body diffusion can also be used to evaluate response of primary tumor and metastases to interval chemotherapy or radiation therapy.[42] After the tumors are depicted, follow-up whole body diffusion can be used to monitor changes in tumor size and ADC values with treatment. Distinguishing residual or recurrent tumor from post-treatment benign changes may be a role for DW imaging but will need to be validated with large patient groups.

One of the most compelling applications of whole-body DW imaging is the evaluation of lymphadenopathy in patients with predominantly nodal metastases.[11] Patients with lymphoma or leukemia are excellent candidates for surveillance with whole body DW imaging (Figs. 9 and 10). Because of suppression of background tissues, the highly cellular lymph nodes are depicted with very high tumor-to-background tissue contrast. Even small nodes are easily depicted. In addition, the volumetric display of the whole-body DW dataset can give a more accurate presentation of the location and distribution of nodal tumor than can routine planar anatomic MR images. Follow-up whole-body DW imaging very quickly displays any interval

change in nodal status. Interpretation of whole-body DW examination for lymphadenopathy is simplified by the predictable locations of lymph nodes in the neck, chest, abdomen, and pelvis. In contrast, the volumetric display of other disseminated tumors involving the peritoneum, bowel, and mesentery can be confusing. In the later situation, thin section multiplanar reformatted images or subvolume MIPs may be a more effective way to display data from whole-body DW imaging.

Comparisons of whole-body DW imaging and PET have been favorable. Ohno and colleagues[43] found that in patients with non-small cell lung cancer (NSCLC), whole-body MR imaging with DW imaging can be used for M-stage assessment with accuracy as good as that of PET/CT. In a comparison of DWIBS and FDG PET, Komori and colleagues[45] found 25 (92.6%) of the 27 malignant lesions were detected visually with DWIBS imaging in contrast to 22 malignant tumors (81.5%) with ^{18}F-FDG PET/CT imaging. Compared to PET/CT, whole-body DW imaging offers several important advantages, including lack of ionizing radiation and much shorter examination times. Currently, the effective radiation dose per PET/CT examination is about 25 mSv and the examinations require 2–3 hours to complete. Whole-body DW imaging can be performed safely without radiation exposure in a fraction of the time required for PET/CT.

Application of the whole-body DW technique for specific malignancies has also been evaluated. For colorectal cancers, Ichikawa and colleagues.[34] evaluated the usefulness of DWIBS. Visual assessment of the DWIBS images resulted in high sensitivity (91%, 20/22) and specificity (100%, 15/15) for detection of the primary tumor.

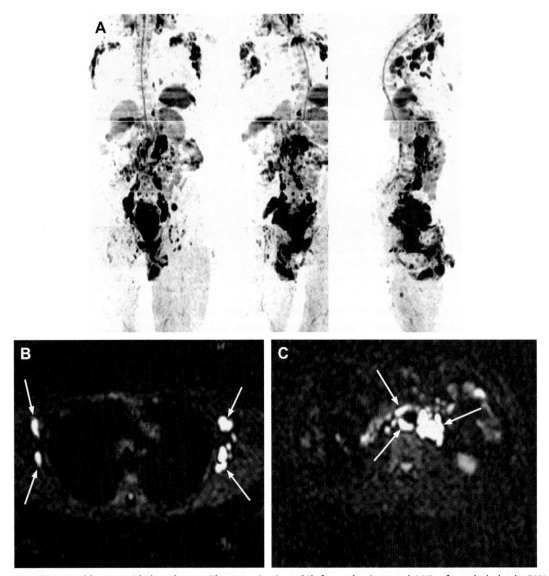

Fig. 9. 82-year-old man with lymphoma. Three projections (*A*) from the inverted MIP of a whole-body DW imaging examination show bulky lymphadenopathy in the neck, chest, abdomen and pelvis. Source DW image (*B*) b-value 500 s/mm² obtained through the chest shows bilateral axillary lymph nodes (*arrows*). Note the marked high contrast of the lymph nodes. DW image (*C*) b-value 500 s/mm² obtained through the abdomen depicts moderately bulky retroperitoneal lymphadenopathy (*arrows*).

For pancreatic adenocarcinoma, 26 patients with pathologically proven pancreatic adenocarcinoma and another 23 controls, assessment of the DWIBS images resulted in high sensitivity (96.2%, 75/78) and specificity (98.6%, 68/69).[35]

DEPICTION OF RECURRENT TUMOR

Detecting recurrent tumor is an imaging challenge that demands high levels of sensitivity and specificity. Small-volume tumor recurrence must be accurately distinguished from normal anatomy

was well as from benign sequela of therapy, including surgery, radiation, percutaneous ablation, and chemoembolization (**Fig. 12**). DW imaging provides such a high tumor-background contrast that its sensitivity for small tumors is markedly increased over normal anatomic MR imaging (**Figs. 13** and **14**). In the author's experience, DW images may depict small volume tumor recurrence before other conventional anatomic images are abnormal.[4] The specificity of areas of restricted diffusion on DW imaging is still being evaluated. It is possible that a quantitative analysis

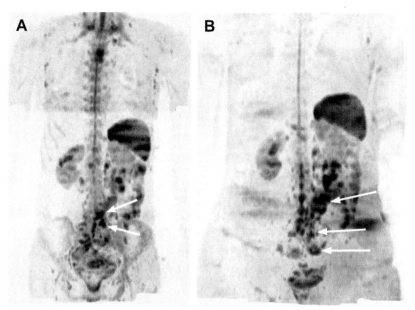

Fig.10. 55-year-old man with lymphoma. Whole-body DW imaging examination performed in December 2007 (*A*) shows small retroperitoneal lymph nodes (*arrows*). Follow-up whole-body DW imaging examination from July 2008 (*B*) shows interval progression of lymphadenopathy (*arrows*).

of DW imaging with ADC values will improve the distinction of small tumors from post therapeutic changes. For neuroimaging, distinguishing recurrent neoplasm from radiation necrosis can be challenging. Using DW imaging, significant differences have been found in maximal ADC values between radiation necrosis and recurrent tumor.[59]

TUMOR CHARACTERIZATION

A quantitative analysis of DW images may allow one to distinguish benign from malignant tumors in the abdomen and pelvis. As a general rule, benign processes would be expected to have a higher ADC than highly cellular malignant

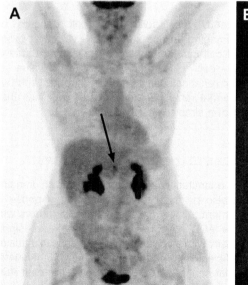
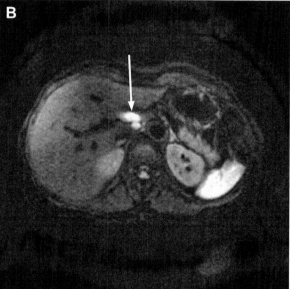

Fig. 11. 55-year-old woman with treated ovarian cancer and a rising serum CA-125 value. Inverted MIP from a whole-body DW imaging acquisition (*A*) shows a small focal lesion in the upper abdomen. Breath-hold DW image (*B*) b-value 400 s/mm^2 shows portal caval lymphadenopathy (*arrow*) representing nodal metastases.

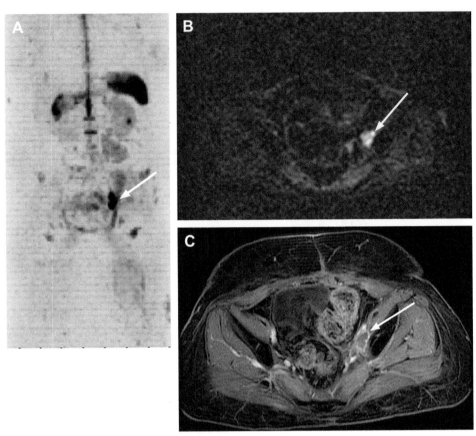

Fig. 12. 65-year-old man with colon cancer. Inverted MIP (*A*) from a whole-body DW imaging examination shows a focal intense area of restricted diffusion in the left pelvic sidewall. DW image (*B*) b-value 600 s/mm² shows a focal tumor in the left side of the pelvis. Fat suppressed, gadolinium-enhanced image (*C*) confirms the 2 cm left iliac nodal metastases (*arrow*).

process, which demonstrates restricted diffusion and lower ADC values. Some of the challenges in implementing this type of analysis include: variations in the ways that DW imaging is implemented on different scanners and obvious differences in DW imaging protocols, all of which will affect the numerical ADC value. It is also not surprising that there is considerable overlap in the ADC values for benign and malignant diseases. However, the ADC values obtained from DW imaging provide an intriguing new tool to characterize abdominal tumors.

In several studies, malignant liver tumors have shown significantly lower ADC values than benign liver cysts and hemangiomas.[15,16] Renal masses may be similarly characterized with quantitative DW imaging. Zhang and colleagues[48] noted that renal tumors had significantly lower ADCs compared with benign cysts and that solid enhancing tumors had significantly lower ADCs compared with nonenhancing necrotic or cystic regions. Cystic renal neoplasms behave differently than solid renal cell cancers on DW imaging. In one study, ADC values of cystic renal cell carcinomas were higher than those of clear cell carcinomas. The ADC value of cystic renal cell carcinomas overlapped with that of normal renal parenchyma but was less than that of a simple renal cyst.[30]

ASSESSMENT OF RESPONSE TO THERAPY

This quantitative approach to diffusion imaging can also be used to assess tumor response to treatment.[21,49–53] Initially, high-signal tumors with a low ADC have been observed to lose signal intensity with a corresponding increase in diffusion coefficient following treatment (**Fig. 15**). Hepatocellular cancer showed an increase in tumor ADC values following trancatheter chemoembolization.[50] Similarly, a significant increase in mean ADC value was observed in liver metastatic lesions that responded to chemotherapy (**Fig. 16**).[20]

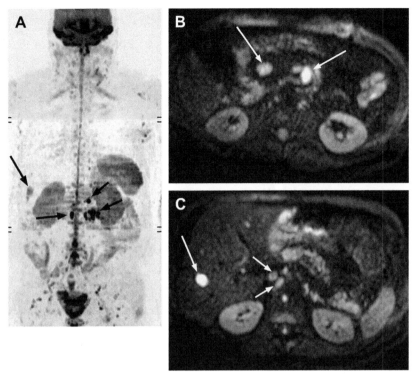

Fig. 13. 59-year-old man with pancreatic cancer status post Whipple procedure. Whole-body DW image (*A*) shows liver metastasis (*long arrow*) and retroperitoneal nodal metastases (*short arrows*). DW image (*B*) b-value 500 s/mm² confirms the moderately bulky retroperitoneal lymphadenopathy (*arrows*). DW image (*C*) b-value 500 s/mm² depicts liver metastasis (*long arrow*) and smaller retroperitoneal lymph nodes (*short arrows*). Findings represent recurrent pancreatic cancer.

PREDICTING RESPONSE TO THERAPY

Evaluating pretreatment ADC values of tumors may also shed light upon which tumors will respond to subsequent therapy. Koh and colleagues[20] noted that for colorectal hepatic metastases, high pretreatment mean ADC values were predictive of poor response to chemotherapy. Similarly, Cui and colleagues[51] evaluated patients with 38 responding and 49 nonresponding metastatic liver lesions from colorectal and gastric cancer. Pretherapy mean ADC values in responding lesions were significantly lower than those of nonresponding lesions (*P* = .003).[51] DW

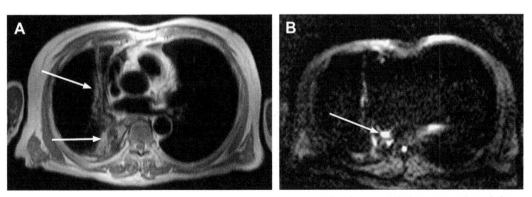

Fig. 14. Patient with lung cancer status post radiation therapy. T1-weighted image (*A*) show parenchymal changes from radiation therapy but no definite evidence of residual tumor. Breath hold DW image (*B*) b-value 500 s/mm² shows a small focal nodule with marked restriction of water diffusion. Findings represent tumor recurrence and correlated with results of subsequent PET scan (not shown).

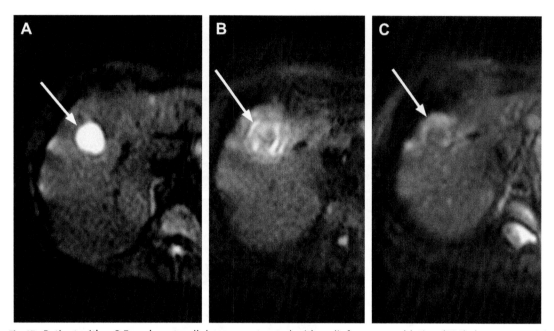

Fig. 15. Patient with a 2.5 cm hepatocellular cancer treated with radiofrequency ablation (RFA) shown on serial MR examinations. Pretreatment DW image (*A*) shows the focal HCC (*arrow*) with marked high signal intensity. Follow up DW image (*B*) obtained 3 months following treatment shows decrease in signal intensity of the treated HCC (*arrow*). Final DW image (*C*) obtained 8 months following treatment shows further loss of signal within the HCC indicating response to RFA. Corresponding increase in ADC value also indicates treatment response.

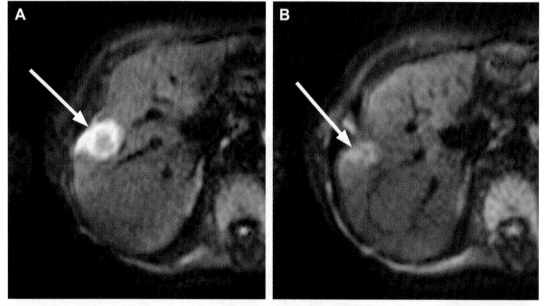

Fig. 16. Patient with metastatic colon cancer. Pretreatment DW image b-value 400 s/mm2 (*A*) shows a 2.5 cm metastasis (*arrow*) in the right hepatic lobe with marked restriction of diffusion. Follow-up DW image b-value 400 s/mm^2 (*B*) obtained following chemotherapy shows decrease size of the metastasis and corresponding loss of signal intensity. Corresponding ADC values for the liver metastasis showed interval increase with treatment indicating response to chemotherapy.

imaging has been advocated as a means to assess tumor necrosis in patients with hepatocellular cancer undergoing chemoembolization[52] with a linear correlation between ADC values and the degree of tumor necrosis at histopathologic evaluation.

SUMMARY

DW imaging provides qualitative and quantitative information that can be critical in the oncology patient. Accurate depiction of the primary tumor and whole-body metastases makes it an ideal sequence for oncologic imaging. Additional information obtained from a quantitative analysis of ADC values can be used to characterize tumors and assess response to treatment. Speculating on the future role of diffusion weighted body imaging compared with PET/CT is intriguing. DW imaging is clearly a powerful new tool that improves the sensitivity and specificity of body MR imaging for oncologic imaging. Because DW imaging does not provide true metabolic information, it seems unlikely to entirely replace PET/CT. Rather these two examinations will play complementary roles. There is growing concern about the radiation exposure and the cost of PET/CT. MR imaging combined with DW imaging is in a unique position to augment the role of PET/CT in cancer imaging. Initial evaluation with PET/CT might be used to identify sites of primary and metastatic tumor. Follow up MR imaging and DW imaging could be performed to monitor the tumor response to therapy. In other clinical settings, the limitations of PET/CT in depicting some tumors, including peritoneal metastases and small liver metastases, makes MR imaging with DW imaging the initial examination of choice. In the author's experience, DW imaging combined with conventional MR imaging leads to more accurate imaging diagnoses, better treatment decisions, and improved patient care.

REFERENCES

1. Ichikawa T, Haradome HH, Hachiya J, et al. Diffusion-weighted MR imaging with single-shot echo-planar imaging in the upper abdomen: preliminary clinical experience in 61 patients. Abdom Imaging 1999;24:456–61.
2. Yamashita Y, Tang Y, Takahashi M. Ultrafast MR imaging of the abdomen: echo planar imaging and diffusion-weighted imaging. J Magn Reson Imaging 1998;8:367–74.
3. Chow LC, Bammer R, Moseley ME, et al. Single breath-hold diffusion-weighted imaging of the abdomen. J Magn Reson Imaging 2003;18:377–82.
4. Low RN, Gurney J. Diffusion-weighted MRI (DWI) in the oncology patient: value of breath hold DWI compared to unenhanced and gadolinium-enhanced MRI. J Magn Reson Imaging 2007;25:848–58.
5. Brammer R, Auer M, Kelling SL, et al. Diffusion tensor imaging using single-shot SENSE-EPI. Mang Reson Med 2002;48:128–36.
6. Murtz P, Flacke S, Traver F, et al. Abdomen: diffusion-weighted MR imaging with pulse-triggered single-shot sequences. Radiology 2002;224:258–64.
7. Koh DM, Collins DJ. Diffusion-weighted MRI in the body: applications and challenges in oncology. AJR Am J Roentgenol 2007;188:1622–35.
8. Tsushima Y, Takano A, Taketomi-Takahashi A. Endo K Body diffusion-weighted MR imaging using high b-value for malignant tumor screening: usefulness and necessity of referring to T2-weighted images and creating fusion images. Acad Radiol 2007;14:643–50.
9. Toney HC, De Keyzer F. Extracranial applications of diffusion weighted magnetic resonance imaging. Eur Radiol 2007;17:1385–93.
10. Provenzale JM, Mukundan S, Barboriak DP. Diffusion weighted and perfusion MR imaging for brain tumor characterization and assessment of treatment response. Radiology 2006;239:632–49.
11. Takahara T, Imai Y, Yamashita T, et al. Diffusion weighted whole body imaging with background body signal suppression (DWIBS): technical improvement using free breathing, STIR and high resolution 3D display. Radiat Med 2004;22:275–82.
12. Bammer R, Keeling RL, Augustin M, et al. Improved diffusion-weighted single-shot echo-planar imaging (EPI) in stroke using sensitivity encoding (SENSE). Magn Reson Med 2001;46:548–54.
13. Sumia M, Sakihamab N, Sumia T, et al. Discrimination of metastatic cervical lymph nodes with diffusion-weighted MR imaging in patients with head and neck cancer. AJNR Am J Neuroradiol 2003;24:1627–34.
14. Kim T, Murakami T, Takahashi S, et al. Diffusion-weighted single-shot echoplanar MR imaging for liver disease. AJR Am J Roengenol 1999;173:393–8.
15. Taouli B, Vilgrain V, Dumont E, et al. Evaluation of liver diffusion isotropy and characterization of focal hepatic lesions with two single-shot echo-planar MR imaging sequences: prospective study in 66 patients. Radiology 2003;226:71–8.
16. Nakimoto T, Yamashia Y, Sumi S, et al. Focal liver masses: characterization with diffusion-weighted echo-planar MR imaging. Radiology 1997;204:739–44.
17. Taouli B, Martin AJ, Qayyum A, et al. Parallel imaging and diffusion tensor imaging for diffusion-weighted MRI of the liver: preliminary experience in healthy volunteers. Am J Roentgenol 2004;183:677–80.
18. Gourtsoyianni S, Papanikolaou N, Yarmenitis S, et al. Respiratory gated diffusion-weighted imaging of the

liver: value of apparent diffusion coefficient measurements in the differentiation between most commonly encountered benign and malignant focal liver lesions. Eur Radiol 2008;18:486–92.

19. Bruegel M, Holzapfel K, Gaa J, et al. Characterization of focal liver lesions by ADC measurements using a respiratory triggered diffusion-weighted single-shot echo-planar MR imaging technique. Eur Radiol 2008;18:477–85.

20. Koh DM, Scurr E, Collins D, et al. Predicting response of colorectal hepatic metastasis: value of pretreatment apparent diffusion coefficients. AJR Am J Roentgenol 2007;188:1001–8.

21. Liapi E, Geschwind JF, Vossen JA, et al. Functional MRI evaluation of tumor response in patients with neuroendocrine hepatic metastasis treated with transcatheter arterial chemoembolization. AJR Am J Roentgenol 2008;190:67–73.

22. Nasu K, Kuroki Y, Nawano S, et al. Hepatic metastases: diffusion weighted sensitivity-encoding versus SPIO-enhanced MR imaging. Radiology 2006;239:122–30.

23. Parikh T, Drew SJ, Lee VS, et al. Focal liver lesion detection and characterization with diffusion-weighted MR imaging: comparison with standard breath-hold T2-weighted imaging. Radiology 2008;246:812–22.

24. Ries M, Jones RA, Basseau F, et al. Diffusion tensor MRI of the human kidney. J Magn Reson Imaging 2001;14:42–9.

25. Squillaci E, Manenti G, Cova M, et al. Correlation of diffusion-weighted MR imaging with cellularity of renal tumours. Anticancer Res 2004;24:4175–9.

26. Cova M, Squillaci E, Stacul F, et al. Diffusion-weighted MRI in the evaluation of renal lesions: preliminary results. Br J Radiol 2004;77:851–7.

27. Chan JH, Tsui EY, Luk SH, et al. MR diffusion-weighted imaging of kidney: differentiation between hydronephrosis and pyonephrosis. Clin Imaging 2001;25:110–3.

28. Namimoto T, Yamashita Y, Mitsuzaki K, et al. Measurement of the apparent diffusion coefficient in diffuse renal disease by diffusion-weighted echo-planar MR imaging. J Magn Reson Imaging 1999;9:832–7.

29. Fukuda Y, Ohashi I, Hanafusa K, et al. Anisotropic diffusion in kidney: apparent diffusion coefficient measurements for clinical use. J Magn Reson Imaging 2000;22:156–60.

30. Squillaci E, Manenti G, Di Stefano F, et al. Diffusion-weighted MR imaging in the evaluation of renal tumours. J Exp Clin Cancer Res 2004;23:39–45.

31. Hosseinzadeh K, Schwartz SD. Endorectal diffusion-weighted imaging in prostate cancer to differentiate malignant and benign peripheral zone tissue. J Magn Reson Imaging 2004;20:654–61.

32. Issa B. In vivo measurements of the apparent diffusion coefficient in normal and malignant prostatic tissues using echo-planar imaging. J Magn Reson Imaging 2002;16:196–200.

33. Nasu K, Kuroki Y, Kuroki S, et al. Diffusion-weighted single shot Echo planar imaging of colorectal cancer using a sensitivity-encoding technique. Jpn J Clin Oncol 2004;34:620–6.

34. Ichikawa T, Erturk SM, Motosugi U, et al. High-B-value diffusion weighted MRI in colorectal cancer. AJR Am J Roentgenol 2006;187:181–4.

35. Ichikawa T, Erturk SM, Motosugi U, et al. High-b value diffusion-weighted MRI for detecting pancreatic adenocarcinoma: preliminary results. AJR Am J Roentgenol 2007;188:409–14.

36. Fujii S, Matsusue E, Kigawa J, et al. Diagnostic accuracy of the apparent diffusion coefficient in differentiating benign from malignant uterine endometrial cavity lesions: initial results. Eur Radiol 2008;18:384–9.

37. Tamai K, Koyama T, Saga T, et al. Diffusion-weighted MR imaging of uterine endometrial cancer. J Magn Reson Imaging 2007;26:682–7.

38. Naganawa S, Sato C, Kumada H, et al. Apparent diffusion coefficient in cervical cancer of the uterus: comparison with the normal uterine cervix. Eur Radiol 2005;15:71–8.

39. Nakayama T, Yoshimitsu K, Irie H, et al. Diffusion-weighted echo-planar MR imaging and ADC mapping in the differential diagnosis of ovarian cystic masses: usefulness of detecting keratinoid substances in mature cystic teratomas. J Magn Reson Imaging 2005;22:271–8.

40. Fuji S, Matsusue E, Kanasaki Y, et al. Detection of peritoneal dissemination in gynecological malignancy: evaluation by diffusion-weighted MR imaging. Eur Radiol 2008;18:18–23.

41. Matoba M, Tonami H, Kondou T, et al. Lung carcinoma: diffusion-weighted MR imaging—preliminary evaluation with apparent diffusion coefficient. Radiology 2007;243:570–7.

42. Kwee TC, Takahara T, Ochiai R, et al. Diffusion-weighted whole-body imaging with background body signal suppression (DWIBS): features and potential applications in oncology. Eur Radiol 2008;18:1937–52.

43. Ohno Y, Koyama H, Onishi Y, et al. Non–Small cell lung cancer: Whole-body MR examination for M-stage assessment—utility for whole-body diffusion-weighted imaging compared with integrated FDG PET/CT. Radiology 2008;248:643–54.

44. Mürtz P, Krautmacher C, Träber F, et al. Diffusion-weighted whole-body MR imaging with background body signal suppression: a feasibility study at 3.0 Tesla. Eur Radiol 2007;17:3031–7.

45. Komori T, Narabayashi I, Matsumura K, et al. 2-[Fluorine-18]-fluoro-2-deoxy-D-glucose positron

emission tomography/computed tomography versus whole-body diffusion-weighted MRI for detection of malignant lesions: initial experience. Ann Nucl Med 2007;21:209–15.

46. Li S, Sun F, Jin ZY, et al. Whole-body diffusion-weighted imaging: technical improvement and preliminary results. J Magn Reson Imaging 2007; 26:1139–44.

47. Ballon D, Watts R, Dyke JP, et al. Imaging therapeutic response in human bone marrow using rapid whole-body MRI. Magn Reson Med 2004;52: 1234–8.

48. Zhang J, Tehrani YM, Wang L, et al. Renal masses: characterization with diffusion-weighted MR imaging—a preliminary experience. Radiology 2008;247:458–64.

49. Yoshikawa T, Kawamitsu H, Mitchell DG, et al. ADC measurement of abdominal organs and lesions using parallel imaging technique. AJR 2006;187: 1521–30.

50. Chen C-Y, Li C-W, Kuo Y-T, et al. Early response of hepatocellular carcinoma to transcatheter arterial chemoembolization: choline levels and MR diffusion constants—initial experience. Radiology 2006;239: 448–56.

51. Cui Y, Zhang X-P, Sun Y-S, et al. Apparent diffusion coefficient: potential imaging biomarker for prediction and early detection of response to chemotherapy in hepatic metastases. Radiology 2008; 248:894–900.

52. Kamel IR, Bluemke DA, Ramsey D, et al. Role of diffusion-weighted imaging in estimating tumor necrosis after chemoembolization of hepatocellular carcinoma. AJR 2003;181:708–10.

53. Hamstra DA, Rehemtulla A, Ross BD. Diffusion magnetic resonance imaging: a biomarker for treatment response in oncology. J Clin Oncol 2007;25:4104–9.

54. Naganawa S, Sato C, Nakamura T, et al. Diffusion-weighted images of the liver: Comparison of tumor detection before and after contrast enhancement with superparamagnetic iron oxide. J Magn Reson Imaging 2005;21:836–40.

55. Chan JHM, Tsui EYK, Luk SH, et al. Diffusion-weighted MR imaging of the liver: distinguishing hepatic abscess from cystic or necrotic tumor. Abdom Imaging 2001;26:161–5.

56. Sukru M, Erturk SM, Ichikawa T, et al. Diffusion-weighted MR imaging in the evaluation of pancreatic exocrine function before and after secretin stimulation. Am J Gastroenterol 2006;101:133–6.

57. Magnetic resonance imaging of benign spinal lesions simulating metastasis: role of diffusion-weighted imaging. Top Magn Reson Imaging 2000;11:224–34.

58. Tsuchiya K, Katase S, Yoshino A, et al. Diffusion-weighted MR imaging of encephalitis. Am J Roentgenol 1999;173:1097–9.

59. Asao C, Korogic Y, Kitajima M, et al. Diffusion-weighted imaging of radiation-induced brain injury for differentiation from tumor recurrence. AJNR Am J Neuroradiol 2005;26:1455–60.

Diffusion-Weighted MR Imaging in Musculoskeletal Radiology: Applications in Trauma, Tumors, and Inflammation

Thorsten A. Bley, MD[a],[*], Oliver Wieben, PhD[a],[b], Markus Uhl, MD[c]

KEYWORDS

- Diffusion-weighted imaging • Musculoskeletal radiology
- Tumor • Osteomyelitis • Trauma

Diffusion-weighted (DW) imaging is a noninvasive magnetic resonance technique that is capable of measuring microscopic movement of water molecules (ie, random or Brownian motion) within biologic tissues. Diffusion weighting is achieved with a pulsed-field-gradient[1] that leaves "static" spins unaffected but causes dephasing of spin ensembles that experience different motion histories according to their diffusion paths, with respect to the direction of the gradient. Using this approach, the movement of intracellular water molecules can be differentiated from movement of water molecules from extracellular space, which tend to diffuse in a less restricted manner. For example, in a fluid-filled cyst, water molecules have a far greater freedom of movement than in a solid tumor that restricts the molecule's movement because of its high cellularity.

The diffusion coefficient of water observed in biologic tissues greatly differs from that of pure water because of the presence of fibers, cell membranes, macromolecules, and so forth. Therefore, the apparent diffusion coefficient (ADC) will have spatial anisotropy, which can be measured by using orthogonal diffusion-encoding in three spatial dimensions.[2] Because most DW imaging sequences are based on a T_2-weighted sequence, the "T_2-shine-through" effect must be taken into account.[3,4] For obtaining a pure diffusion image, the diffusivity needs to be calculated. Then, an ADC or ADC map are calculated using images of the same slice acquired with different gradient encoding settings, usually referred to as "b-values."[5]

Water diffusion values relate to the ratio of intracellular and extracellular water, and changes in ADC maps are inversely correlated with changes in cellularity. Increased mobility of water represents an increase in extracellular water or loss of cell membrane integrity (eg, because of effective tumor treatment in oncology). Conversely, decrease in water diffusivity reflects decreasing extracellular water content or increasing cell number or size: for example, in tumor progression, fibrosis, or edema.[6] In tumors with very densely packed tumor cells, such as a neuroblastoma or Ewing sarcoma, reduced diffusion may arise from their specific cellular anatomy with small

[a] Department of Radiology, University of Wisconsin, 600 Highland Avenue, Madison, WI 53792, USA
[b] Department of Medical Physics, University of Wisconsin, 600 Highland Avenue, Madison, WI 53792, USA
[c] Division of Pediatric Radiology, Department of Diagnostic Radiology, University of Freiburg, Freiburg, Germany
* Corresponding author.
E-mail address: tbley@uwhealth.org (T.A. Bley).

Magn Reson Imaging Clin N Am 17 (2009) 263–275
doi:10.1016/j.mric.2009.01.005

cytoplasms and large nuclei. This results in a high nuclear-to-cytoplasm ratio, which limits intracellular diffusion (Fig. 1).[7]

DW imaging has found widespread use in neuro imaging, particularly in the diagnosis of acute brain ischemia, where changes in cellularity can be observed within minutes in ischemic regions. Used in conjunction with perfusion imaging diffusion, perfusion mismatches can be used to identify patients with stroke who are likely to benefit from reperfusion therapy.[8–11] While other articles in this special issue discuss further details of DW imaging and its applications in various radiology subspecialties, this review focuses on the interesting opportunities of its use in the diagnosis of musculoskeletal diseases, including trauma, tumor, and inflammation. The utility of DW imaging has been described for various musculoskeletal

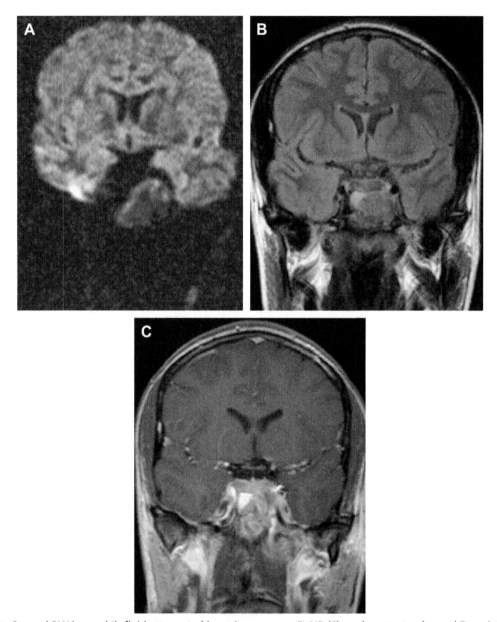

Fig. 1. Coronal DW image (*A*), fluid-attenuated inversion recovery FLAIR (*B*), and contrast enhanced T_1-weighted image (*C*) of the head of a 22-year-old man with Ewing sarcoma of the clivus. The DW images help delineate the tumor. Because of the chemotherapy, the signal of the sarcoma becomes more and more hypointense in diffusion-weighted images.

applications, such as imaging of muscle,[12] carti-lage,[13] synovial fluids for differentiation of inflam-matory versus degenerative arthritis,[14] treatment response in oncology,[15–17] and assessment of bone marrow and vertebral fractures.[5,18–20]

DIFFUSION-WEIGHTED IMAGING TECHNIQUES IN MUSCULOSKELETAL RADIOLOGY

Many routine MR imaging sequences can be sensi-tized to diffusion by the addition of diffusion gradi-ents after the rf excitation and before the readout gradient. However, the presence of strong diffusion gradients may lead to inadvertent effects, such as artifacts from motion, eddy currents, and concom-itant gradient terms.[5] Artifacts from motion occur because the diffusion gradients sensitize the acqui-sition not only to molecular movements at the microscopic level but also to voluntary and involun-tary and physiologic motion at the macroscopic level. For example, bulk patient motion, blood flow, and cerebral spinal fluid pulsation in the spinal canal can be sources of such artifacts, especially with multishot sequences.

The most commonly used acquisition strategy for DW imaging is single or multishot echo-planar (EP) imaging because of its efficiency in terms of scan time. The rapid acquisition within seconds makes this technique fast and less sensitive to patient motion, while large volume coverage is feasible. EP imaging sequences usually achieve a comparably high signal-to-noise ratio (SNR) with low power deposition because several echoes are acquired after a single excitation pulse. Unfortunately, echo-planar DW images are prone to artifacts just as regular EP images, particularly magnetic susceptibility artifacts, especially at tissue interfaces such as air and soft tissue or bone and soft tissue, and geometric distortions created by eddy currents, particularly in large fields of view.

Alternatively, diffusion weighting can be incor-porated into spin echo (SE) and stimulated echo acquisitions, which are less prone to artifacts. Both sequences provide high SNRs and are robust to field inhomogeneities. However, they require relatively long acquisition times and the likelihood of patient movements during the acquisition with subsequent motion artifacts is significantly increased. Several approaches have been proposed to overcome motion-related artifacts in DW imaging, including the use of navigator echoes.[21,22] Non-Cartesian acquisitions, including radial sampling, the PROPELLER technique, and line scanning, have been explored for DW imaging because of their advantageous properties for dealing with motion. Dietrich and colleagues[23]

developed a diffusion-weighted SE sequence with a radial k-space trajectory to obtain ADC values in the spine in a more robust fashion and with higher quality. The spine is known to be a diffi-cult region for DW imaging, as susceptibility effects occur at interfaces from bone to soft tissue, and artifacts from cardiac and respiratory motion degrade image quality. The PROPELLER tech-nique[24] has been successfully adapted to DW imaging of spinal hematoma and other DW imaging applications.[25] Another method for reli-able quantitative diffusion measurements, despite physiologic motion, is line-scan diffusion imaging. In this approach, multiple diffusion-weighted SE column excitations are used to construct a two-dimensional image. As line-scan diffusion imaging is not as sensitive to susceptibility artifacts as EP imaging, it is considered a reliable method for imaging of the spinal column.[26]

Other sequences that have been explored for DW imaging include a non-Carr-Purcell-Mei-boom-Gill single-shot fast spin-echo sequence that produced significantly higher SNR compared with the EP imaging-based DW imaging technique ($P<.01$) when imaging the appendicular skeleton and the spine.[27,28] Jeong and colleagues[29] have introduced a segmented three-dimensional steady-state free precession (SSFP) high-resolu-tion diffusion-weighted MR imaging technique with DW equilibrium inserted between each segment. Utilizing a tip-up pulse that converted microscopic motions into amplitude errors at the end of the DW segment, motion artifacts caused by small bulk motions were avoided. Dietrich and colleagues[30] introduced a centric-reordered modi-fied rapid acquisition with relaxation enhancement (mRARE) sequence for single-shot DW imaging in soft-tissue tumors in the musculoskeletal system. This mRARE sequence rendered less distorted images than those acquired with the single-shot EP imaging sequence. Considerably higher muscle and fat signals than in the single-shot EP imaging sequence were beneficial for anatomic information. This technique also provides a reliable tool for determining quantitative ADCs in vertebral bone marrow with adequate image quality. The ADC values of bone marrow lesions, such as edema, tumor, or inflammation were significantly higher than in healthy bone marrow ($1.27 \pm 0.32 \times 10^{-3}$ mm^2 per second versus $0.21 \pm 0.10 \times 10^{-3}$ mm^2 per second).[31] With its relatively low diffusivity, the high-fat signal is b-value-indepen-dent and may superimpose onto the b-value-dependent water signal within the same voxel. Therefore, it can be beneficial to use fat suppres-sion techniques in areas with high fat and low water content, such as the vertebral bodies.

DIFFUSION-WEIGHTED IMAGING IN ASSESSMENT OF TUMOR RESPONSE

MR imaging plays an important role in the detection and staging of primary bone tumors, as well as in postoperative monitoring. Assessment of tumor size before, during, or after therapeutic intervention is a traditional measure of treatment efficacy. In some tumor entities, such as osteosarcomas, treatment success is not necessarily reflected by a reduced tumor size. Despite having a favorable impact on the event-free survival, neoadjuvant chemotherapy may not lead to the reduction of tumor size, as it has no significant impact on the mineralized matrix of the tumor. In this regard, assessment of treatment response may be difficult with conventional imaging strategies that rely on measuring the size of the tumor. In those sites where response cannot be measured by RECIST (response evaluation criteria in solid tumors)

criteria, no accepted method exists for assessing tumor response to treatment of primary or metastatic skeletal tumors.[32] In fact, tumor size may increase during treatment because of edematous changes or ossification, and therefore may not be an accurate predictor of tumor response.

Changes in tumor volume or structure detected on radiography or CT have failed to predict histologic tumor response.[33–35] Catheter-based angiography was found to be an accurate method for assessing the response of osteosarcoma to chemotherapy.[36,37] Furthermore, this method is invasive and unfavorable as a means of routine follow-up examinations. Conventional MR criteria may not be helpful in the early identification of good responders, and nested foci of residual viable tumor may be overseen.[38,39] Instead, detection of necrosis has been recognized as a prognostic factor of tumor response to chemotherapy in Ewing sarcoma and osteogenic sarcoma.[40]

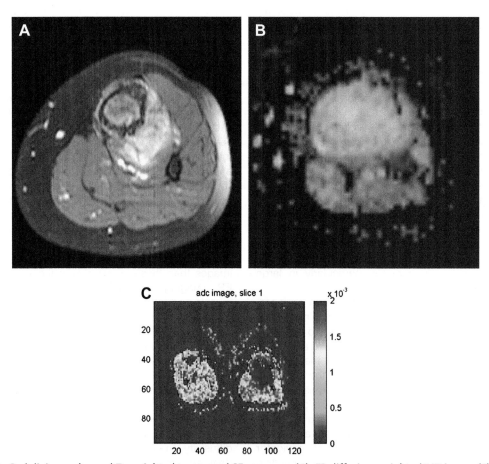

Fig. 2. Gadolinium-enhanced T_1-weighted transversal SE sequence (A), EP diffusion-weighted MR image (B), and ADC map (C) of the left lower extremity of a 12-year-old boy with histologically proven osteosarcoma after chemotherapy. Contrast-enhanced T_1-weighted imaging readily reveals an enhancing mass but fails to reliably distinguish vital tumor from necrotic residuals. High ADC values (C) indicate necrosis rather than vital tumor, which was proven by histology after resection.

Greater than 90% necrosis after chemotherapy resembles a positive response to treatment and is associated with a favorable prognosis.[41] However, bone marrow lesions may show nonspecific changes in signal intensity under treatment, and conventional MR imaging may fail to identify tumor response. In this setting, where response to treatment cannot be assessed accurately with conventional imaging, DW imaging represents a noninvasive biomarker of treatment response by identifying necrotic regions within a tumor.

Viable tumors demonstrate high cellularity with intact cell membranes and, therefore exhibit restricted diffusion (high DW-imaging signal). In contrast, the cellularity within the tumor decreases with successful antineoplastic therapy, cell membranes lose their integrity, and eventually tumor necrosis allows for an increased diffusion of water, with larger mean free-path lengths of diffusing molecules (low DW-imaging signal). Clinical examples of an osteosarcoma after chemotherapy and a metastasis of renal cell carcinoma to the skull are shown in **Figs. 2** and **3**.

DW imaging has been shown to be a useful tool to monitor tumor response to treatment, as it displays decreased signal intensity, for example, of primary bone sarcomas[16,42,43] and of metastatic disease of the vertebral bone marrow.[44] In

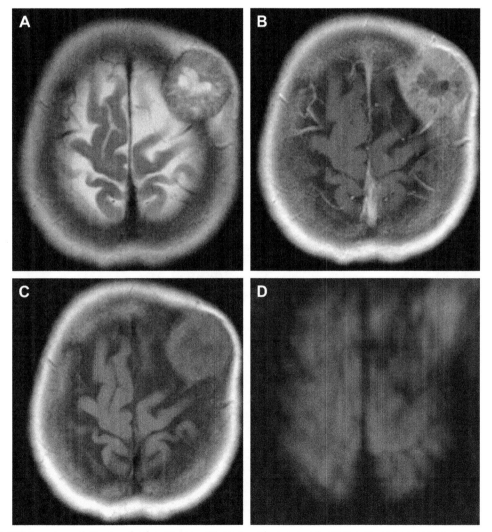

Fig. 3. MR imaging of the head of a 65-year-old man with renal cell carcinoma and metastasis to the skull. T_2-weighted turbo-spin echo (TSE) (*A*) and T_1-weighted SE with (*B*) and without (*C*) contrast enhancement demonstrate the extent of the bony metastasis. The "cystic" areas within the metastasis appear hyperintense on the T_2-weighted image, hypointense on the T_1-weighted image, and do not enhance. They demonstrate hypointense signal on DWI with a *b*-value of 900 mm² per second (*D*), consistent with necrotic areas.

this regard, DW imaging may help in assessing response to tumor therapy rather than differentiating tumor entities.

DW imaging was used to evaluate a series of patients with osteosarcomas after chemotherapy, and results were compared with macroscopic and histologic examination.[41] Areas with histologically proven necrosis displayed increased values of ADC at 2.3 plus or minus 0.2 when compared with viable areas with mean ADC values of 0.8 plus or minus 0.3. In a series of patients with osteosarcoma and Ewing sarcoma, ADC values of tumors with less than 90% necrosis after treatment (poor response group) demonstrated a mean increase of 25%, compared with the responding group (tumors with at least 90% necrosis after treatment) with mean increase of ADC values of 95% (P<.003).[42]

Diffusion-weighted MR imaging has also been used to assess treatment response in metastatic disease of the vertebral bone marrow. The signal intensity changed from hyperintense relative to normal vertebral bodies before treatment to hypointense in patients with clinical improvement.[44] These studies support the strategy of using DW imaging as an early biomarker for tumor response. However, because diffusion MR imaging data can be collected and analyzed with various techniques, uniform standards for data acquisition, timing, postprocessing, and so forth are needed.[45]

DW IMAGING IN ASSESSMENT OF THE SPINE

The spinal column is a challenging anatomic region for DW imaging. Acquisition of robust DW images with sufficient spatial resolution and a reasonable scan time is challenging. Artifacts can be induced by physiologic patient motion, pulsation of the closely surrounding vasculature, and by pulsations from the cerebrospinal fluid.[46]

Baur and colleagues[18,47] have demonstrated that diffusion-weighted MR imaging provided excellent distinction between pathologic and benign vertebral fractures, and can be reliably performed using quantitative diffusion measurements.[48] Metastatic fractures tend to display hypointensity in DW imaging, whereas fractures caused by malignant processes typically display a hyperintense signal on DW imaging (Figs. 4 and 5). With increased diffusion weighting, the number of false-positive hyperintense osteoporotic fractures was reduced and the hypointensity associated with osteoporotic fractures was found to be more conspicuous.[47] Other groups have confirmed the utility of DW imaging for differentiating benign from malignant acute, vertebral body compression fractures.[19,49,50] For this application, b values of 300 mm^2 per second were recommended, taking into account both SNR and diffusion weighting of water molecules.[51] However, Maeda and colleagues[52] found considerable overlap in ADC values of

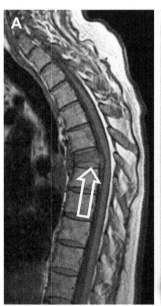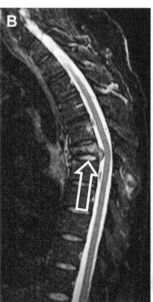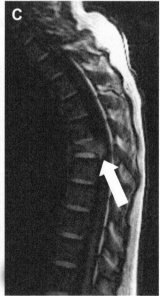

Fig. 4. A 63-year-old patient with colon carcinoma. T$_1$-weighted (A) and short TI inversion recovery (STIR) imaging (B) readily reveal a vertebral lesion in the sixth thoracic vertebral body (open arrows). (C) Hyperintense signal in SSFP DW image is consistent with malignancy (arrow). (Courtesy of A. Baur-Melnyk, MD, Munich, Germany.)

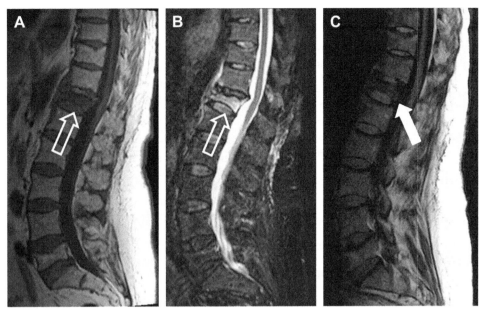

Fig. 5. A 69-year-old woman with no history of trauma or malignancy. T_1-weighted (A) and STIR imaging (B) readily reveal a fractured 12-thoracic vertebral body (*open arrows*). (C) Hypointense signal in SSFP DW image is suggestive of edema/acute osteoporotic fracture (*arrow*). (*Courtesy of* A. Baur-Melnyk, MD, Munich, Germany.)

malignant and benign fractures. They concluded that even quantitative vertebral diffusion assessment may not always permit a clear distinction between benign and malignant compression fractures. Furthermore, Raya and colleagues[31] found a higher variability of ADC values in pathologic bone marrow conditions (edema, tumor, and inflammation) than in healthy tissues [$(1.27 \pm 0.32) \times 10^{-3}$ mm^2 per second versus $(0.21 \pm 0.10) \times 10^{-3}$ mm^2 per second]. Different stages of the disease and variable composition of the affected cells may explain the discrepancy in ADC values in the studied pathologic bone marrow conditions.

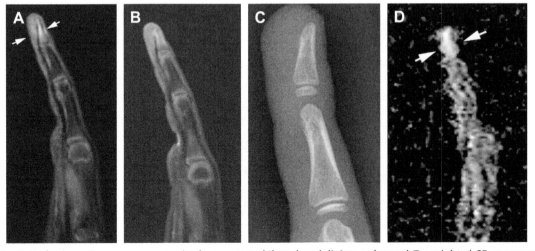

Fig. 6. Turbo-inversion recovery magnitude sequence (A) and gadolinium-enhanced T_1-weighted SE sequence (B) of the middle finger reveals increased signal intensity (*arrows in A*) and contrast enhancement within the distal phalanx. Lateral radiography is inconspicuous (C). (D) Increased ADC values (*arrows*) are indicative of osteomyelitis, as compared with reduced values in malignancies.

DIFFUSION-WEIGHTED IMAGING IN ASSESSMENT OF INTERVERTEBRAL DISCS

Several studies have evaluated the usefulness of DW imaging in the assessment of intervertebral discs.[53–57] In general, degenerated discs have lower water content and thus demonstrate decreased diffusivity and lower ADC values. DW imaging may be helpful to detect those changes in the content of the nucleus pulposus and may act as an early indicator of disk degeneration and precursor to disk herniation.[53,54,57]

DIFFUSION-WEIGHTED IMAGING IN ASSESSMENT OF INFECTION/OSTEOMYELITIS

Differentiating osteomyelitis from osseous tumor can be challenging, as osteomyelitis may display increased diffusion with low ADC values, mimicking malignancy.[18,49] The role of DW imaging in osteomyelitis has been viewed controversially.

Normal marrow is depleted and the water content and the extracellular volume fraction are increased when fibrovascular degenerative changes occur. This results in low signal intensity in diffusion-weighted MR imaging and high ADC values. In osteomyelitis, the extracellular volume is decreased because of dense infiltrate of inflammatory cells, which results in decreased ADC values and high signal intensity on DW imaging (Fig. 6).[58] The same mechanism accounts for tuberculous spondylitis, where restricted diffusivity and increased signal on DW imaging has been found.[59] In tuberculous spondylitis, overlapping ADC values with malignant fractures have also been reported.[49]

Pui and colleagues[60] examined the efficacy of DW imaging in discriminating infection from tumor in 51 consecutive patients with suspected spinal infection or malignancy. ADC values of infectious and malignant vertebral marrow lesions were significantly higher than ADCs of normal marrow. However, DW imaging had only limited utility in

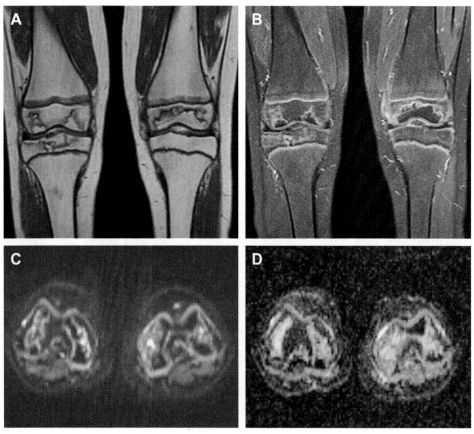

Fig. 7. An 11-year-old girl with avascular necrosis of both knees. Coronal T_1-weighted SE sequence before (A) and after (B) gadolinium-based contrast agent application readily reveal band-like signal alterations of the left tibial and bilateral femoral epiphyses. Hyperintense signal on the ADC map (C and D) represents increased ADC values that are indicative of osteonecrosis.

distinguishing infection from malignancy, with a sensitivity of 60.3% and specificity of 66% at a cutoff ADC of 1.02×10^{-3} mm^2 per second for bone marrow. Herneth and colleagues[48] found increased diffusivity in patients with aggressive osteomyelitis. This was indistinguishable from malignancy in conventional radiography and routine MR imaging.

Bozgeyik and colleagues[61] used diffusion-weighted MR imaging for detection of active inflammatory changes in the sacroiliac joints of patients with early axial spondyloarthritis. In a study of 42 patients with lower back pain, ADC values in patients with sacroiliitis were significantly higher than in patients with low back pain of mechanical origin. It was concluded that DW imaging may help to discern normal from involved subchondral bone.

Gaspersic and colleagues[62] recently reported that the use of DW imaging was effective in quantifying changes in inflammation in skeletal lesions during the treatment of ankylosing spondylitis. After 12 months of infliximab treatment, the ADC diminished from an average of 1.31 to 0.88×10^{-3} mm^2 per second. The decrease in diffusion correlated with the effectiveness of treatment according to clinical and laboratory parameters, indicating the usefulness of DW imaging for assessing treatment efficacy.

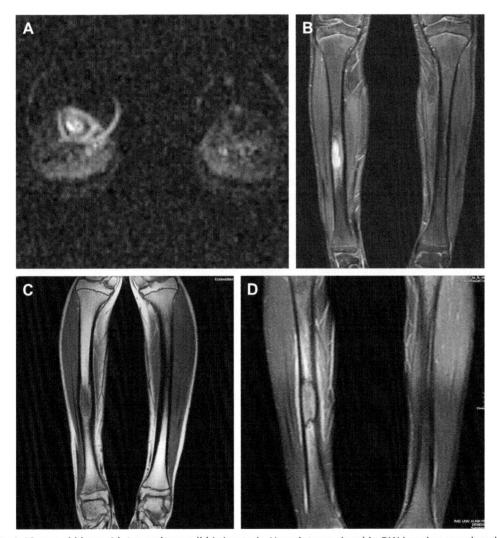

Fig. 8. A 16-year-old boy with Langerhans cell histiocytosis. Hyperintense signal in DW imaging reveals reduced perfusion because of high density of cells, no necrosis visible (A). The lesion is hyperintense on STIR imaging (B) and hypointense on T$_1$-weighted TSE sequence (C). Note the paraossal inflammatory reaction revealed on contrast-enhanced T$_1$-weighted SE imaging (D).

DIFFUSION-WEIGHTED IMAGING IN ASSESSMENT OF AVASCULAR NECROSIS

Skeletal ischemia can present as bone destruction on radiography, abnormal signal behavior of bone marrow in MR imaging, or abnormal contrast uptake in scintigraphy. Alterations in femoral head perfusion have also been investigated using gadolinium-enhanced MR imaging.[63–65] However, assessment of the clinical relevance of altered blood flow is complex. In this scenario, DW imaging may serve as a prognostic marker of skeletal ischemia before gross anatomic changes depicted by conventional means (**Figs. 7** and **8**).

Jaramillo and colleagues[53] evaluated changes in diffusion characteristics in the femur in piglets during femoral head ischemia. They found that diffusion was initially restricted with decreased blood flow as the mean ADC value decreased by 26% after 3 hours of maximal abduction. However, 3 and 96 hours after femoral neck ligation, diffusivity increased as the mean ADC values increased by 27% and 75%, respectively. These findings were confirmed in another animal study that assessed diffusion changes with ischemia of increasing duration, and also compared DW imaging with gadolinium-enhanced imaging findings. DW imaging was found to be sensitive to early ischemia. Interestingly, ADC values remained elevated despite the spontaneous partial restoration of blood flow seen on gadolinium-enhanced images.[66]

Increased ADC values were also seen in patients with avascular necrosis (AVN). Hong and colleagues[67] have used DW imaging to evaluate diffusion properties of the femoral head in patients with AVN. They reported significantly higher ADC values in femoral heads with AVN (mean 1.66×10^{-3} mm^2 per second ± 0.20) than in the normal femoral heads (mean 0.47×10^{-3} mm^2 per second ± 0.082; $P<.0001$). Of note, they did not encounter overlaps between the normal and AVN femoral heads.

DIFFUSION-WEIGHTED IMAGING IN ASSESSMENT OF TRAUMA

Bone bruises represent posttraumatic bone marrow hemorrhage and edema in the absence of cortical disruption. While T_2-weighted, fat-suppressed images are commonly used to identify bone bruises, they may not be able to evaluate the severity of bone trauma. Ward and colleagues[20] analyzed the diffusion characteristics of normal and posttraumatic bone marrow, and found that diffusivity of interstitial water increased after trauma when trabecular damage was present. They also showed that the magnitude of diffusion change correlated with the severity of marrow injury.

It seems to be of importance to define the correct inclusion criteria for using DW imaging when trying to discern benign from malignant fractures. Acute fractures may be suitable before soft callus grows and diffusivity decreases. In cases of malignancy, therapy effects may lead to increased diffusivity. Therefore, DW imaging should be performed early in treatment, before therapy-related increase of diffusivity occurs and DW imaging results become false-negative.

SUMMARY

DW imaging adds important additional information to conventional MR imaging studies of musculoskeletal diseases. It has been proven useful in the assessment of tumor response to treatment in osteosarcoma and Ewing sarcoma: two tumor entities in which response to treatment is difficult to assess with conventional MR imaging, and the presence of necrosis rather than change in size and enhancement pattern determines a positive response. In addition, DW imaging offers potential in differentiating malignant from benign vertebral body fractures, especially early in the treatment and early after trauma before regenerative changes and therapy-related effects come into play. Furthermore, DW imaging may be used in differentiating osteomyelitis from osseous tumors. However, these applications have been found controversial. DW imaging offers potential to assess presence of avascular necrosis as well as posttraumatic bone bruise. In fact, DW imaging can be used as a prognostic marker of skeletal ischemia before gross anatomic changes. Although currently not universally applied, these applications of DW imaging offer great potential to enhance the diagnostic utility of MR imaging in musculoskeletal radiology.

REFERENCES

1. Stejskal E, Tanner J. Spin diffusion measurements: spin echoes in the presence of a time-dependent field gradient. J Chem Phys 1965;42:288–92.
2. Schaefer PW, Grant PE, Gonzalez RG. Diffusion-weighted MR imaging of the brain. Radiology 2000;217:331–45.
3. Le Bihan D, Breton E, Lallemand D, et al. MR imaging of intravoxel incoherent motions: application to diffusion and perfusion in neurologic disorders. Radiology 1986;161:401–7.
4. Provenzale JM, Engelter ST, Petrella JR, et al. Use of MR exponential diffusion-weighted images to

eradicate T2 "shine-through" effect. AJR Am J Roentgenol 1999;172:537–9.

5. Raya JG, Dietrich O, Reiser MF, et al. Methods and applications of diffusion imaging of vertebral bone marrow. J Magn Reson Imaging 2006;24:1207–20.

6. Armitage PA, Schwindack C, Bastin ME, et al. Quantitative assessment of intracranial tumor response to dexamethasone using diffusion, perfusion and permeability magnetic resonance imaging. Magn Reson Imaging 2007;25:303–10.

7. Uhl M, Altehoefer C, Kontny U, et al. MRI-diffusion imaging of neuroblastomas: first results and correlation to histology. Eur Radiol 2002;12:2335–8.

8. Lansberg MG, Thijs VN, Bammer R, et al. The MRA-DWI mismatch identifies patients with stroke who are likely to benefit from reperfusion. Stroke 2008;39:2491–6.

9. Wang X, Fan YH, Lam WW, et al. Clinical features, topographic patterns on DWI and etiology of thalamic infarcts. J Neurol Sci 2008;267:147–53.

10. Bristow MS, Poulin BW, Simon JE, et al. Identifying lesion growth with MR imaging in acute ischemic stroke. J Magn Reson Imaging 2008;28:837–46.

11. Schellinger PD, Kohrmann M. MRA/DWI mismatch: a novel concept or something one could get easier and cheaper? Stroke 2008;39:2423–4.

12. Cleveland GG, Chang DC, Hazlewood CF, et al. Nuclear magnetic resonance measurement of skeletal muscle: anisotrophy of the diffusion coefficient of the intracellular water. Biophys J 1976;16:1043–53.

13. Knauss R, Schiller J, Fleischer G, et al. Self-diffusion of water in cartilage and cartilage components as studied by pulsed field gradient NMR. Magn Reson Med 1999;41:285–92.

14. Eustace S, DiMasi M, Adams J, et al. In vitro and in vivo spin echo diffusion imaging characteristics of synovial fluid: potential non-invasive differentiation of inflammatory and degenerative arthritis. Skeletal Radiol 2000;29:320–3.

15. Baur A, Huber A, Arbogast S, et al. Diffusion-weighted imaging of tumor recurrences and post-therapeutical soft-tissue changes in humans. Eur Radiol 2001;11:828–33.

16. Uhl M, Saueressig U, Koehler G, et al. Evaluation of tumour necrosis during chemotherapy with diffusion-weighted MR imaging: preliminary results in osteosarcomas. Pediatr Radiol 2006;36:1306–11.

17. Hamstra DA, Galban CJ, Meyer CR, et al. Functional diffusion map as an early imaging biomarker for high-grade glioma: correlation with conventional radiologic response and overall survival. J Clin Oncol 2008;26:3387–94.

18. Baur A, Stabler A, Bruning R, et al. Diffusion-weighted MR imaging of bone marrow: differentiation of benign versus pathologic compression fractures. Radiology 1998;207:349–56.

19. Spuentrup E, Buecker A, Adam G, et al. Diffusion-weighted MR imaging for differentiation of benign fracture edema and tumor infiltration of the vertebral body. AJR Am J Roentgenol 2001;176:351–8.

20. Ward R, Caruthers S, Yablon C, et al. Analysis of diffusion changes in posttraumatic bone marrow using navigator-corrected diffusion gradients. AJR Am J Roentgenol 2000;174:731–4.

21. Anderson AW, Gore JC. Analysis and correction of motion artifacts in diffusion weighted imaging. Magn Reson Med 1994;32:379–87.

22. Ordidge RJ, Helpern JA, Qing ZX, et al. Correction of motional artifacts in diffusion-weighted MR images using navigator echoes. Magn Reson Imaging 1994;12:455–60.

23. Dietrich O, Herlihy A, Dannels WR, et al. Diffusion-weighted imaging of the spine using radial k-space trajectories. MAGMA 2001;12:23–31.

24. Pipe JG, Farthing VG, Forbes KP. Multishot diffusion-weighted FSE using PROPELLER MRI. Magn Reson Med 2002;47:42–52.

25. Fujiwara H, Oki K, Momoshima S, et al. PROPELLER diffusion-weighted magnetic resonance imaging of acute spinal epidural hematoma. Acta Radiol 2005; 46:539–42.

26. Bammer R, Herneth AM, Maier SE, et al. Line scan diffusion imaging of the spine. AJNR Am J Neuroradiol 2003;24:5–12.

27. Oner AY, Aggunlu L, Akpek S, et al. Diffusion-weighted imaging of the appendicular skeleton with a non-Carr-Purcell-Meiboom-Gill single-shot fast spin-echo sequence. AJR Am J Roentgenol 2007;189:1494–501.

28. Oner AY, Tali T, Celikyay F, et al. Diffusion-weighted imaging of the spine with a non-Carr-Purcell-Meiboom-Gill single-shot fast spin-echo sequence: initial experience. AJNR Am J Neuroradiol 2007;28:575–80.

29. Jeong EK, Kim SE, Parker DL. High-resolution diffusion-weighted 3D MRI, using diffusion-weighted driven-equilibrium (DW-DE) and multishot segmented 3D-SSFP without navigator echoes. Magn Reson Med 2003;50:821–9.

30. Dietrich O, Raya JG, Sommer J, et al. A comparative evaluation of a RARE-based single-shot pulse sequence for diffusion-weighted MRI of musculoskeletal soft-tissue tumors. Eur Radiol 2005;15: 772–83.

31. Raya JG, Dietrich O, Birkenmaier C, et al. Feasibility of a RARE-based sequence for quantitative diffusion-weighted MRI of the spine. Eur Radiol 2007; 17:2872–9.

32. Therasse P, Arbuck SG, Eisenhauer EA, et al. New guidelines to evaluate the response to treatment in solid tumors. European Organization for Research and Treatment of Cancer, National Cancer Institute of the United States, National Cancer Institute of Canada. J Natl Cancer Inst 2000;92:205–16.

33. Smith J, Heelan RT, Huvos AG, et al. Radiographic changes in primary osteogenic sarcoma following

intensive chemotherapy. Radiological-pathological correlation in 63 patients. Radiology 1982;143: 355–60.

34. Holscher HC, Hermans J, Nooy MA, et al. Can conventional radiographs be used to monitor the effect of neoadjuvant chemotherapy in patients with osteogenic sarcoma? Skeletal Radiol 1996;25:19–24.

35. Mail JT, Cohen MD, Mirkin LD, et al. Response of osteosarcoma to preoperative intravenous high-dose methotrexate chemotherapy: CT evaluation. AJR Am J Roentgenol 1985;144:89–93.

36. Kumpan W, Lechner G, Wittich GR, et al. The angiographic response of osteosarcoma following preoperative chemotherapy. Skeletal Radiol 1986;15: 96–102.

37. Carrasco CH, Charnsangavej C, Raymond AK, et al. Osteosarcoma: angiographic assessment of response to preoperative chemotherapy. Radiology 1989;170:839–42.

38. Holscher HC, Bloem JL, van der Woude HJ, et al. Can MRI predict the histopathological response in patients with osteosarcoma after the first cycle of chemotherapy? Clin Radiol 1995;50:384–90.

39. Pan G, Raymond AK, Carrasco CH, et al. Osteosarcoma: MR imaging after preoperative chemotherapy. Radiology 1990;174:517–26.

40. Meyers PA, Gorlick R, Heller G, et al. Intensification of preoperative chemotherapy for osteogenic sarcoma: results of the Memorial Sloan-Kettering (T12) protocol. J Clin Oncol 1998;16:2452–8.

41. Uhl M, Saueressig U, van Buiren M, et al. Osteosarcoma: preliminary results of in vivo assessment of tumor necrosis after chemotherapy with diffusion- and perfusion-weighted magnetic resonance imaging. Invest Radiol 2006;41:618–23.

42. Hayashida Y, Yakushiji T, Awai K, et al. Monitoring therapeutic responses of primary bone tumors by diffusion-weighted image: initial results. Eur Radiol 2006;16:2637–43.

43. Lang P, Wendland MF, Saeed M, et al. Osteogenic sarcoma: noninvasive in vivo assessment of tumor necrosis with diffusion-weighted MR imaging. Radiology 1998;206:227–35.

44. Byun WM, Shin SO, Chang Y, et al. Diffusion-weighted MR imaging of metastatic disease of the spine: assessment of response to therapy. AJNR Am J Neuroradiol 2002;23:906–12.

45. Hamstra DA, Rehemtulla A, Ross BD. Diffusion magnetic resonance imaging: a biomarker for treatment response in oncology. J Clin Oncol 2007;25: 4104–9.

46. Holder CA. MR diffusion imaging of the cervical spine. Magn Reson Imaging Clin N Am 2000;8: 675–86.

47. Baur A, Huber A, Ertl-Wagner B, et al. Diagnostic value of increased diffusion weighting of a steady-state free precession sequence for differentiating

acute benign osteoporotic fractures from pathologic vertebral compression fractures. AJNR Am J Neuroradiol 2001;22:366–72.

48. Herneth AM, Friedrich K, Weidekamm C, et al. Diffusion weighted imaging of bone marrow pathologies. Eur J Radiol 2005;55:74–83.

49. Chan JH, Peh WC, Tsui EY, et al. Acute vertebral body compression fractures: discrimination between benign and malignant causes using apparent diffusion coefficients. Br J Radiol 2002;75:207–14.

50. Matoba M, Tonami H, Yokota H, et al. Role of diffusion-weighted MRI and ^{31}P-MRS in differentiating between malignant and benign vertebral compression fractures. Presented at the Proceedings of the 7th Annual Meeting of the ISMRM. Philadelphia, May 24-28, 1999.

51. Tang G, Liu Y, Li W, et al. Optimization of b value in diffusion-weighted MRI for the differential diagnosis of benign and malignant vertebral fractures. Skeletal Radiol 2007;36:1035–41.

52. Maeda M, Sakuma H, Maier SE, et al. Quantitative assessment of diffusion abnormalities in benign and malignant vertebral compression fractures by line scan diffusion-weighted imaging. AJR Am J Roentgenol 2003;181:1203–9.

53. Jaramillo D, Connolly SA, Vajapeyam S, et al. Normal and ischemic epiphysis of the femur: diffusion MR imaging study in piglets. Radiology 2003; 227:825–32.

54. Kurunlahti M, Kerttula L, Jauhiainen J, et al. Correlation of diffusion in lumbar intervertebral disks with occlusion of lumbar arteries: a study in adult volunteers. Radiology 2001;221:779–86.

55. Tokuda O, Okada M, Fujita T, et al. Correlation between diffusion in lumbar intervertebral disks and lumbar artery status: evaluation with fresh blood imaging technique. J Magn Reson Imaging 2007;25:185–91.

56. Kealey SM, Aho T, Delong D, et al. Assessment of apparent diffusion coefficient in normal and degenerated intervertebral lumbar disks: initial experience. Radiology 2005;235:569–74.

57. Beattie PF, Morgan PS, Peters D. Diffusion-weighted magnetic resonance imaging of normal and degenerative lumbar intervertebral discs: a new method to potentially quantify the physiologic effect of physical therapy intervention. J Orthop Sports Phys Ther 2008;38:42–9.

58. Buyn W. Diffusion-weighted MRI of vertebral bone marrow: differentiation of degenerative spines and spondylitis involving bone marrow adjacent to end plates. Presented at the Proceedings of the 9th Annual Meeting of the ISMRM. Glasgow (Scotland), April 21–27, 2001.

59. Stabler A, Doma AB, Baur A, et al. Reactive bone marrow changes in infectious spondylitis: quantitative assessment with MR imaging. Radiology 2000; 217:863–8.

60. Pui MH, Mitha A, Rae WI, et al. Diffusion-weighted magnetic resonance imaging of spinal infection and malignancy. J Neuroimaging 2005;15:164–70.
61. Bozgeyik Z, Ozgocmen S, Kocakoc E. Role of diffusion-weighted MRI in the detection of early active sacroiliitis. AJR Am J Roentgenol 2008;191:980–6.
62. Gaspersic N, Sersa I, Jevtic V, et al. Monitoring ankylosing spondylitis therapy by dynamic contrast-enhanced and diffusion-weighted magnetic resonance imaging. Skeletal Radiol 2008;37:123–31.
63. Lang P, Mauz M, Schorner W, et al. Acute fracture of the femoral neck: assessment of femoral head perfusion with gadopentetate dimeglumine-enhanced MR imaging. AJR Am J Roentgenol 1993;160:335–41.
64. Tsukamoto H, Kang YS, Jones LC, et al. Evaluation of marrow perfusion in the femoral head by dynamic magnetic resonance imaging. Effect of venous occlusion in a dog model. Invest Radiol 1992;27:275–81.
65. Cova M, Kang YS, Tsukamoto H, et al. Bone marrow perfusion evaluated with gadolinium-enhanced dynamic fast MR imaging in a dog model. Radiology 1991;179:535–9.
66. Menezes NM, Connolly SA, Shapiro F, et al. Early ischemia in growing piglet skeleton: MR diffusion and perfusion imaging. Radiology 2007;242:129–36.
67. Hong N, Du X, Nie Z, et al. Diffusion-weighted MR study of femoral head avascular necrosis in severe acute respiratory syndrome patients. J Magn Reson Imaging 2005;22:661–4.

Fundamentals of Quantitative Dynamic Contrast-Enhanced MR Imaging

Michael J. Paldino, MD*, Daniel P. Barboriak, MD

KEYWORDS

- Dynamic contrast-enhanced MR imaging
- Perfusion • Physics • Oncology

The development of small molecular weight paramagnetic contrast agents for MR imaging has had a major impact on the practice of oncology. These agents pass from the intravascular space into the extracellular extravascular space, thereby improving both detection and characterization of malignant tumors by MR imaging. Many factors contribute to the uptake of gadolinium-based contrast agents in tumor tissue, including blood flow, microvascular density, vessel permeability, and the fractional volume of the extracellular extravascular space. Estimation of the relative contribution of each of these factors with MR imaging has, until recently, been beyond the technical capabilities of the technique. With the advent of faster imaging techniques in MR, temporal resolution has now become sufficient to characterize the dynamic patterns of gadolinium uptake in tumors over time. Using pharmacokinetic modeling, this dynamic enhancement data can be used to provide quantitative information regarding specific functional and anatomic characteristics of tumor vasculature. For this reason, these techniques have the capacity to improve both the detection and characterization of malignant diseases. The purpose of this article is to review the pathophysiologic basis and technical aspects of dynamic contrast-enhanced MR imaging (DCE-MR imaging) techniques.

PATHOPHYSIOLOGIC BASIS FOR ENHANCEMENT

Neoplasms are not capable of generating blood vessels on their own.[1] As a result, early malignant lesions are avascular and rely on diffusion to provide substrates for metabolism and for the elimination of waste. Although tumorigenesis is a diverse process involving a wide range of cell types and genetic alterations, all tumors eventually require a blood supply to grow to a size greater than a few millimeters.[2] Furthermore, it is believed that induction of tumor vasculature is a rate-limiting step in tumor progression.[3] Development of tumor vasculature depends on formation of blood vessels by the host, a process known as angiogenesis. This process is directed by the mitogenic effects of a diverse group of local mediators elaborated by neoplastic cells, the most studied of which is vascular endothelial growth factor (VEGF). VEGF is produced by tumor cells and acts by way of specific receptors to stimulate endothelial migration and proliferation. Although the exact process by which malignant cells become angiogenically competent is yet to be determined, it is clear that expression of these mediators can be modulated by oncogenes, transcription factors such as p53, and hypoxia.[4,5]

Although the process of angiogenesis may result in tumors with higher vascularity than that of normal tissues, the resultant neovasculature is both structurally and functionally abnormal.[6] Tumor microcirculatory architecture consists of tortuous, irregular vessels with excessive branching and extensive arteriovenous shunting.[7] Furthermore, tumor neovasculature is spatially heterogeneous and, in many regions, inadequate, contributing to a microenvironment characterized

Division of Neuroradiology, Department of Radiology, Duke University Medical Center, Box 3808, Erwin Road, Durham, NC 27710, USA
* Corresponding author.
E-mail address: paldi001@mc.duke.edu (M.J. Paldino).

Magn Reson Imaging Clin N Am 17 (2009) 277–289
doi:10.1016/j.mric.2009.01.007
1064-9689/09/$ – see front matter © 2009 Elsevier Inc. All rights reserved.

by hypoxia and acidosis.[8] Tumor vessels are further characterized by the absence of muscularis propria, widened interendothelial junctions, and a widely discontinuous or absent basement membrane, all of which contribute to increased permeability.[7] Vesiculo-vascular organelles (VVOs), an intracellular network of vesicles and vacuoles that span the vascular endothelium, provide an additional mechanism of transendothelial transport and may be an important pathway for the gadolinium-chelate contrast agent leakage.[9,10] The number and permeability of these VVOs are regulated by several local mediators, most notably VEGF.[11]

Human tumors display diverse combinations of these abnormalities along a spectrum that seems to depend on the degree to which structural maturation can keep pace with vascular proliferation.[3] Therefore, highly differentiated tumors may have nearly normal vascular architecture, while highly anaplastic tumors tend to demonstrate extremely disorganized and heterogeneous networks of vascular spaces without recognizable mature elements.[12]

DCE-MR imaging is a noninvasive imaging technique that can be used to derive quantitative parameters that reflect microcirculatory structure and function in imaged tissues. Since abnormalities in these parameters, including blood volume and vascular permeability, are inherent to tumor neovasculature, such information is of great potential value to the practice of oncology. In addition, agents which inhibit tumor angiogenesis, for example the anti-VEGF antibody bevacizumab, have become important weapons in the anticancer armamentarium.[13] Noninvasive techniques that can provide information about angiogenesis and serve as early biomarkers of drug activity in drug trials are, therefore, in great demand.[14] For these reasons, DCE-MR imaging has been investigated for a wide range of oncologic applications, including cancer detection, staging or prognosis, and for assessment of treatment response.

FUNDAMENTALS OF DYNAMIC-CONTRAST MR IMAGING

After intravenous administration of a contrast agent, it travels through the vascular system reaching the neoplastic tissues and will start to leak from the tumor vasculature, accumulating in the extracellular extravascular space (EES) by passive diffusion. As the plasma concentration falls because of renal excretion, backflow of contrast agent from the EES to plasma will continue until the contrast agent has been eliminated.[11]

There are two main approaches for the acquisition of dynamic MR imaging data. Relaxivity-based methods such as DCE-MR imaging use T_1-weighted acquisitions, while susceptibility-based techniques such as dynamic susceptibility contrast-enhanced MR imaging (DSC-MR imaging) use T2*-based sequences. Both methods have advantages and disadvantages and historically they have tended to be used in different applications. DCE-MR imaging is the focus of this article.

DCE-MR imaging uses T_1-weighted images to detect the relaxivity effects of contrast agents during dynamic data collection. In solutions of gadolinium contrast agents, the increase in the rate of T_1 relaxation is proportional to the concentration of the contrast agent. It is therefore possible to relate signal enhancement in T_1-weighted images to the tissue contrast agent concentration.[15] A time-concentration function can then be generated which describes the concentration of gadolinium within tumor tissue over time.

For most analysis techniques, it is important to include a large blood vessel in the field of view. This practice allows the measurement of the contrast agent concentration in plasma over time, commonly referred to as the vascular input function (VIF). The VIF can be used to estimate the contrast agent concentration changes occurring within the tumor vasculature and, therefore, to allow estimation of the contrast agent concentration gradient between blood and the tumor EES. It is the combined information from time-concentration curves of both tumor and the VIF that allows for mathematical modeling of contrast agent distribution (**Fig. 1**).

DYNAMIC CONTRAST-ENHANCED MR IMAGING ACQUISITION

DCE-MR imaging data is generally acquired in three basic steps. First, images are obtained which provide anatomic information including localization of tumor. Next, sequences are performed that allow for calculation of baseline T_1 values. Finally, dynamic data are acquired, typically every few seconds for a total duration of 5 to 10 minutes.

Baseline T_1 Mapping

Pharmacokinetic modeling of tissue contrast agent distribution requires accurate measurement of the concentration of gadolinium at each time point during the imaging procedure. The first step is to use the signal changes observed in the dynamic MR acquisition to calculate contrast agent concentration at each time point. In order

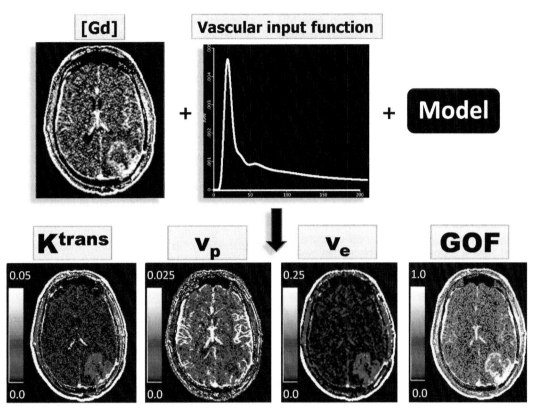

Fig.1. DCE-MR imaging analysis performed in a patient with a left parietal-occipital glioblastoma multiforme. The results of T1 mapping techniques and dynamic MR images are used to create a set of images estimating gadolinium concentration for each location and time point (a single image, marked [Gd], is shown in the top row, left). This image set is combined with an estimate of the gadolinium contrast agent concentration-time function in the plasma space, or vascular input function (VIF, top row, middle), and a pharmacokinetic model to produce a series of parameter maps (bottom row). In this example analysis, parametric K^{trans} (transfer constant.), v_p (fractional plasma volume), and v_e (fractional volume of the extracellular extravascular space) maps are derived. Goodness of fit images (GOF; bottom row, right) are also calculated to demonstrate how well the model predicted the contrast agent concentration-time curve at each image location.

to simplify this process, it is sometimes assumed that the change in T_1 is directly proportional to the tissue contrast agent concentration.[16] Unfortunately, the relationship between contrast agent concentration and signal intensity is not always linear and will be affected by the underlying native T_1 of the tissues.[17]

Although there is some disagreement on this issue,[18] expert groups have recommended baseline mapping of T_1 and equilibrium magnetization as a preliminary step in DCE-MR imaging analysis to correct for the nonlinear relationship between signal intensity on dynamically acquired DCE-MR imaging images and underlying gadolinium-based contrast agent concentration.[17,19,20] Several techniques have been used to acquire imaging data for T_1 mapping[19] including: variable nutation angle technique,[21,22] inversion-recovery technique,[23,24] and Look-Locker technique.[25,26] The variable nutation angle technique is probably the most widely used in clinical DCE-MR imaging because T_1 can be estimated with reasonable accuracy in a relatively short acquisition time.[27]

Dynamic Acquisition

DCE-MR imaging is most commonly acquired using gradient echo (GRE) sequences. Standard gradient echo sequences have high T2 sensitivity. This behavior is not optimal since T2-mediated signal decreases secondary to tissue gadolinium will oppose the desired T_1-mediated increase in signal.[28] Many dynamic studies have therefore used spoiled gradient echo sequences that are more specifically sensitive to T_1 effects. The lower signal-to-noise ratio of these techniques can be compensated to some extent by the use of three-dimensional acquisitions.[29]

There is significant interest in using new MR imaging techniques to more rapidly acquire images for DCE-MR imaging. Rapid imaging allows the vascular input function obtained from image data after bolus contrast agent injection to be more accurately sampled. In addition, more sophisticated pharmacokinetic models can be used if the vascular input function and tissue contrast agent concentrations are measured using higher temporal resolution.

Parallel imaging is one method by which temporal resolution in DCE-MR imaging can potentially be improved. This technique uses multiple receiver coils to simultaneously receive separate spatial components of the MR signal.[30] Although variation in signal-to-noise across the field of view is a potential drawback, this method can increase temporal resolution by several-fold, making this technique very attractive for DCE-MR imaging.[31]

Three-dimensional time-resolved imaging of contrast kinetics and time-resolved angiography with stochastic trajectories are K-space subsampling techniques that (in contrast to older rapid imaging techniques such as keyhole imaging) sample both the center and periphery of K-space during the dynamic image acquisition, allowing for high spatial resolution. Temporal acceleration is achieved by sampling the periphery of K-space less frequently than the center. These promising techniques have been used to characterize dynamic enhancement patterns in human tumors,[32–34] and are likely to be further evaluated in future studies. Highly constrained back-projection reconstruction methods have great potential to further improve temporal resolution in undersampled MR sequences.[35,36] These methods exploit the spatial and temporal redundancy involving any serial change in an imaging variable, including time. The result is significantly reduced streak artifacts and increased signal-to-noise ratios, permitting decreased numbers of projections to be used when acquiring each image in the image time series. Preliminary data suggest such methods may improve the accuracy of parameters derived from DCE-MR imaging.[37]

As seen from the discussion above, the specific sequence chosen will usually represent a compromise between multiple imaging quality factors. Furthermore, the optimal balance between these factors will depend on the characteristics of the specific organ system being imaged.

ANALYSIS OF DYNAMIC DATA

A large range of techniques has been applied to the analysis of the signal-enhancement curves observed in DCE-MR imaging. These range from simple visual inspection to complex quantification using pharmacokinetic models. Although the former methods will be briefly addressed, methods of contrast agent curve analysis that provide quantitative information are the focus of this article.

Visual Inspection and Semiquantitative Analysis

One commonly used analysis of dynamic enhancement patterns is subjective evaluation of the time-signal intensity curve. In such methods, the generated curve is classified in accordance with a grading system. This approach has used successfully in differentiating malignant from benign breast lesions.[38]

Semiquantitative parameters characterize tissue enhancement using a number of different measures derived from time-signal intensity curves, often using normalization of postcontrast signal intensities to surrounding normal tissue or to the precontrast signal intensity of the lesion in question.[39] These parameters include onset time (time from injection to the first increase in tissue signal enhancement), initial and mean gradient of the upsweep of enhancement curves, maximum signal intensity, and washout gradient.[6]

Although semiquantitative parameters have the advantage of being relatively straightforward to calculate they have a number of limitations. First, they do not accurately reflect contrast medium concentration in the tissue of interest and can therefore be influenced by scanner settings. As a result, these methods may show considerable variation between acquisition method and individual examinations, making direct comparison between studies difficult.[14] Furthermore, it is unclear what these parameters reflect physiologically and how robust they are to variations in patient factors (for example, cardiac output) that may not be directly related to tumor physiology.[20] Despite their limitations, these subjective or semiquantitative curve analyses can be extremely valuable, particularly in their application to tumor characterization.[40,41] This may reflect the fact that differences in tumor vasculature between benign and malignant tumors are substantial and, therefore, are evident despite relatively crude analysis techniques.[17]

Quantitative Analysis

Quantitative parameters are more complicated to derive than those derived semiquantitatively. Nevertheless, quantitative approaches may be beneficial for several reasons. First, the ability to produce measurements that reflect the physio-logic and anatomic structure of the tumor micro-vasculature is of great potential value for improving the characterization of tumors before treatment (see above) and for detecting the effects of novel therapies on tumor vascular function. Second, quantitative approaches offer the poten-tial for development of more precise and repro-ducible measures, independent of scanner acquisition and tissue type.[42] Such measures might then be used to guide treatment in individual patients or as surrogate markers of therapeutic efficacy in multicenter drug trials.

The simplest method for quantifying the kinetics of contrast agent accumulation is an integration of the concentration of contrast agent observed in the tissue of interest over time, the initial area under curve (IAUC).[42] The IAUC is easy to calcu-late and has been shown to be relatively reproduc-ible.[14] Furthermore, when normalized to surrounding normal tissue, IAUC has been demon-strated to parallel parameters of vessel perme-ability obtained using more complex mathematical modeling.[17] One disadvantage of using IAUC is that the parameter represents a conglomerate of physiologic processes, including blood flow, blood volume, endothelial permeability, and the volume of the EES.[20] As a result, modeled parameters have the capacity to provide more physiologically meaningful information.[14]

Pharmacokinetic modeling

A wide range of pharmacokinetic models have been applied to the analysis of DCE-MR imaging data, most of which use curve-fitting methods to estimate the parameters of the pharmacokinetic models being studied. These iterative approaches alter the modeled parameters until the combina-tion that best describes the observed relationship between the VIF curve and the tumor voxel curve is found.

All tissues, including neoplastic ones, can be described as being comprised of three compart-ments: the vascular plasma space, the EES, and the intracellular space. All clinically used MR imaging contrast agents do not pass into the intra-cellular space.[43] Hence, for the purposes of most DCE-MR imaging modeling, the anatomic param-eters that influence contrast agent distribution are assumed to be limited to the vascular plasma space and the EES (Fig. 2). Relevant functional parameters include blood flow, the endothelial permeability, and vascular surface area.

In theory, an optimal analysis would allow inde-pendent assessment of each anatomic and func-tional variable. Unfortunately, even with rapid MR

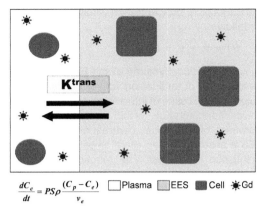

$$\frac{dC_e}{dt} = PS\rho \frac{(C_p - C_e)}{v_e}$$ ☐ Plasma ▨ EES ■ Cell ☀ Gd

Fig. 2. Two compartment model of contrast agent distribution. Gadolinium-based contrast agents (Gd) distribute across the endothelium within the plasma space and EES, but do not enter intact cells. The rate of change of contrast agent concentration in the EES is related to the difference in concentrations across the endothelium ($C_p - C_e$), the fractional volume of the EES (v_e), capillary permeability (P), capillary surface area (S) and the tissue density (ρ). K^{trans} (the volumetric transfer coefficient between the plasma space and the EES) is defined, under condi-tions of adequate contrast-agent supply, as $PS \rho$. C_p and C_e represent the concentration of contrast agent in the plasma space and EES, respectively.

imaging, temporal resolution may not be adequate to extract every parameter accurately. In practice, a range of simplified pharmacokinetic models that combine the effects of several parameters into one have been used to analyze DCE-MR imaging data. The volumetric transfer constant between blood plasma and EES (K^{trans}) is the parameter of interest in most studies.[43]

Kinetic modeling of contrast agent distribution is based on diffusion of solute across a semiperme-able membrane. Flux of solute is determined by the difference in concentration of that substance between the two compartments and the freedom with which the membrane allows molecules of that substance to diffuse. In normal tissues, the vascular volume is a small fraction of the total tissue volume, typically less than 5%.[44] Therefore, it has been assumed by some kinetic models that contrast agent concentration in the tissue as a whole is not influenced significantly by the intra-vascular contrast agent.[45] An example of such a simplified model is presented first.

Models that ignore the contribution of intravascular contrast agent With respect to the distribution of gadolinium, the total amount of contrast agent in the EES (ET) can be expressed as a product of the gadolinium concentration within the EES (C_e), as follows:

$$ET = v_e \times V_t \times C \qquad (1)$$

v_e is the fractional volume of the EES (expressed as a fraction of total lesion volume), V_t is the total volume of the tissue of interest, and C_e is the gadolinium concentration within the EES. For the purposes of this model, contrast agent within the EES is assumed to represent all gadolinium within the tissue of interest. The function of contrast agent concentration over time can be described by the following formula:

$$\frac{dC_t(t)}{dt} = v_e \frac{dC_e(t)}{dt} = PS\rho[C_p(t) - C_e(t)] \qquad (2)$$

where v_e is the fractional volume of the EES (expressed as a fraction of total lesion volume), C_t is the gadolinium concentration within the tissue, C_e is the gadolinium concentration within the EES, C_p is the concentration of tracer in plasma, P is the permeability coefficient, S is the endothelial surface area and ρ is the tissue density. This equation can be rewritten:

$$\frac{dC_t(t)}{dt} = K^{trans}\left(C_p(t) - \left(\frac{C_t(t)}{v_e}\right)\right) \qquad (3)$$

where the transfer coefficient, K^{trans}, is defined by the equation:

$$K^{trans} = PS\rho \qquad (4)$$

This relationship only holds when rate of inflow of contrast agent by way of perfusion is high compared with the rate of contrast agent flux across the capillary endothelium. When inflow of contrast agents by way of perfusion is insufficient to replenish the gadolinium that has diffused into the EES, flux of contrast agent across the endothelium is flow limited and K^{trans} is equal to the blood plasma flow per unit volume of tissue:

$$K^{trans} = F\rho(1 - Hct) \qquad (5)$$

where F equals total blood flow (ie, perfusion), Hct is the hematocrit, and ρ is the tissue density.

Models such as this one provide estimates only of v_e and of K^{trans}. In turn, the value of K^{trans} at any location will reflect local blood flow, endothelial permeability, endothelial surface area, and the proportional blood volume within a given voxel; the individual effects of each component cannot be distinguished. Despite its physiologic nonspecificity, this parameter is relatively reproducible and has been widely used in clinical studies.[43]

Models that incorporate intravascular contrast agent The contribution of intravascular contrast agent to the MR imaging signal remains a significant challenge for current modeling strategies. Neglecting it may be reasonable in some instances, for example in the case of a freely diffusible tracer, when the volume of distribution is large compared with the blood volume.[46] However, this approximation is less appropriate for gadolinium-based contrast agents, which remain solely within the extracellular space and therefore have a smaller volume of distribution. Such inaccuracy can be exaggerated under pathologic circumstances, especially in the case of malignant tumors that have substantially increased blood volume.[8] The situation is further complicated by the fact that intravascular tracer is likely to be in slow or intermediate exchange with tissue water, making it partially invisible to the tissue water by MR imaging.[47] This reduces its influence on the T_1 of tissue water to an extent that depends on the particular T_1-weighted sequence that is used.[47] To date, the degree to which intravascular gadolinium affects contrast enhancement remains controversial.

By estimating an additional parameter, the fractional volume of the plasma space, models that account for the effects of intravascular gadolinium estimate a more physiologically specific K^{trans}. In the simplest of these models, the total tissue contrast agent (C_t) is considered to be the sum of both the intravascular and extracellular extravascular compartments according to the following equation:

$$C_t = v_p C_p + v_e C_e \qquad (6)$$

v_e and C_e represent the fractional volume and gadolinium concentration within the EES. v_p and C_p represent the fractional volume and gadolinium concentration within the plasma. Substituting this new concentration term into the previous equation results in a new expression for tissue concentration:

$$\frac{dC_t(t)}{dt} = v_p * \frac{dC_p(t)}{dt} + K^{trans}\left(C_p(t) - \left(\frac{C_t(t) - v_p * C_p(t)}{v_e}\right)\right) \qquad (7)$$

This equation is solved by the integral equation:

$$C_t(t) = v_p C_p + K^{trans}\int_0^t C_p(t')\exp\left[-K^{trans}\frac{t-t'}{v_e}\right]dt' \qquad (8)$$

Models such as this one are capable of estimating the fractional volume of the plasma compartment (v_p), v_e, and K^{trans}. In this case, K^{trans}

will be affected by flow, capillary surface area, and endothelial permeability and less affected by changes in plasma volume. It is important to note, however, that estimates of K^{trans} by models that estimate v_p are not truly independent of plasma volume. This is because capillary surface area remains to some extent dependent on v_p. The precise relationship of surface area to v_p depends on the size distribution of the underlying vessels.

For certain applications, it may be desirable to separate the effects of flow on K^{trans} from those of capillary endothelial permeability and surface area.[43,48] For example, it may be of interest in studying the mechanism of action of antiangiogenic drugs to determine whether the drugs affect tumor tissue perfusion independently of effects on capillary endothelium. Recent work by St. Lawrence and Lee[49] has attempted to extend the pharmacokinetic models presented above to account for blood flow. This model also divides tissue into plasma and extracellular extravascular compartments, but defines the intravascular tracer concentration as a function of both time and distance along the length of the capillary. As a result, this model can provide information regarding blood flow and allows the permeability-surface area product to be estimated independently. It must be considered that complex models such as this one place more stringent constraints on image acquisition as the vascular input function must be measured with temporal resolution in the range of 1 second to detect tracer entering and passing through the capillary bed.[17] Despite such constraints, Buckley and colleagues[50] have demonstrated not only the feasibility of such a modeling technique but also the potential value of blood flow measurements to distinguish tumor from peripheral zone in patients with prostate cancer.

It must be remembered that the pharmacokinetic models discussed above provide only an approximation of complex pathophysiologic features of the underlying tumor microvasculature. As a corollary to this statement, simpler models are associated with greater degrees of approximation. Over-simplification may result in systematic errors in the physiologic parameters being assessed and a degradation of the correlation between the true parameter and its modeling analog.[48] This results from distortion of the fitted parameters to compensate for effects that are caused by an omitted factor. Such inaccuracies have been shown to result in artifactually high values of K^{trans} by models that ignore the contribution of blood pool contrast to tissue enhancement.[42] More complex models may, in addition, be able to reduce bias in parameter estimates of v_e and v_p.[51] However, the loss of accuracy caused by the use of simpler models may be accompanied by an increase in precision as fitting processes become more stable.[48] Thus, the model chosen for a particular analysis often represents a compromise between parameters that are more physiologically meaningful and those that are reproducible.

As a final note, although quantification of contrast agent kinetics in absolute terms offers the potential for interstudy comparability, in practice this is rarely the case. For example, it should now be clear that the physiologic meaning of K^{trans}, commonly considered synonymous with endothelial permeability, depends greatly on the pharmacokinetic model being applied. Hence, transfer coefficients derived by two different models are rarely directly comparable. In addition, a wide range of technical limitations in image acquisition make direct comparison of published K^{trans} parameters difficult. These technical factors include temporal resolution, T_1 contrast dynamic range, and spatial resolution.[48,52] The last factor can lead to differences in partial volume averaging, potentially a significant issue in spatially heterogeneous tumors. Therefore, even results derived with the same model may not be comparable if they were obtained using disparate image acquisition techniques.

ADDITIONAL TECHNICAL ISSUES
Vascular Input Function

Although most models used in DCE-MR imaging have been shown to be theoretically compatible, many disparate assumptions have been used in their application.[42,44] Often such differences reflect limitations imposed by data acquisition on modeling assumptions.[43] Perhaps the most significant constraint on model assumptions is the ability to measure the VIF noninvasively for each patient.[15] Though now more practical than ever before owing to improvements in MR sequences and hardware, accurate measurement of the VIF remains a great technical challenge. For this reason, some models make an assumption of a specific input function for all individuals. For example, the model proposed by Tofts and Kermode[45] derived a theoretical VIF using biexponential decay drawn from literature regarding elimination of gadolinium in the normal population. While such assumptions may allow analyses to proceed in the absence of the technical resources required for more sophisticated acquisition, modeling under these conditions is likely to produce less accurate and less reproducible kinetic parameters.[14,53] This is because the VIF is related to multiple dynamic physiologic factors including cardiac output, vascular tone, and renal function and, therefore, varies between patients and over time.[14] Since many chemotherapeutic regimens potentially alter cardiac output and renal function, an assumed VIF would be a particular limitation in studies of treatment response as apparent changes in fitted parameters could be wholly or in part due to undetected alterations in the VIF. In addition, it has been demonstrated in studies of CT arteriography, contrast-enhanced CT, and contrast-enhanced MR arteriography that left arm injections lead to reflux of contrast agent into venous structures.[54–56] It stands to reason that inconsistencies in the arm that is injected could therefore lead to variability in the shape of the VIF, further exaggerating the potential inaccuracy of an assumed input function.

For these reasons, direct measurement of the VIF in each patient during each study is highly desirable. It should be realized, however, that a nearby large artery might not provide all or even the majority of blood to the tissue of interest. Furthermore, even if the VIF can be accurately measured in the sole large artery responsible for tumor perfusion, such an input still might not accurately reflect the time-concentration curve that would be observed in the microcirculation providing direct supply to the tumor of interest because of the effects of flow delay and dispersion.[57] These phenomena may introduce significant inaccuracies into parameter estimation by dynamic contrast-enhanced methods.[58]

Measurement of the VIF requires that the image acquisition method has adequate spatial resolution and volume coverage to identify a suitably large vascular structure. In some organ systems, it may be difficult, or even impossible, to include both the tissue of interest and a satisfactory blood vessel. Temporal resolution of the dynamic acquisition is an additional technical constraint in the measurement of the VIF and must be sufficient to sample the shape of the initial bolus passage.[17] Significant inaccuracies in the measurement of the VIF may still occur in the setting of high temporal resolution, however, highlighting the importance of stringent acquisition.[15] Finally, the selected MR sequence must be capable of accurately measuring the signal intensities associated with a very broad range of contrast agent concentration, including the peak concentrations present in vascular structures. Despite these technical constraints, direct measurement of the VIF is not only feasible but has been shown to be relatively reproducible given a suitable image acquisition protocol.[59,60]

In order to address the challenges presented when direct imaging of appropriate vascular structures is impractical, methods that provide indirect measurements of VIFs for each patient have been developed. For example, Brix and colleagues[16] included the VIF as a free-fitted parameter in their pharmacokinetic model. Reference tissue- or region-based approaches, which provide vascular input based on measured data from multiple regions within the tissues of interest, provide an additional alternative to direct measurement.[61] These methods, however, have their own limitations, including the potential for large errors in parameter estimates when using complicated pharmacokinetic models.[61] At this time, although most experts would agree that it would be advantageous to directly measure the VIF during every DCE-MR imaging examination, the best methods to use for this purpose remain to be determined.

Data Presentation

Many analysis techniques are based on measurements taken from user-defined regions of interest. This technique has the advantage of simplicity but is incapable of identifying or quantifying significant heterogeneity within the tumor microvasculature that may occur within the region of interest. Furthermore, since functional parameters estimated by DCE-MR imaging may vary in different proportions in different areas of tumor, calculating parameters to fit the observed dynamic enhancement averaged over the entire tumor may therefore be erroneous.[41] These limitations are of particular relevance to the evaluation of malignant lesions, which are likely to be spatially heterogeneous.[12]

These shortcomings can be addressed by the production of parametric images that allow pixel-by-pixel analysis of the calculated microvascular parameters. This method depicts kinetic enhancement information as maps coregistered with anatomic images on a pixel-by-pixel basis. Such displays have been successfully used to demonstrate spatially heterogeneous distributions of kinetic parameters in tumors.[62–64]

Unfortunately, the use of parametric images imposes further demands on data acquisition and analysis. First, since a typical voxel size is on the order of 1 milllimeter in size, even small degrees of motion can have a significant impact on the calculated parameters.[43] Pixel mapping is therefore especially challenging in areas with significant physiologic motion, including the chest and abdomen.[42] Second, although visual appreciation of heterogeneity is improved by pixel mapping displays, quantification of this heterogeneity presents an additional challenge.[39] Summary statistics, histogram analysis, and pixel scatter plots have all been used to quantify the heterogeneous distribution of parameters derived from DCE-MR imaging.[48,64–67] Although these quantification techniques are promising, they have yet to be validated in a clinical setting, and none are widely accepted. Additional disadvantages of pixel mapping techniques include poor signal-to-noise and further requirements for specialized software.[48]

Changes in physiologic parameters that occur after treatment also tend to be spatially heterogeneous. Image registration can be extremely valuable, not only by permitting visual appreciation of interval changes, but also by allowing assessment of interval change on a pixel-by-pixel basis (Fig. 3). Such an analysis has been shown to provide prognostic information in patients with high-grade primary brain tumors evaluated by diffusion-weighted imaging.[68]

Contrast Agent Administration

A major source of variability in the DCE-MR imaging literature relates to the method of contrast agent administration. The dose and method of administration of contrast agent is of considerable importance and may affect modeling procedures and clinical results.[6] Typically a single dose (0.1 mmol/kg) of a standard gadolinium chelate will be administered at a rate of up to 4 mL/s.[43] The optimal contrast agent dose for a given application, however, remains controversial. For example, it has been suggested that the accuracy of breast MR imaging is improved increasing the dose to 0.16 mmol/kg of body weight.[69]

Contrast agent administration is performed through a peripheral vein, most commonly using a bolus injection, and it is important that this be administered in a consistent manner.[45] Although some studies have administered contrast agents as an infusion, most often a power injector is used to more reproducibly administer the bolus injection.[16] Recent work suggests that the optimal injection rate depends on the particular pathology and method of acquisition. While short injection times are appropriate when using fast-imaging techniques, especially when evaluating lesions with high permeability, slower infusion methods may be superior when the temporal resolution of the study is longer.[6]

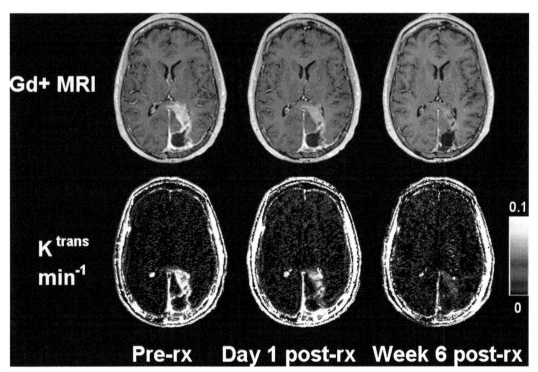

Fig. 3. Serial DCE-MR imaging performed in a patient with a left parietal-occipital glioblastoma multiforme. Co-registered, contrast enhanced T_1-weighted images (top row) and parametric K^{trans} maps (bottom row) performed before treatment (Pre-rx) as well as 1 day (Day 1 post-rx) and 6 weeks (Week 6 post-rx) after initiation of a chemotherapeutic protocol. Appreciation of changes in both enhancement and K^{trans} occurring after therapy is substantially enhanced by image registration.

Finally, the choice of contrast agent injected for DCE-MR imaging may have important effects on the results of the analysis. Although the pharmacokinetics of most low molecular weight contrast media (LMCM) such as gadolinium diethylene triamine penta acetic acid (Magnevist), gadoteridol (Prohance), and gadobutrol (Gadovist) are thought to be comparable, gadobenate dimeglumine (Multihance) shows increased protein binding compared with the other agents. Because increased protein binding leads to increases in relaxivity and presumably alterations of pharmacokinetics of this agent, DCE-MR imaging parameters obtained when using gadobenate dimeglumine may not be comparable to those of other agents.[27,70]

In the future, macromolecular agents, which have plasma half lives on the order of several hours owing to their large molecular weights, may become available for clinical use.[71–73] Because these agents do not pass through normal endothelial surfaces, DCE-MR imaging using macromolecular contrast media (MMCM) may more accurately depict the hyperpermeability of tumor vasculature than the same technique using LMCMs, which leak rapidly through the capillary endothelium of both normal (noncerebral) and neoplastic tissues.

A number of MMCMs have been investigated, many of which are Gd-based. Albumin-gadolinium diethylene triamine penta acetic acid, the prototype MMCM, has been shown to correlate with microvessel density[74] and may provide superior tumor characterization compared with LMCMs in some settings.[75] Prolonged retention of this agent and a theoretical risk of toxicity have prompted the development of additional Gd-chelates which bind reversibly to albumin, allowing for more rapid clearance.[73] Although results have varied,[76] preliminary data suggest potential utility for such agents in DCE-MR imaging.[77]

Iron oxide agents are paramagnetic compounds and therefore provide tissue contrast by shortening T2 relaxation time. In particular, ultrasmall superparamagnetic iron oxide (USPIO) particles are small enough to avoid rapid sequestration by the reticuloendothelial system, allowing their use as blood pool agents. There is some evidence to suggest that the pathologic grade of tumors can be characterized using permeability estimates derived from dynamic MR imaging performed with USPIOs.[78]

In addition to the advantages listed above, blood pool contrast agents have the potential to significantly reduce constraints on the temporal resolution required for dynamic acquisition. If these theoretical advantages can be validated, such agents could play a crucial role in the future of DCE-MR imaging.

SUMMARY

Quantitative analysis of DCE-MR imaging has the power to provide information regarding physiologic characteristics of the microvasculature and is therefore of great potential value to the practice of oncology. In particular, these techniques could have significant impact on the development of novel anticancer therapies as a promising biomarker of drug activity. DCE-MR imaging also has the capacity to guide patient management by improving tumor characterization. In fact, noninvasive characterization of tumor vascularity may improve on traditional pathologic methods of tumor grading with regard to patient prognosis.[79] Perhaps the greatest obstacle to realization of this potential will be standardization of DCE-MR imaging acquisition and analysis to provide more reproducible measures of tumor vessel physiology.

REFERENCES

1. Folkman J. The role of angiogenesis in tumor growth. Semin Cancer Biol 1992;3:65–71.
2. Knopp MV, Giesel FL, Marcos H, et al. Dynamic contrast-enhanced magnetic resonance imaging in oncology. Top Magn Reson Imaging 2001;12:301–8.
3. Dadiani M, Furman-Haran E, Degani H. The application of NMR in tumor angiogenesis research. Progress in Nuclear Magnetic Resonance Spectroscopy 2006;49:27–44.
4. Jubb AM, Oates AJ, Holden S, et al. Predicting benefit from anti-angiogenic agents in malignancy. Nat Rev Cancer 2006;6:626–35.
5. Mukhopadhyay D, Tsiokas L, Zhou XM, et al. Hypoxic induction of human vascular endothelial growth factor expression through c-Src activation. Nature 1995;375:577–81.
6. Padhani AR. Dynamic contrast-enhanced MRI in clinical oncology: current status and future directions. J Magn Reson Imaging 2002;16:407–22.
7. Carmeliet P, Jain RK. Angiogenesis in cancer and other diseases. Nature 2000;407:249–57.
8. Gaustad JV, Brurberg KG, Simonsen TG, et al. Tumor vascularity assessed by magnetic resonance imaging and intravital microscopy imaging. Neoplasia 2008;10:354–62.
9. Delorme S, Knopp MV. Non-invasive vascular imaging: assessing tumour vascularity. Eur Radiol 1998;8:517–27.
10. Dvorak AM, Kohn S, Morgan ES, et al. The vesiculovacuolar organelle (VVO): a distinct endothelial cell structure that provides a transcellular pathway for

macromolecular extravasation. J Leukoc Biol 1996; 59:100–15.

11. Knopp MV, Weiss E, Sinn HP, et al. Pathophysiologic basis of contrast enhancement in breast tumors. J Magn Reson Imaging 1999;10:260–6.

12. Kaur B, Tan C, Brat DJ, et al. Genetic and hypoxic regulation of angiogenesis in gliomas. J Neurooncol 2004;70:229–43.

13. Hurwitz H, Fehrenbacher L, Novotny W, et al. Bevacizumab plus irinotecan, fluorouracil, and leucovorin for metastatic colorectal cancer. N Engl J Med 2004; 350:2335–42.

14. O'Connor JP, Jackson A, Parker GJ, et al. DCE-MRI biomarkers in the clinical evaluation of antiangiogenic and vascular disrupting agents. Br J Cancer 2007;96:189–95.

15. Cheng HL. Investigation and optimization of parameter accuracy in dynamic contrast-enhanced MRI. J Magn Reson Imaging 2008;28:736–43.

16. Brix G, Semmler W, Port R, et al. Pharmacokinetic parameters in CNS Gd-DTPA enhanced MR imaging. J Comput Assist Tomogr 1991;15:621–8.

17. Evelhoch JL. Key factors in the acquisition of contrast kinetic data for oncology. J Magn Reson Imaging 1999;10:254–9.

18. Ashton E, Durkin E, Kwok E, et al. Conversion from signal intensity to Gd concentration may be unnecessary for perfusion assessment of tumors using DCE-MRI. Presented at the Proceedings of the International Society for Magnetic Resonance in Medicine. Berlin, 2007.

19. Evelhoch JL. Consensus recommendations for acquisition of dynamic contrasted-enhanced MRI data in oncology. In: Jackson A, Buckley DL, Parker GJ, editors. 1st edition, Dynamic contrast-enhanced magnetic resonance imaging in oncology, vol 1. Berlin/Heidelberg (NY): Springer; 2005. p. 109–13.

20. Leach MO, Brindle KM, Evelhoch JL, et al. The assessment of antiangiogenic and antivascular therapies in early-stage clinical trials using magnetic resonance imaging: issues and recommendations. Br J Cancer 2005;92:1599–610.

21. Wang HZ, Riederer SJ, Lee JN. Optimizing the precision in T1 relaxation estimation using limited flip angles. Magn Reson Med 1987;5:399–416.

22. Deoni SC, Rutt BK, Peters TM. Rapid combined T1 and T2 mapping using gradient recalled acquisition in the steady state. Magn Reson Med 2003;49:515–26.

23. Jahng GH, Stables L, Ebel A, et al. Sensitive and fast T1 mapping based on two inversion recovery images and a reference image. Med Phys 2005;32:1524–8.

24. Ogg RJ, Kingsley PB. Optimized precision of inversion-recovery T1 measurements for constrained scan time. Magn Reson Med 2004;51:625–30.

25. Karlsson M, Nordell B. Analysis of the Look-Locker T(1) mapping sequence in dynamic contrast uptake studies: simulation and in vivo validation. Magn Reson Imaging 2000;18:947–54.

26. Freeman AJ, Gowland PA, Mansfield P. Optimization of the ultrafast Look-Locker echo-planar imaging T1 mapping sequence. Magn Reson Imaging 1998;16: 765–72.

27. Buckley DL, Parker GJ. Measuring contrast agent concentration in T1-weighted dynamic contrast enhanced MRI. In: Jackson A, Buckley DL, Parker GJ, editors. 1st edition, Dynamic contrast-enhanced magnetic resonance imaging in oncology, vol 1. Berlin/-Heidelberg (NY): Springer; 2005. p. 69–79.

28. Haase A. Snapshot FLASH MR imaging. Applications to T1, T2, and chemical-shift imaging. Magn Reson Med 1990;13:77–89.

29. Cercignani M, Symms MR, Schmierer K, et al. Three-dimensional quantitative magnetisation transfer imaging of the human brain. Neuroimage 2005;27: 436–41.

30. Heidemann RM, Ozsarlak O, Parizel PM, et al. A brief review of parallel magnetic resonance imaging. Eur Radiol 2003;13:2323–37.

31. Tsao J, Boesiger P, Pruessmann KP. k-t BLAST and k-t SENSE: dynamic MRI with high frame rate exploiting spatiotemporal correlations. Magn Reson Med 2003;50:1031–42.

32. Storey P, Ko JP, Nonaka D, et al. Dynamic 3D contrast-enhanced perfusion imaging of lung cancer with one-second temporal resolution. Presented at a meeting of the International Society for Magnetic Resonance in Medicine. Toronto, 2008.

33. Rijpkema M, Kaanders JH, Joosten FB, et al. Method for quantitative mapping of dynamic MRI contrast agent uptake in human tumors. J Magn Reson Imaging 2001;14:457–63.

34. Ramsay E, Causer P, Hill K, et al. Adaptive bilateral breast MRI using projection reconstruction time-resolved imaging of contrast kinetics. J Magn Reson Imaging 2006;24:617–24.

35. Mistretta CA, Wieben O, Velikina J, et al. Highly constrained backprojection for time-resolved MRI. Magn Reson Med 2006;55:30–40.

36. O'Halloran RL, Wen Z, Holmes JH, et al. Iterative projection reconstruction of time-resolved images using highly-constrained back-projection (HYPR). Magn Reson Med 2008;59:132–9.

37. Knoll F, Ebner F, Keeling S, et al. Assessment of image reconstruction methods for subsampled DCE-MRI. Presented at a meeting of the International Society for Magnetic Resonance in Medicine. Toronto, 2008.

38. Daniel BL, Yen YF, Glover GH, et al. Breast disease: dynamic spiral MR imaging. Radiology 1998;209: 499–509.

39. Parker GJ, Suckling J, Tanner SF, et al. MRI: parametric analysis software for contrast-enhanced dynamic MR imaging in cancer. Radiographics 1998;18:497–506.

40. Kuhl CK, Mielcareck P, Klaschik S, et al. Dynamic breast MR imaging: are signal intensity time course data useful for differential diagnosis of enhancing lesions? Radiology 1999;211:101–1010.

41. Gribbestad IS, Nilsen G, Fjosne HE, et al. Comparative signal intensity measurements in dynamic gadolinium-enhanced MR mammography. J Magn Reson Imaging 1994;4:477–80.

42. Jackson A, O'Connor JP, Parker GJ, et al. Imaging tumor vascular heterogeneity and angiogenesis using dynamic contrast-enhanced magnetic resonance imaging. Clin Cancer Res 2007;13:3449–59.

43. Gribbestad IS, Gjesdal KI, Nilsen G, et al. An introduction to dynamic contrast-enhanced MRI in oncology. In: Jackson A, Buckley DL, Parker GJ, editors. 1st edition. Dynamic contrast-enhanced MRI in oncology, vol 1. Berlin/Heidelberg (NY): Springer; 2005. p. 3–22.

44. Tofts PS, Brix G, Buckley DL, et al. Estimating kinetic parameters from dynamic contrast-enhanced T(1)-weighted MRI of a diffusible tracer: standardized quantities and symbols. J Magn Reson Imaging 1999;10:223–32.

45. Tofts PS, Kermode AG. Measurement of the blood-brain barrier permeability and leakage space using dynamic MR imaging. 1. Fundamental concepts. Magn Reson Med 1991;17:357–67.

46. Brix G, Bahner ML, Hoffmann U, et al. Regional blood flow, capillary permeability, and compartmental volumes: measurement with dynamic CT–initial experience. Radiology 1999;210:269–76.

47. Donahue KM, Weisskoff RM, Burstein D. Water diffusion and exchange as they influence contrast enhancement. J Magn Reson Imaging 1997;7:102–1010.

48. Parker GJ, Buckley DL. Tracer kinetic modelling for T1-weighted DCE-MR imaging. In: Jackson A, Parker GJ, Buckley DL, editors. 1st edition. Dynamic contrast-enhanced magnetic resonance imaging in oncology, vol 1. Berlin/Heidelberg (NY): Springer; 2005. p. 81–92.

49. St Lawrence KS, Lee TY. An adiabatic approximation to the tissue homogeneity model for water exchange in the brain: I. Theoretical derivation. J Cereb Blood Flow Metab 1998;18:1365–77.

50. Buckley DL, Roberts C, Parker GJ, et al. Prostate cancer: evaluation of vascular characteristics with dynamic contrast-enhanced T1-weighted MR –initial experience. Radiology 2004;233:709–15.

51. Buckley DL. Uncertainty in the analysis of tracer kinetics using dynamic contrast-enhanced T1-weighted MRI. Magn Reson Med 2002;47:601–6.

52. Henderson E, Rutt BK, Lee TY. Temporal sampling requirements for the tracer kinetics modeling of breast disease. Magn Reson Imaging 1998;16:1057–73.

53. Ashton E, Raunig D, Ng C, et al. Scan-rescan variability in perfusion assessment of tumors in MRI using both model and data-derived arterial input functions. J Magn Reson Imaging 2008;28:791–6.

54. Tseng YC, Hsu HL, Lee TH, et al. Venous reflux on carotid computed tomography angiography: relationship with left-arm injection. J Comput Assist Tomogr 2007;31:360–4.

55. You SY, Yoon DY, Choi CS, et al. Effects of right-versus left-arm injections of contrast material on computed tomography of the head and neck. J Comput Assist Tomogr 2007;31:677–81.

56. Lee YJ, Chung TS, Joo JY, et al. Suboptimal contrast-enhanced carotid MR angiography from the left brachiocephalic venous stasis. J Magn Reson Imaging 1999;10:503–9.

57. Calamante F, Gadian DG, Connelly A. Quantification of perfusion using bolus tracking magnetic resonance imaging in stroke: assumptions, limitations, and potential implications for clinical use. Stroke 2002;33:1146–51.

58. Calamante F. Bolus dispersion issues related to the quantification of perfusion MRI data. J Magn Reson Imaging 2005;22:718–22.

59. Harrer JU, Parker GJ, Haroon HA, et al. Comparative study of methods for determining vascular permeability and blood volume in human gliomas. J Magn Reson Imaging 2004;20:748–57.

60. van Osch MJ, Vonken EJ, Viergever MA, et al. Measuring the arterial input function with gradient echo sequences. Magn Reson Med 2003;49:1067–76.

61. Yang C, Karczmar GS, Medved M, et al. Multiple reference tissue method for contrast agent arterial input function estimation. Magn Reson Med 2007;58:1266–75.

62. Teifke A, Behr O, Schmidt M, et al. Dynamic MR imaging of breast lesions: correlation with microvessel distribution pattern and histologic characteristics of prognosis. Radiology 2006;239:351–60.

63. Gaustad JV, Benjaminsen IC, Graff BA, et al. Intratumor heterogeneity in blood perfusion in orthotopic human melanoma xenografts assessed by dynamic contrast-enhanced magnetic resonance imaging. J Magn Reson Imaging 2005;21:792–800.

64. Jackson A, Kassner A, Annesley-Williams D, et al. Abnormalities in the recirculation phase of contrast agent bolus passage in cerebral gliomas: comparison with relative blood volume and tumor grade. AJNR Am J Neuroradiol 2002;23:7–14.

65. de Lussanet QG, Backes WH, Griffioen AW, et al. Dynamic contrast-enhanced magnetic resonance imaging of radiation therapy-induced microcirculation changes in rectal cancer. Int J Radiat Oncol Biol Phys 2005;63:1309–15.

66. Li KL, Wilmes LJ, Henry RG, et al. Heterogeneity in the angiogenic response of a BT474 human breast cancer to a novel vascular endothelial growth factor-receptor tyrosine kinase inhibitor: assessment by voxel analysis of dynamic contrast-enhanced MRI. J Magn Reson Imaging 2005;22:511–9.

67. Rose CJ, Mills S, O'Connor JP, et al. Quantifying heterogeneity in dynamic contrast-enhanced MRI parameter maps. In: Ayache N, Ourselin A, Maeder A, editors. Lecture notes in computer science. Vol 4792. Verlag/Berlin/Heidelberg (NY): Springer; 2007. p. 376–84.

68. Hamstra DA, Chenevert TL, Moffat BA, et al. Evaluation of the functional diffusion map as an early biomarker of time-to-progression and overall survival in high-grade glioma. Proc Natl Acad Sci U S A 2005;102:16759–64.

69. Heywang-Kobrunner SH, Haustein J, Pohl C, et al. Contrast-enhanced MR imaging of the breast: comparison of two different doses of gadopentetate dimeglumine. Radiology 1994;191:639–46.

70. Sardanelli F, Iozzelli A, Fausto A, et al. Gadobenate dimeglumine-enhanced MR imaging breast vascular maps: association between invasive cancer and ipsilateral increased vascularity. Radiology 2005;235:791–7.

71. Roberts TP, Noseworthy MD. Contrast agents for magnetic resonance. In: Jackson A, Buckley DL, Parker GJ, editors. 1st edition. Dynamic contrast-enhanced magnetic resonance imaging in oncology, vol 1. Berlin/Heidelberg (NY): Springer; 2005. p. 23–37.

72. Barrett T, Brechbiel M, Bernardo M, et al. MRI of tumor angiogenesis. J Magn Reson Imaging 2007; 26:235–49.

73. Barrett T, Kobayashi H, Brechbiel M, et al. Macromolecular MRI contrast agents for imaging tumor angiogenesis. Eur J Radiol 2006;60:353–66.

74. Marzola P, Degrassi A, Calderan L, et al. Early antiangiogenic activity of SU11248 evaluated in vivo by dynamic contrast-enhanced magnetic resonance imaging in an experimental model of colon carcinoma. Clin Cancer Res 2005;11: 5827–32.

75. Daldrup H, Shames DM, Wendland M, et al. Correlation of dynamic contrast-enhanced MR imaging with histologic tumor grade: comparison of macromolecular and small-molecular contrast media. AJR Am J Roentgenol 1998;171:941–9.

76. Turetschek K, Floyd E, Helbich T, et al. MRI assessment of microvascular characteristics in experimental breast tumors using a new blood pool contrast agent (MS-325) with correlations to histopathology. J Magn Reson Imaging 2001;14: 237–42.

77. Preda A, Novikov V, Moglich M, et al. MRI monitoring of Avastin antiangiogenesis therapy using B22956/ 1, a new blood pool contrast agent, in an experimental model of human cancer. J Magn Reson Imaging 2004;20:865–73.

78. Turetschek K, Roberts TP, Floyd E, et al. Tumor microvascular characterization using ultrasmall superparamagnetic iron oxide particles (USPIO) in an experimental breast cancer model. J Magn Reson Imaging 2001;13:882–8.

79. Law M, Young RJ, Babb JS, et al. Gliomas: predicting time to progression or survival with cerebral blood volume measurements at dynamic susceptibility-weighted contrast-enhanced perfusion MR imaging. Radiology 2008;247:490–8.

Diffusion and Perfusion MR Imaging of Acute Ischemic Stroke

Ashley D. Harris, PhD[a,b,c,d,e], Shelagh B. Coutts, MBChB, MD, FRCPC[b,d,e,f], Richard Frayne, PhD[a,b,c,d,e,g],*

KEYWORDS

- Diffusion • Perfusion • Ischemia • Infarction
- Hyperacute ischemic stroke • Thrombolysis
- Transient ischemic attack • Diffusion-perfusion mismatch

Ischemic stroke is an interruption in cerebral blood flow as a result of an arterial occlusion. The decrease in cerebral perfusion causes an inadequate supply of oxygen and nutrients to cerebral tissue that is required maintain normal neurologic function. The arterial blockage is typically caused by a thrombus, a clot that forms in place, or an embolus that breaks off a plaque and travels with the arterial flow until it lodges in a smaller vessel. Irrespective of thrombotic or embolic origin, stroke causes focal neurologic symptoms that depend on the part of the brain that is affected. For this article, we are specifically interested in the early phase of stroke, the acute phase, defined as within 24 hours of stroke onset and the hyperacute phase, defined as within 6 hours of onset.

STROKE PATHOPHYSIOLOGY

There are a variety of processes acting over different time periods that contribute to cell damage and death after the onset of ischemia and are often referred to as the ischemic cascade. Briefly, the occluded arterial vessel prevents blood flow, thereby limiting the delivery of oxygen and nutrients and causing excessive accumulation of metabolic by-products. In ischemic tissue, anaerobic metabolism replaces aerobic metabolism, producing lactate and tissue acidosis. Once energy stores are depleted, all energy-dependent processes are compromised. An early result of this energy failure is extensive ion disequilibrium, as up to 70% of the cerebral energy requirement is consumed by Na^+/K^+-ATPase in the plasma membrane of cells.[1] Without functioning ion pumps, potassium ions leak out of the cells, and sodium and calcium ions enter the cells. Water follows the osmotic gradient into cells, resulting in cytotoxic edema. Excitotoxic damage occurs in surrounding tissue as Ca^{2+} imbalances cause cell depolarization. Later, the resulting neuronal injury causes a recruitment of white blood cells,

A.D.H. received funding from the Natural Sciences and Engineering Research Council of Canada, the Informatics Circle of Research Excellence and Alberta Heritage Foundation for Medical Research (AHFMR). R.F. is a Canada Research Chair in Image Science and an AHFMR Senior Medical Scholar. Operational support for our stroke imaging program is provided by the Canadian Institutes for Health Research and the Heart and Stroke Foundation of Alberta.

[a] Department of Radiology, University of Calgary, Calgary, Alberta, T2N 2T9 Canada
[b] Clinical Neurosciences, University of Calgary, Calgary, Alberta, T2N 2T9 Canada
[c] Department of Biomedical Engineering, University of Calgary, Calgary, Alberta, T2N 2T9 Canada
[d] Hotchkiss Brain Institute, University of Calgary, Calgary, Alberta, T2N 2T9 Canada
[e] Seaman Family MR Research Centre, Foothills Medical Centre, 1403 29th Street NW, Calgary, Alberta T2N 2T9, Canada
[f] Calgary Stroke Program, C1246, Foothills Medical Centre, 1403 29th Street NW, Calgary, Alberta T2N 2T9, Canada
[g] Department of Electrical Engineering, University of Calgary, Calgary, Alberta, T2N 2T9 Canada
* Corresponding author. Seaman Family MR Research Centre, Foothills Medical Centre, 1403 29th Street NW, Calgary, Alberta T2N 2T9, Canada.
E-mail address: rfrayne@ucalgary.ca (R. Frayne).

initiating the inflammatory process. Apoptosis is initiated as mitochondrial membranes are compromised and various apoptotic enzymes and pathways are activated.

ISCHEMIC TISSUES DESCRIPTIONS

With advances in neuroimaging, tissue fate and tissue properties can be predicted; however, improved descriptions and interpretations are still desired, as well as definitive definitions that are not modality dependent or observer subjective. The following tissue descriptions are now commonly applied and used in clinical descriptions of ischemic stroke, although before being able to characterize tissue physiology with imaging, they had limited use. Perfusion and diffusion imaging provide the required information for operational definitions of tissue types.[2]

A stroke causes a focus of irreversible damage, in which cell death is inevitable, and is referred to as the stroke core or *infarcted core* (Fig. 1). In this core, the cerebral blood volume (CBV) and cerebral blood flow (CBF) are both reduced. The

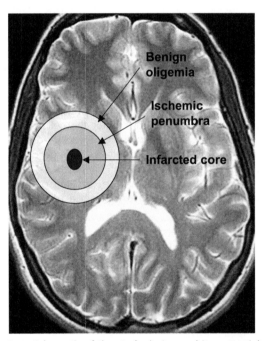

Fig. 1. Schematic of the stroke lesion and its potential progression. The infarcted core has such severe blood flow reductions that it is irreversibly damaged. Surrounding the infarcted core is the ischemic penumbra that is experiencing critically limited perfusion. If blood flow is quickly restored this tissue is salvageable; however, as time progresses this tissue is less likely to be recovered. Surrounding the ischemic penumbra is hypoperfused tissue, but it will not progress to infarction.

ischemic penumbra is the area immediately surrounding the infarcted core that is *at risk* of being infarcted if blood flow is not quickly restored. This tissue experiences decreased CBF, but blood flow is not as low as in the infarcted core. In early stroke, this potential for damage is thought to be reversible, as long as blood flow is restored quickly. The length of time that a tissue potentially remains viable depends on multiple factors (eg, collateral blood flow, clot location, tissue type). The ischemic penumbra exhibits dysfunction (eg, is electrically silent) because of metabolic and ionic imbalances; however, the cellular structural integrity is maintained. This damage is reversible, but recovery becomes less likely over time as ion pumps fail.[1] It is when the membrane functions (ie, maintaining ion gradients, acting as a barrier between the cell and the external environment, and so forth) fail, as CBF is decreased and/or CBF has been decreased for too long of a time period that ischemic damage becomes irreversible and the tissue is no longer considered salvageable. Over time, if blood flow is not restored, the infarcted core expands into the penumbral region. *Benign oligemia* is used to describe the third region in which cerebral blood flow is decreased but not to the extent of putting this tissue at risk for infarction. Normal neural function is maintained in this region and this tissue does not progress to infarction. In some ways, this term is misleading, as CBV may be increased, decreased, or be unchanged from the normal state. This above analysis and categorization of tissue into infarcted, penumbral, and benignly oligemic regions is a gross oversimplification, as the ongoing cellular processes are complex, interrelated, and vary depending on a variety of factors. Nevertheless, this model provides a useful methodology when understanding the role of MR imaging in acute ischemic stroke.

CEREBRAL PERFUSION

There are varying degrees of ischemia depending on the part of the brain affected and the metabolic, functional, or morphologic definition of ischemia in use. Often with imaging, CBF indicating the volume of blood (in mL) passing through a mass of tissue (typically 100 g) over time (min) is used to describe and quantify cerebral perfusion.

The CBF in gray and white matter is approximately 65 mL min^{-1} (100 g)$^{-1}$ and 20 mL min^{-1} (100 g)$^{-1}$, respectively, according to positron emission tomography results.[3,4] A generally accepted threshold for ischemia is a CBF of less than 20 mL 100 g^{-1} min^{-1}. It is at this level that autoregulation, the ability of the brain to respond to a drop in blow flow, is reduced such that autoregulation alone is unable to meet tissue demands, and the oxygen extraction fraction increases. This is the threshold defining the ischemic penumbra; proper neuronal electrical function is decreased because energy supplies are limited, and cells are unable to maintain normal metabolic processes. Specifically, cellular ion-exchange and signaling mechanisms that require continual energy supplies begin to shut down. A second, even lower CBF threshold of approximately 10 mL min^{-1} (100 g)$^{-1}$, demarcates the blood flow at which cell membrane function is compromised and mitochondrial metabolism shuts down and irreversible damage occurs; ie, the threshold for infarction, where parenchymal tissue will eventually die and vasogenic edema will occur. However, these thresholds are highly debatable. Not only do they vary between people, as well as between vascular territories, but the amount of time with reduced blood flow mediates tissue damage and is not explicitly included in any of these definitions.[5] Also, different techniques and technologies may impact results. For example, some results indicate that early neurologic signs appear when CBF falls below 29 mL min^{-1} (100 g)$^{-1}$ and hemiparesis develops as early as when cortical CBF drops by 30% (ie, to 45 mL min^{-1} [100 g]$^{-1}$ for GM or 14 mL min^{-1} [100 g]$^{-1}$ for WM).[3] However, others have found that tissue with CBF less than 12 mL min^{-1} (100 g)$^{-1}$ may be salvaged with thrombolysis.[6–8] Umemura and colleagues[9] found that tissue with CBF less than 20 mL min^{-1} (100 g)$^{-1}$ will likely infarct. The threshold inconsistencies and lack of information regarding time at different levels of CBF further serve to illustrate the complex and heterogeneous nature of acute ischemic stroke.

THROMBOLYSIS

Until 1995, there was no specialized treatment for ischemic stroke. In 1995, the National Institute of Neurologic Disease and Stroke (NINDS) tPA Stroke Trial[10] demonstrated that thrombolysis with tissue plasminogen activator (tPA), when administered intravenously (IV) within 3 hours of stroke onset was effective in treating ischemic stroke. tPA is an endogenous enzyme that degrades blood clots; for stroke treatment, it is administered to degrade the thrombus that is occluding a cerebral artery, thus restoring flow to cerebral tissue. Early recanalization is associated with an improved clinical outcome.[11] More recently, off-label intra-arterial (IA) administration of tPA treatment has become a potential treatment option, and evidence suggests that the time

window can be extended to 6 hours from stroke onset.[12] IA-tPA is typically used to lyse large clots that are generally not successfully lysed with IV administration.

The integrity of the blood brain barrier (BBB) is essential for successful stroke treatment with tPA. Although the mechanism(s) of hemorrhagic transformation are not completely understood, entry of tPA into the parenchyma will likely result in intracerebral hemorrhage. Additionally, tPA may exacerbate any BBB damage present; therefore, if tPA cannot immediately enter the parenchyma, its damaging effects on the BBB may enable it to subsequently enter the parenchyma. The major concern with thrombolysis is causing hemorrhage, which in the brain could be fatal. Specifically, BBB disruption presents a problem for administering tPA because tPA will not be confined to the intravascular space, which will induce hemorrhage.[13,14]

Noncontrast CT and time from onset alone cannot predict outcome because patients are heterogeneous, and factors such as autoregulation and collateral flow are not considered in either of these two measures. Imaging can, and in many centers does, play a greater role in the individual selection of stroke patients for thrombolysis.[8,15–19] Imaging-based stroke treatment strategies are designed to improve the risk-benefit ratio by selecting patients who will benefit from thrombolysis, while excluding patients at high risk for hemorrhage as a result of thrombolytic therapy.

Imaging, using MR perfusion and diffusion imaging, can identify characteristics of physiology and pathology to make more informed treatment decisions. Although it is well established that the risk of hemorrhage increases and the potential benefit of thrombolysis decreases with time,[10] information from imaging may enable the treatment of patients who would normally be excluded on the basis of a simple time window. Also, imaging may be used to exclude patients from receiving thrombolysis who are assessed within 3 hours of stroke onset, but who will not respond favorably to thrombolysis.[2,8,15–17,19–22] Moreover, imaging for patient selection and surrogate outcome measures is becoming increasingly used and accepted in stroke trials and by regulatory bodies.

DIFFUSION IMAGING
Theory

The theoretical and technical aspects of diffusion MR imaging are explained in recent reviews.[23,24] Briefly, Brownian motion describes the random motion of particles in a fluid that occurs due to their thermal energy. In biologic tissues, diffusion becomes restricted by boundaries (such as membranes and organelles) and the diffusion distance decreases. Biologic tissues are complex because many of these boundaries are semi-permeable. The result is that in vivo diffusion is more limited than the free diffusion constant; hence the diffusion constant is the apparent diffusion coefficient (ADC).[23]

MR diffusion-weighted pulse sequences are designed to have a high sensitivity to the motion of water through the use of strong magnetic field gradients—called diffusion gradients—that greatly increase sensitivity to diffusion motion. For diffusion-weighted acquisitions, typically a conventional spin-echo sequence is modified to permit accurate diffusion measurements by adding the two identical diffusion gradients around the 180° refocusing pulse. Since the two gradient pulses are the same, if a spin undergoes no motion, the phase accumulation during the first gradient pulse is negated by the 180° radiofrequency pulse and the second gradient pulse yielding a zero net phase (ie, no phase dispersion). When diffusion occurs, however, the second gradient pulse does not perfectly negate the phase accrual during the first gradient pulse. This imperfect refocusing, when averaged over a large number of spins, causes signal attenuation, which is dependent on the level of diffusion. The *b*-value is a diffusion sensitivity factor defined by the diffusion gradient amplitudes and timing. Most frequently, the Stejskal-Tanner diffusion gradient encodings[24] are used and the *b*-value is defined as $b = \gamma^2 G^2 \delta^2 (\Delta - \delta/3)$, where δ is the duration of the diffusion encoding gradient, Δ is the time between the leading edges of the diffusion encoding gradients, G is the gradient strength and γ is the gyromagnetic ratio. This equation is strictly valid only for the spin-echo sequence with square gradient waveforms. However for Δ and δ being longer than the gradient rise and fall times, this equation yields a good approximation to the true *b*-value.

Role in Stroke Imaging

Diffusion imaging is often used to detect the acute ischemic infarct. In the early 1990s, the utility of diffusion imaging was shown in stroke models, and included showing the correlation with perfusion deficits,[25,26] earlier stroke detection than conventional T2-weighted imaging (the previous standard), stroke detection within 1 hour of stroke onset,[25,27] and histologic confirmation of diffusion-weighted imaging (DWI) changes corresponding to cellular death.[28] It was suggested the cause of

restricted diffusion to be related to cytotoxic edema[29] and the disruption of the sodium-potassium transmembrane pump function,[25,26] which was later confirmed.[27] As the net diffusion becomes reduced with the development of cytotoxic edema, the stroke lesion is depicted as an ADC drop or a hyperintensity on DWI. Often, this lesion is thought to represent tissue with irreversible damage.

Challenges

Understanding the diffusion signal

One of the challenges with diffusion imaging is the lack of understanding associated with the biophysical origin of the diffusion signal. The drop in ADC is coincidental with cytotoxic edema, but the mechanism by which it changes is not clear. Simplistically, extracellular water can diffuse more freely than intracellular water and, with the onset of ischemia; the volume shift of water into the intracellular space causes the drop in the observed ADC. However, the 30% to 50% drop in ADC that is seen in ischemic stroke cannot be explained by a water volume shift alone. An evaluation of the proposed biophysical explanations for the mechanisms of the ADC drop is beyond the scope of this review, but some of the alternatives models will be summarized.[30]

The interaction of water with structures may contribute to the diffusion signals. In this model, the diffusion of water is affected by interactions with cellular structures. With more interactions, water diffusion becomes more restricted. With cellular swelling, time between interactions decreases; therefore, diffusion is seen as more restricted. Similarly, extracellular water tortuosity has been used to explain the changes in water diffusion with cerebral pathologies. Tortuosity is defined by the ratio of the free and the effective extracellular water diffusion; thus the extracellular diffusion pathways and the fraction of extracellular water are considered. Cell swelling and changes in cellular morphology causes the extracellular water to become trapped into multiple smaller areas (reducing the water fraction) and increasing the diffusion pathway. These two effects increase the tortuosity, thereby decreasing the apparent diffusion.

Examining the intra- and the extracellular compartments and water exchange suggests another mechanism that may explain the changes seen in water diffusion signals. The exchange between these two compartments is related to the life of a water molecule in each compartment. Using this analysis, fast and slow decay curves are observed and these curves are simultaneous with changes in the intra- and extracellular space fractions. However, the observed fraction changes do not correspond to physiologic values. Nevertheless, the fast decay is thought to represent the extracellular space and the slow decay is thought to be associated with the intracellular diffusion. Finally, the cell membrane permeability has been proposed as a mechanism by assuming that diffusion across healthy membranes is relatively high, and it becomes decreased in ischemic conditions.

An improved biophysical understanding of the diffusion signal and the ADC maybe useful and, in fact, necessary to develop a better understanding of the underlying pathophysiology of ischemic stroke and to extend the utility of DWI beyond its current use.

Diffusion reversal

The diffusion lesion is often considered to be predictive of the final lesion; however, there is some evidence that reversal of the diffusion lesion can occur.[31] Although it is not completely clear in what circumstances diffusion reversal occurs, it is likely associated with *rapid* recanalization and reperfusion of the affected tissue. The fraction of patients who show evidence of diffusion reversal appears to be quite small and it is unlikely that the circumstances in which diffusion lesion reversal occurs will significantly affect the commonly accepted premise that the acute diffusion lesion is predictive of the final lesion.

Technical issues

As described in more detail in recent reviews,[23,24] the *b*-value is a parameter that is used to manipulate the diffusion sensitivity. It is based on the diffusion gradient amplitudes, timing, and duration and is most often set to 1000 s mm^{-2}. Although collecting multiple *b*-values for acute stroke is unlikely to provide substantial information that warrant the time expense of longer acquisition times, choosing an optimal *b*-value for improved image characteristics does not affect the acquisition time, as the same number of images are acquired. A mathematical derivation followed by phantom- and patient-imaging analyses concluded that the optimal *b*-value for hyperacute ischemic stroke was 1500 s mm^{-2} (**Fig. 2**).[32] A subsequent comparative patient imaging study, however, showed no diagnostic improvement of using the *b* = 1500 s mm^{-2} over *b* = 1000 s mm^{-2}.[33]

A further modification of the standard diffusion acquisition is to include a 180° preparation pulse for cerebrospinal fluid (CSF) suppression.[34] By performing CSF suppression diffusion imaging (also known as fluid inversion prepared (FLIP-D) imaging, **Fig. 2**), CSF contamination of diffusion measurements is avoided; therefore ADC measurements should be more accurate for tissue. With FLIP-D, the measured ADC values are significantly smaller than with conventional diffusion-weighted imaging,[35] which is expected as the high ADC of CSF can no longer affect ADC values through partial volume averaging. Additionally, the ADC measurements are relatively unaffected with FLIP-D when the parenchyma tissue fraction (fraction of brain tissue in a voxel) is changed compared with a conventional DWI ADC measurement that depends on the parenchymal volume fraction. However, for acute stroke, when evaluated in terms of contrast- and signal-to-noise, FLIP-D images are inferior to the conventional DWI for visual conspicuity of ischemic strokes.[36] These findings were further confirmed when FLIP-D imaging was shown to have a negative prognostic value and a lower sensitivity than conventional diffusion imaging for acute ischemic stroke.[33] FLIP-D may have an increased accuracy in identifying reversible ADC lesions[37]; however, an improvement for outcome prediction has not yet been demonstrated.

PERFUSION IMAGING
Theory

Perfusion imaging depicts blood flow at the microvascular level in the parenchyma. In stroke, perfusion-weighted imaging (PWI) is useful to identify tissue with reduced cerebral blood flow, thus it can theoretically be used to define the ischemic tissue exactly, including benign oligemia, the ischemic penumbra and the infarct. The most common MR technique to examine cerebral perfusion is dynamic susceptibility contrast (DSC) perfusion imaging. Arterial spin labeling is another perfusion technique, but it does not currently have substantial application in ischemic stroke and will not be considered here. DSC-PWI requires the injection of a paramagnetic contrast agent, in standard clinical use a gadolinium chelate, and uses a multiphase, single-shot T2*-weighted echo-planar imaging technique. The contrast agent causes local magnetic field changes by causing spins to dephase, resulting in T2* and susceptibility signal loss as the contrast agent passes through the brain (**Fig. 3**). The multiphase imaging acquisition "visualizes" the passage of the contrast agent through the brain by rapidly acquiring multiple image volumes over the acquisition time—for example, 45 to 90 temporal phases (each phase is a data volume) over 90 seconds.

The simplest parametric maps are relative perfusion maps, such as relative mean transit time, relative cerebral blood volume, and relative

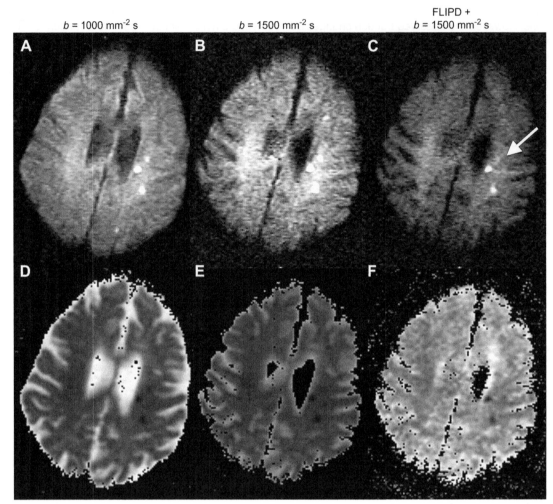

Fig. 2. Acute stroke diffusion images with different *b*-values and (*A, B, D, E*) with and (*C, F*) without CSF suppression. At different *b*-values (*A, D*: 1000 mm^{-2} s and *B, C, E, F*: 1500 mm^{-2} s), lesion conspicuity changes, while the addition of a CSF suppression pulse additionally can increase lesion conspicuity. (Imaging performed at 3 T.)

cerebral blood flow (rMTT, rCBV, and rCBF, respectively). Assuming that the signal losses are proportional to the contrast agent concentration and therefore blood flow, these maps are based on the signal characteristics as the contrast agent passes through the brain relative to the baseline characteristics (see **Fig. 3**). However, these maps have limited use beyond showing large-scale differences in the level of perfusion of one area of the brain relative to another area. To compare different patient examinations or defined thresholds, more quantitative methods are required (**Fig. 4**).

Quantitative perfusion data are complex, but likely to be necessary in order to define thresholds for salvageable and infarcted tissues and treatment guidelines; hence, absolute measurement of brain perfusion is required.[38] Semi-quantitative

maps can be constructed for comparisons between imaging sessions; however, as of yet, none of these maps are fully quantitative, in such a way that universal CBF thresholds could guide treatment decisions.[4,38,39] In addition to assuming contrast agent concentration is directly related to signal losses, quantitative perfusion MR imaging is based on bolus tracer kinetics and assumes blood flow through the brain is a linear time-invariant system. The three components to this system are (1) the arterial input function AIF(*t*), (2) the residue function, *R*(*t*), and (3) the transport function, *h*(*t*). The arterial input function is the function describing blood input to the system and is often defined by an observer as a voxel on the middle cerebral artery. The residue function is the instantaneous fraction of tracer remaining in a voxel. The transport function is a probability

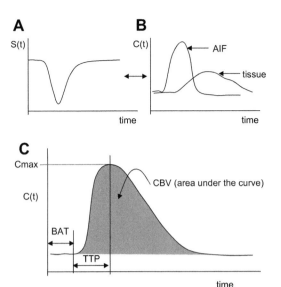

Fig. 3. Perfusion map development and definitions. The perceived signal drop (*A*) is assumed to be directly translated to the (*B*) contrast agent concentration within the voxel. The concentration-time curve is used to develop (*C*) summary characteristics of tissue perfusion. The deconvolution of TTP with the input = Tmax. Other summary parameters (ie, CBF) require more complex mathematical algorithms. AIF, arterial input function; BAT, bolus arrival time; CBV, cerebral blood volume; Cmax, maximum contrast agent concentration; C(t), concentration as a function of time; S(t), signal as a function of time; TTP, time to peak.

density function of the tracer's time-passage through the vasculature, ie, the fraction of tracer exiting a voxel at any point in time. The residue function is related to the transport function by $R(t) = [1 - \int h(t)dt]$.[40] The contrast agent entering the tissue, the contrast agent remaining in the tissue, and the contrast agent leaving the tissue allow for all components of flow through the parenchymal tissue to be calculated.

Cerebral blood flow in the brain tissue is determined from the deconvolution of the AIF from the residue function: $C_{VOI}(t) = \rho/k_H \cdot CBF \cdot [AIF(t) \otimes R(t)]$, where $C_{VOI}(t)$ is the concentration of the contrast agent in a voxel at time t, ρ, and k_H are constants for the blood density and hematocrit. The mean transit time (MTT) is the time it takes for the contrast agent to pass through the tissue of examination, and is mathematically defined by the transport function, $MTT = \int t \times h(t)dt / \int h(t)dt$, and is the area under the residue function curve. CBV is the area under the tissue concentration curve. CBF is the peak of the *CBF·R(t)* curve. By the central volume theorem, all blood flow parameters are related by $CBF = CBV/MTT$.

There are many additional parameters that can be calculated, and depending on the post-processing involved, they may be relative or quantitative. Time-to-peak (TTP) is the delay between the arrival of the contrast agent bolus arrival time (BAT) and the peak of the concentration curve. The full-width half-maximum of the contrast agent concentration curve and the first moment of the concentration-time curve are used as other characterizations of the transit time through the tissue without requiring deconvolution. The T_{max} is "the time of the maximum of the tissue residue function," and reflects the lag between the tissue response and the arterial input and will be used in the following discussion.

Role in Stroke Imaging

As stated previously, ischemic stroke is a result of perfusion deficits; thus a depiction of these deficits should be highly useful in the diagnosis and treatment plan; however, because of the limitations associated with perfusion imaging, the full benefits have yet to be realized. Nevertheless, relative cerebral blood flow maps are used to compare the ipsilateral to the contralateral perfusion characteristics. Current quantitative methods are used to enable the comparisons of results and are used in the definition of tissue experiencing a reduction in perfusion. However, when examining these results, it is important to realize that the mathematical algorithms and selected thresholds used often vary between research groups, and that these differences can greatly impact results. Perfusion imaging can be useful in the confirmation of stroke diagnosis and is a standard method to determine reperfusion status. Additionally, reperfusion may be a useful surrogate for clinical trials.[17]

Challenges

Clinical interpretation

During acute ischemic stroke, perfusion is highly dynamic and is continually changing. Perfusion-weighted imaging only gives a snapshot in time of the perfusion characteristics. Even in the absence of thrombolysis or any other treatment, tissue perfusion may change greatly within a short amount of time, thus translating and combining information gained from perfusion imaging with other clinical information, even diffusion imaging, requires caution. For example, in our experience, even during the short time delay between CT imaging and MR imaging, perfusion characteristics may change, which confounds comparisons needed for diagnosis and treatment decisions.

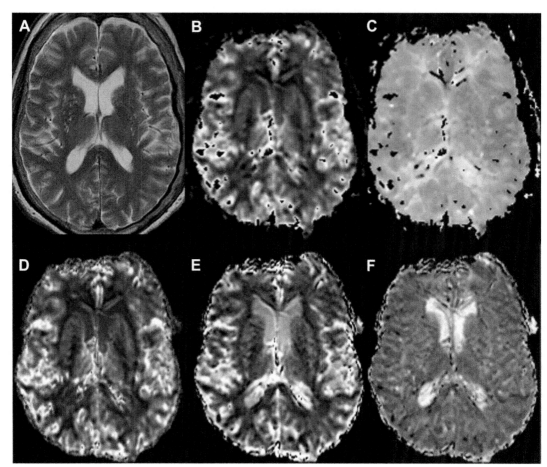

Fig. 4. Typical perfusion maps comparing qualitative and quantitative estimates. Qualitative maps include (*B*) negative enhancement integral, corresponding to relative CBV and (*C*) mean time to enhance or relative MTT. Quantitative maps include (*D*) CBF, (*E*) CBV and (*F*) MTT. (*A*) T2 map shown for anatomic reference. (Imaging performed at 3 T.)

Perfusion imaging postprocessing

Ideally, quantitative perfusion would enable comparisons between different acquisitions, either separate examinations performed on the same patient or between different patients, as well as providing information to assist in diagnosis and treatment decisions and providing a means to compare perfusion data from different sites, which may have protocol differences. As stated earlier, perfusion is not fully quantitative for assisting in treatment decisions. There are multiple issues associated with perfusion-weighted imaging, which will be reviewed here.

First, not only is the selection of the AIF a subjective process, but it is also highly subject to error through partial volume effects. Most often, the AIF is estimated by selecting a voxel on the middle cerebral artery of the hemisphere contralateral to the ischemic tissue. The MCA is approximately 2 mm in diameter. If the MCA is perpendicular to the imaging slice, it may be well represented in a single voxel; however, it is more likely that the MCA is divided between multiple voxels. Additionally, it is likely that the MCA runs within the para-axial imaging slice, which further augments the error in the AIF estimation. If the selected AIF voxel is half artery and half surrounding tissue (ie, 50% partial volume effect), the CBF can be overestimated by a factor of 4. The CBF overestimation increases to over 15 times if the AIF voxel is only 20% artery.[41] Ideally, the AIF would be the input to each voxel; however, that is not possible, therefore, there is delay and dispersion before the AIF reaches each voxel (and the measurement site).[42] Even the slice ordering (ie, interleaved slices) and the delay between adjacent slices when selecting an AIF can introduce perfusion characteristic errors.[43]

To have comparable values in a single patient and across patients, a cross-calibration step is necessary. The most common calibration is based on normal white matter, which is assumed to have a CBF of 22 mL $(100 \text{ g})^{-1}$ min^{-1}. In quantitative perfusion, a region of normal white matter is selected and all voxels are normalized to that white matter volume having a CBF of 22 mL 100 g^{-1} min^{-1}. However, this cross-calibration process can introduce biases and mask other errors in perfusion measurements, which are dependent on the algorithms used for the perfusion deconvolution as well as the tissue characteristics. The errors that are introduced during the deconvolution procedure may be increased or decreased with the cross-calibration depending on the deconvolution procedure and how errors become incorporated into parameters, specifically the MTT.[33] Finally, the deconvolution algorithm implemented may introduce errors, which can vary based on the cerebral blood flow characteristics.[44]

Two of the key assumptions associated with tracer kinetic methods are (1) the contrast agent remains within the vasculature and (2) the contrast agent does not recirculate. Both of these assumptions may be violated during PWI for acute ischemic stroke. With ischemic stroke, blood brain barrier disruption may allow the contrast agent to exit the vascular space. MR contrast agent half-life is on the order of hours; therefore, the contrast agent continues to circulate and reenter the cerebral tissue.[42] Although these two sources of error are introduced in PWI, the errors associated with the AIF and with subsequent cross-calibration processes are more likely to cause larger errors.

COMBINING DIFFUSION-WEIGHTED IMAGING AND PERFUSION-WEIGHTED IMAGING IN STROKE IMAGING
Mismatch Hypothesis

One of the most widely used concepts when using advanced MR techniques for acute ischemic stroke is the perfusion-diffusion mismatch theory (Figs. 1 and 5). The principle behind this hypothesis is that MR DWI and PWI can help identify a "tissue window" for thrombolysis rather than relying solely on time from onset to guide treatment. This hypothesis relies on information gained from both perfusion and diffusion imaging to predict which tissue has irreversible damage and which tissue is potentially salvageable with rapid thrombolysis. Irreversible tissue is defined by the region with reduced diffusion, as identified on the diffusion-weighted image or the ADC map. Tissue that is at risk of infarction but potentially salvageable with thrombolysis is the tissue experiencing reduced perfusion, but lying outside the diffusion lesion. This region is the ischemic penumbra (see

Fig. 1) and is the volumetric mismatch between the PWI and DWI lesions. Currently, no imaging model allows for effective acute differentiation of tissue that is benignly oligemic and will not progress to infarction; it is only at follow-up imaging that this distinction can be estimated.

Numerous studies have examined the mismatch hypothesis, and in some centers MR imaging is routinely used to choose patients for thrombolysis in the 0-hour to 3-hour and later time windows.[45] Two recent clinical trials have specifically evaluated mismatch as a method to select patients for thrombolysis in the time frame of 3 hours to 6 hours after onset. The DEFUSE trial[16] (Diffusion and Perfusion Imaging Evaluation for Understanding Stroke Evolution) examined the potential of the diffusion-perfusion mismatch to guide thrombolysis treatment decisions. In this study, patients who presented with stroke within 3 hours to 6 hours of onset received a baseline CT and MR imaging and were then treated with IV tPA within 6 hours of stroke onset. A second MR was performed 3 to 6 hours after tPA and radiologic outcome was defined using the 30-day MR scan. The perfusion abnormality was defined according to the T_{max} maps, with any voxel showing at least a 2-second delay being classified as ischemic. This study showed that patients with a diffusion-perfusion mismatch who reperfused had more favorable clinical outcomes compared with patients who did not have a diffusion-perfusion mismatch.

In addition, the DEFUSE trial defined a target mismatch profile, which describes the most favorable mismatch characteristics for patients who receive the greatest benefit from reperfusion after thrombolysis and a malignant profile. Importantly, the investigators identified a malignant profile that was characterized by a DWI lesion 100 mL or larger and/or PWI lesion 100 mL or larger, with T_{max} = 8 seconds or greater. These investigators defined a target mismatch as all patients with mismatch, but excluded patients who displayed the malignant profile. In the DEFUSE trial, the malignant profile was indicative of patients with an increased risk of symptomatic hemorrhage after tPA despite the fact these patients typically had a large mismatch volume.[16] Identifying patients who were at high risk of a poor outcome with thrombolysis is one area that is not specifically evaluated with DWI-PWI mismatch. It is not surprising, however, that patients with larger imaging abnormalities (ie, the malignant profile) at baseline have worse outcomes, whether it is a poor clinical outcome or a hemorrhagic transformation. Results from the DEFUSE study indicated that a large diffusion lesion is predictive of a symptomatic hemorrhage,[46] and this result has been

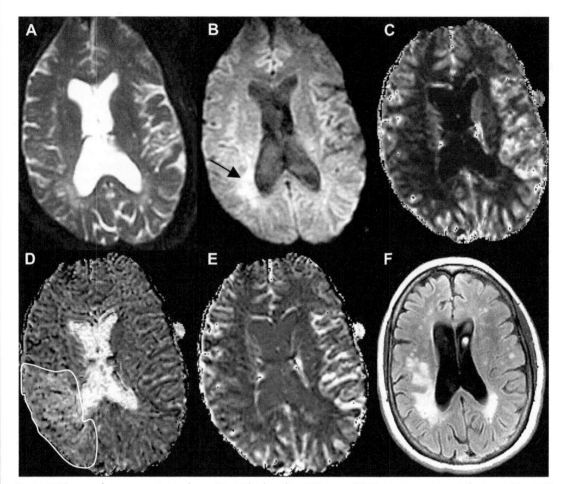

Fig. 5. MR images from an acute stroke patient. The baseline T2 image (*A*) illustrates anatomic features. The DWI hyperintensity (*B, arrow*) shows the acute infarct. Quantitative perfusion maps of cerebral blood flow (CBF, *C*) mean transit time (MTT, *D*), cerebral blood volume (CBV, *E*) show perfusion deficits. MTT is increased in the right hemisphere (*outlined*) while CBV and CBF are reduced. The difference between the DWI hyperintensity and the perfusion deficits—the diffusion-perfusion mismatch— indicates the penumbra that is potentially salvageable. The 30-day FLAIR (*F*) shows the final lesion grew from the initial diffusion lesion but did now extend into the entire perfusion deficit. (Imaging performed at 3 T.)

confirmed in other studies.[22,47–50] This finding is not surprising, as symptomatic hemorrhage likely occurs in more severe stroke and increasing lesion size is one component of increasing stroke severity. Nonetheless, there are likely patients with small infarcts and a small area at risk that should not be considered for thrombolysis and the mismatch hypothesis as it currently stands does not present a method to identify these patients.

The Echoplanar Imaging Thrombolytic Evaluation Trial (EPITHET)[17] was a phase II prospective, randomized, double-blinded, placebo-controlled trial in which the effect of intravenous tPA was administered 3 to 6 hours after stroke onset and reperfusion, infarct growth, and clinical outcome were analyzed compared with the baseline

penumbra. The diffusion-perfusion mismatch was used to define the penumbral region, and a couple of different perfusion deficit definitions were explored. The original analyses of the attenuation of infarct growth in patients with diffusion-perfusion mismatch when treated with tPA resulted in a negative result;[17] however, a number of subsequent secondary analyses performed showed statistically significant differences.[18] It was shown that patients with a DWI-PWI mismatch who were treated with tPA showed a better outcome than those who received the placebo.[17] Treatment with tPA also showed increased reperfusion rate and less infarct expansion, both of which were associated with a better outcome according to functional and neurologic scores. Additionally, this trial supported the use of reperfusion as a surrogate marker for outcome.[17] The results of EPITHET, while not significant for the primary outcome, concur with the results of DEFUSE. Also, the malignant profile in EPITHET (same as in DEFUSE, DWI lesion ≥ 100 mL, PWI lesion ≥ 100 mL, with $T_{max} \geq 8$ s), while indicative of a poor clinical outcome, did not show an increased risk of hemorrhage.[17]

When examining these studies, it is important to realize that differences in patient populations exist, specifically when examining PWI-DWI mismatch at different times and before and after therapy, as it has been shown that thrombolysis alters the evolution of perfusion and diffusion patterns and their mismatch.[51] One of the challenges associated with DWI-PWI mismatch is the appropriateness of the PWI lesion definition. It appears that perfusion maps tend to overestimate the tissue at risk; however, in some cases the tissue at risk is underestimated.[38] Additionally, it is likely that thresholds for infarct may vary between patients. As such, there is likely no mismatch definition that can be universally applied to always predict patient outcome.[52] As stated previously, perfusion maps can also be subjective, contain biases and systematic errors that vary depending on the techniques used for quantitative measures. Additionally, different perfusion maps may show significantly different volumes of ischemia.[38] Some advocate use of perfusion maps that are more quantitative, as they are more accurate; however, these maps may be more prone to threshold-induced errors.[52] In the DEFUSE and EPITHET trials, T_{max}, a simpler, less biased map, was used to define the perfusion abnormality. The selection of T_{max} + 2 seconds, was based on a preliminary analysis of 40 patients of the EPITHET trial.[52] While T_{max} + 2 seconds was an appropriate parameter for these studies, caution must be used when using this result, as the patients in this study were assessed between 3 and 6 hours after stroke onset and randomized to thombolysis (which alters patient outcome);[51] hence, there may be a bias in the selection of this parameter. With a combined analysis of DEFUSE and EPITHET planned, this perfusion lesion definition can be refined for improved outcome predictions.

The results of both EPITHET and DEFUSE are exciting and the scene is now set for a large phase III randomized controlled trial based on mismatch. Despite the varying definitions of mismatch used in the various studies and case series, the ability to safely and successfully choose patients for thrombolysis on the basis of a tissue window rather than time seems likely. The planned pooled analysis of the EPITHET and DEFUSE studies will help clarify the optimal tissue-based definition of mismatch.[53] In addition, technological developments, including decreased acquisition and post-processing times, increased spatial resolution, and improved computer algorithms will likely further improve the ability to develop and to interpret perfusion maps.[53]

Research Developments and Interests

Surrogate measures and study comparisons

One of the challenges associated with ischemic stroke is the heterogeneity of the disease, including differences in pathophysiology and mechanism; the affected neurovascular territory and the resulting differences in disability, perceived severity, and ischemic thresholds; and differences in systemic and intracranial hemodynamics and risk factors.[54] Not only does stroke heterogeneity present challenges in treatment decisions, but it also imposes challenges to clinical research and therefore development of improved clinical practices, as it can severely limit study enrollment, comparisons between patients at baseline, and outcome and study results significance as outcome measures can be biased depending on the nature of stroke. Imaging is one technique to enable comparisons between acute ischemic stroke patients. As stroke is a heterogeneous disease, appropriate references for comparison are required and imaging provides one such method.

Often the 3-month follow-up (either conventional MR imaging or clinical assessment) is used for efficacy trial end points; however, many stroke trials have failed to meet this end point even though they had important findings at earlier points. This observation provides an argument for more relevant surrogate end points.[54] The definition of surrogate outcomes is not trivial, as the technical success of thrombolytic therapy (recanalization) does not guarantee clinical success in terms of improved deficits.[55]

For example, cerebral reperfusion has been proposed as a surrogate for stroke outcome.[17] The diffusion lesion is useful in the definition of the infarcted core and irreversible damage, and has been shown to be a valid surrogate end point because it is strongly correlated with poor clinical outcome.[17] Diffusion and perfusion imaging have been used in the development and evaluation of animal models of stroke,[56] and these data can likely assist in the translation of results from animal studies to the clinical situation, particularly in combination with imaging surrogate references.

Stroke pathophysiology

The clinical-diffusion mismatch compares the extent of the clinical deficit and the diffusion lesion

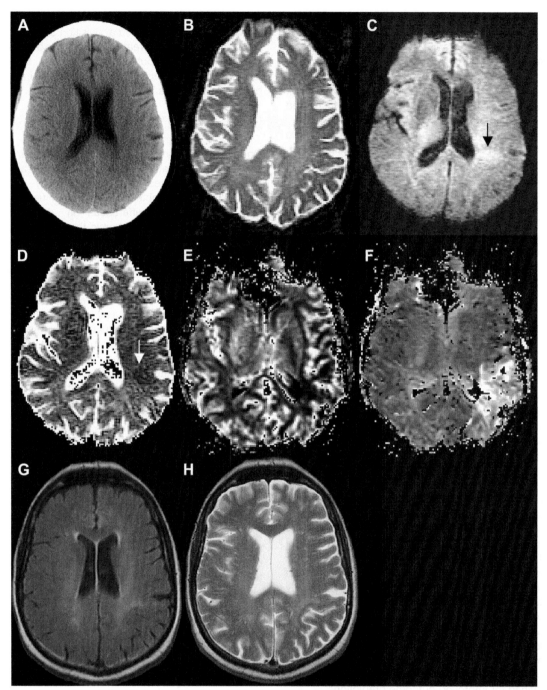

Fig. 6. This patient was diagnosed with TIA after an episode of aphasia that lasted 18 hours and then completely resolved. The CT (A), and the T2 image (B) for this patient show no evidence of pathology. On diffusion imaging (C), confirmed on the ADC map (D), there is a region of restricted diffusion (arrows). The relative cerebral blood volume (E) and the relative mean transit time maps (F) show a large region of reduced perfusion. Follow-up FLAIR (G) and T2 (H) imaging performed at 30 days from symptom onset shows a small area of infarction, not at large as the perfusion abnormality at baseline. (Imaging performed at 3 T.)

and theorizes that patients with an extensive clinical deficit and a small diffusion lesion are likely to have a large penumbra. Perfusion-diffusion mismatch was shown to be more accurate in selecting patients who would benefit from thrombolysis compared with the clinical-diffusion mismatch.[49] In another study, clinical-CT mismatch was evaluated as an alternative to diffusion-perfusion mismatch; with the premise that clinical deficits can indicate potential chronic deficits (ie, the perfusion lesion) while subtle CT changes are indicative of infarcted tissue (ie, the diffusion lesion). However, there was no correlation between clinical-CT mismatch and DWI-PWI mismatch.[57] These two studies serve as an example of the potential utility of imaging to better understand ischemic stroke pathophysiology. Although a small stroke in a critical area can have devastating consequences, the lack of concordance between clinical deficits and ischemic volume remains paradoxic and better

understanding in this area may assist the understanding of stroke pathophysiology and future treatment options. One group has developed atlases to quantify stroke severity based on subacute stroke lesions and National Institutes of Health Stroke Score (NIHSS).[58] The potential of stroke severity maps in combination with perfusion-diffusion mismatch will be an interesting investigation into stroke evolution.

Tissue, physiology, and time windows
Stroke can progress very rapidly and to emphasize the importance of rapid medical assessment and intervention, the phrase "time is brain" was coined. Since the initial use of "time is brain," other phrases, including "physiology is brain"[21] have been developed, again to stress the acute deterioration that can occur, especially in the absence of treatment, while recognizing that there are multiple factors to consider. Although time is critical in stroke therapy, a more complete

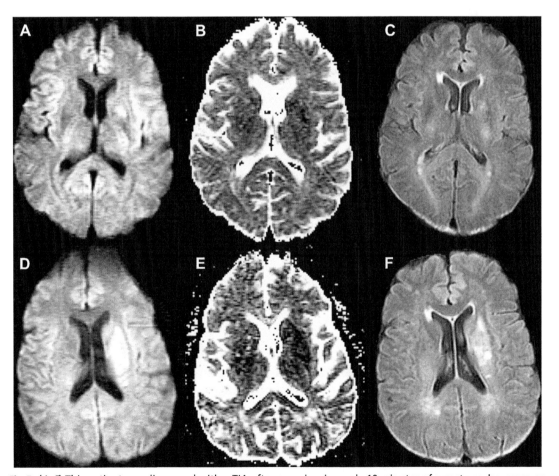

Fig. 7. (A–F) This patient was diagnosed with a TIA after experiencing only 10 minutes of symptoms; however, on the acute DWI (A) a diffusion lesion is apparent, as confirmed by the ADC (B). At the 3-week follow-up, this lesion had extended on both DWI (D) and ADC (E) and was also seen on FLAIR. (Imaging performed at 3 T.)

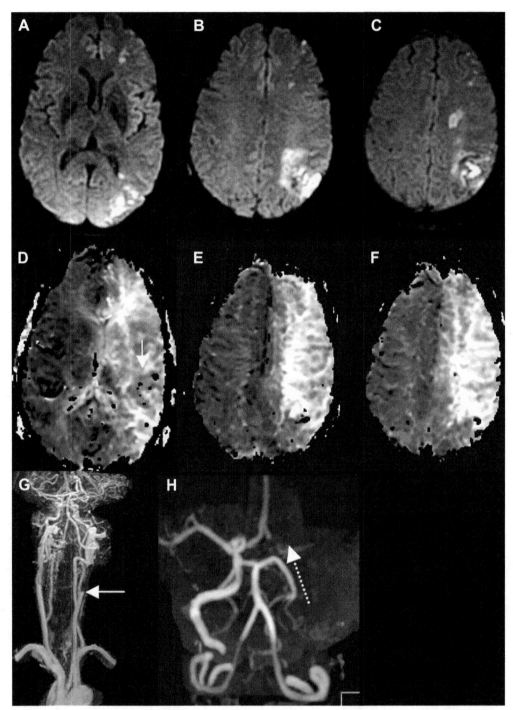

Fig. 8. This patient presented with very mild right-sided weakness (NIHSS = 1) and had a normal CT. However, on diffusion and perfusion imaging, there was extensive damage and abormalities. DWI shows a pattern consistent with both the anterior MCA-ACA watershed region and the posterior MCA-ACA-PCA watershed (*A–C*). There also is evidence of extensive rMTT delay throughout the left MCA and ACA territories (*D–F*). MR angiography shows an occlusion at its origin of the left internal carotid artery (*G, arrow*) and little flow in the left MCA (*H, dotted arrow*). There was concern that despite these mild symptoms that much of the left MCA and ACA territories were at risk for infarction. She, however, did not deteriorate and had a good outcome. (Imaging performed at 3 T.)

understanding of the underlying pathophysiology is also necessary, and this understanding should enable better treatment decisions. Diffusion and perfusion imaging are key elements in the assessment and description of underlying tissue physiology in stroke. These imaging techniques will likely enable a transition from strict time windows to administer treatment to tissue-based characteristics and physiology (tissue-window) to guide treatment decisions.

The interaction of reduced perfusion and time is an important consideration. Extreme reductions in CBF progress to infarction essentially immediately, while less extreme CBF drops take longer to progress to infarction. One group that examined CBF thresholds compared with ADC as an index of infarction showed that patient who were imaged earlier (≤ 4 hours after onset) had lower CBF thresholds for infarction compared with patients who were imaged later (>4 hours but <6 hours).[5] Others have examined the relationships between

WM and GM infarction thresholds and their dependencies on time, CBF, and ADC finding that all of these variables have a significant effect on tissue outcome and should be accordingly considered when examining ischemic stroke progression and defining thresholds of infarction or for treatment guidelines.[48,59] While the diffusion-perfusion mismatch is useful in defining potential benefit of thrombolysis, an accurate tissue window is complex and likely requires more information than T_{max} lesions and ADC lesions; CBF and time from onset must also be given consideration.

Clinical Issues and Implications

Correlations with other imaging techniques

Diffusion-weighted imaging has a much higher accuracy, sensitivity, and specificity for the detection of acute ischemic stroke compared with conventional MR or CT imaging (Fig. 6A–C).[60] This finding has been reconfirmed in the combined

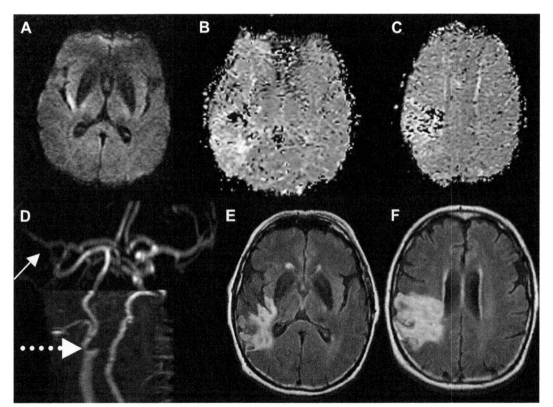

Fig. 9. This patient presented with mild left-sided deficits (NIHSS = 1), and a small area of restricted diffusion (A). There is a larger region of rMTT delay in the right MCA territory (B and C). Magnetic resonance angiography of the neck and the circle of Willis (D) show a posterior M2 occlusion (*solid arrow*) and an occluded right internal carotid artery just past the bifurcation. Over the first 24 hours, this patient deteriorated clinically and the FLAIR imaging shows a large stroke at 30 days (E and F). Unfortunately, by day 90, this patient's modified Rankin score = 4. Unlike the patient in the previous figure this patient did deteriorate over the first 24 hours and had a dependent outcome at 90-day follow-up. These two cases show the difficulty in using DWI-PWI mismatch in predicting outcome. (Imaging performed at 3 T.)

analysis of studies comparing DWI and CT that the sensitivity, sensitivity, positive predictive value, and negative predictive value of DWI are superior to CT.[61] It is a relatively simple and fast acquisition, and thus, is included in most, if not all, acute ischemic MR stroke protocols. It has been argued that perfusion imaging using CT is more reliable in terms of measurement accuracy and precision; however, CT perfusion (CTP) has limited brain coverage. Additionally, the high radiation dose and the iodinated contrast agent used for CTP results in substantial risks associated with CTP without a guarantee of additional information being acquired.

Perfusion and diffusion imaging have been used to assist in the diagnosis, treatment monitoring, and follow-up of acute ischemic stroke,[19] as perfusion and diffusion imaging can provide information not apparent on CT (Fig. 7). One study comparing the diagnosis and treatment plans before and after MR imaging found that the initial diagnosis based on clinical assessment and CT imaging was changed in

21% of patients and the treatment plan was changed in 26% of patients after MR imaging.[15] These treatment changes included some patients not receiving thrombolytic therapy and in other patients receiving more aggressive treatment, such as administering thrombolysis or performing IA thrombolysis rather than IV thrombolysis. The efficacy of MR over CT for predicting a favorable outcome in the treatment of ischemic stroke between 3 and 6 hours after onset has been shown.[45]

MILD STROKE AND TRANSIENT ISCHEMIC ATTACKS

Diffusion and perfusion MR imaging may also be highly useful in the diagnosis and treatment options of mild strokes and transient ischemic attacks (TIAs). By classical definitions of TIA, it was assumed that there was no permanent cerebral damage; however, advances in neuroimaging, specifically diffusion imaging, have shown this to be incomplete or invalid (see Figs. 6 and 7).

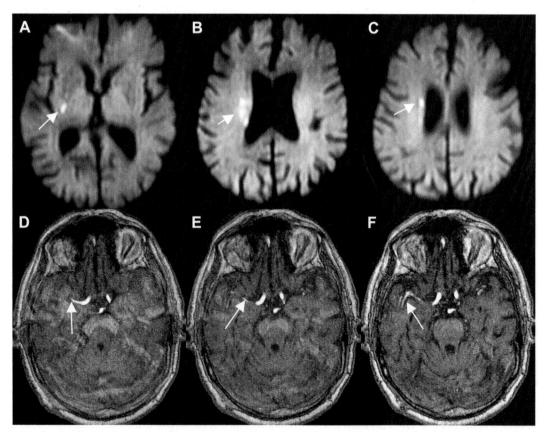

Fig. 10. Acute MR imaging was performed on a 1.5-T scanner. This patient had multiple acute DWI lesions (A–C), which are secondary to a 70% right MCA-M1 stenosis shown by MR angiography (D–F) as there appears to be highly restricted blood flow proximally (D and E); however, there is some flow distally (F), but it is markedly reduced, consistent with a severe stenosis. This patient was initially treated with just aspirin. He re-presented with a further event 3 months later in the same territory and was then treated with dual antiplatelet therapy.

Approximately one third of patients with strokes/ TIA that are too mild for thrombolytic treatment are dependent or dead upon discharge.[62] This indicates there is a need to better triage mild stroke and TIA patients and then be proactive in therapy for those at high risk of stroke progression and diffusion and perfusion imaging may be useful tools.

A substantial proportion of patients with TIA and minor stroke have injury observed on DWI of the brain (**Figs. 6–9**)[63–67] and it was shown that hyperacute MR in TIA and minor stroke patients can stratify the risk of recurrent stroke and disability.[68] In a cohort of 120 patients, the overall 90-day risk of recurrent stroke (using a standard definition of new stroke that included progression of symptoms) was 12%. Patients with no DWI lesion were at a low risk of recurrent events, 4.3%, compared with a rate of 10.8% with a DWI lesion and no large vessel occlusion, and 32.6% in those with a DWI lesion and a large vessel occlusion. There was a trend to increased likelihood of new lesions (symptomatic or asymptomatic) at 30-day follow-up MR with progressing baseline scan lesion number (none [2.2%], solitary [12.9%], multiple [19.8%]: $P = .046$).[62] Not just the patients with DWI lesions were at high risk for subsequent

asymptomatic events, patients with no DWI lesions were at a much *lower* risk for subsequent asymptomatic lesions. These lesions are very likely clinically relevant, as the literature suggests that the accumulation of silent infarcts does not appear to be benign in the longer term.[69–72] Patients with no DWI lesion (ie, no damage on their MR) have a low risk of an actual stroke, but often have recurrent transient events that do not cause any lasting damage.[73] The risk of recurrent stroke also increases with the presence of lesions of varying ages on the baseline MR imaging.[74] It appears that patients with no DWI lesions are at a relatively low risk of recurrent symptomatic and asymptomatic events.[62,68,75–78]

There are many causes of transient neurologic symptoms,[79,80] for example migraine with aura and seizure. It is not clear whether the initial event in patients without DWI lesions is an ischemic event with a more benign prognosis or a nonischemic event, eg, migraine or seizure that was misdiagnosed as stroke or TIA. It is likely that both of these factors contribute to the better prognosis in patients without DWI lesions. Regardless of the underlying pathogenesis, the predictive value of a DWI negative scan for benign outcome is strong. Similarly, another study found only a moderate performance

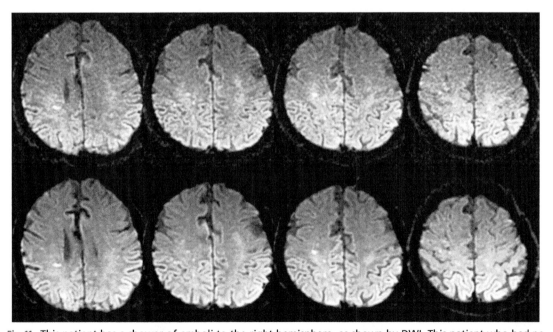

Fig. 11. This patient has a shower of emboli to the right hemisphere, as shown by DWI. This patient who had no significant past medical history presented with transient symptoms of left-sided weakness. He completely resolved but his MR image showed a shower of emboli to the right hemisphere. His neck imaging showed an approximately 40% right ICA stenosis with an ulcerated plaque. This was the likely cause of this embolic shower. The top row shows DWI with 3.0-mm slices while the bottom row DWI are 3.5 mm slices; and more than the minimum three diffusion images, thus an increased signal-to-noise ratio in the acquisition. This increase in image quality can assist in detecting subtle and small lesions. (Imaging performed at 3 T.)

in clinical/CT diagnosis of small deep infarcts.[81] Additionally, the diffusion lesions observed in TIA patients are generally indicative of chronic infarcts as only 21% of TIA-DWI lesions did not progress to infarct on diffusion-weighted, FLAIR, T1 and T2 imaging at follow-up (>4 months).[82]

A substantial proportion of patients with a TIA have been shown to have perfusion deficits (34%), even when symptoms have resolved.[83] Because many patients had had their symptoms resolve at the time of MR imaging (~80%) the actual perfusion deficits of TIA may be underestimated. This is potentially important in confirming the diagnosis of ischemia rather than a TIA mimic.

Clinical diagnosis of the vascular territory of acute-TIA or minor stroke is only moderately reliable.[84] Imaging, and in particular DWI, can improve the reliability of this diagnosis and often for cases of mild stroke and TIA a confident diagnosis is often only reached after DWI.[84] New lesions on repeat

MR in minor stroke and TIA patients may be used as surrogate markers of disease activity for secondary stroke prevention trials.[62,85]

STROKE ETIOLOGY

Determination of the etiology of the event is central to the management of stroke and TIA patients. Diffusion imaging improves stroke subtype diagnosis and the accuracy improves further when DWI is combined with MR angiography.[86] Stroke subtype is important, as it will alter the long-term care of the patient, including secondary stroke prevention, as well as assigning prognosis, identification of patients with increased risk of neurologic worsening, recurrent stroke, and medical complications. Although not supported by clinical trials, many clinicians tailor their acute stroke treatment according to the stroke subtype. Additionally, future stroke trials such as neuro-interventional

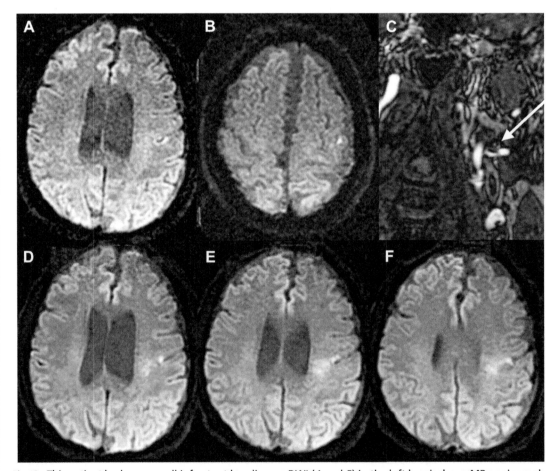

Fig. 12. This patient had some small infarcts at baseline on DWI (*A* and *B*) in the left hemisphere. MR angiography detected less than 50% stenosis, but found an intraluminal thrombus in the left ICA (*C*). The patient was treated for 5 days with heparin, but re-presented 2 weeks later with a recurrent event in the left hemisphere (*D–F*). (Imaging performed at 3 T.)

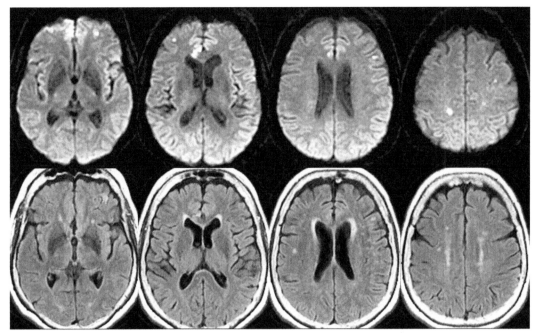

Fig. 13. This patient has a cardiac embolic source (atrial fibrillation) as indicated by multiple infarcts in both hemispheres. The DWI (*top row*) shows the recent events, whereas the FLAIR (*bottom row*) shows evidence of previously undetected or undiagnosed events. (Imaging performed at 3 T.)

studies may rely on early subtype diagnosis.[86] The lesion patterns as shown on DWI have been shown to have significant association with stroke subtype, therefore the acute DWI may assist in determining stroke etiology.[87] Simple patterns on MR such as showers of emboli in one hemisphere secondary to a middle cerebral artery stenosis (**Fig. 10**) or an internal carotid artery stenosis (**Figs. 11** and **12**), multiple emboli in multiple arterial territories secondary to atrial fibrillation (**Fig. 13**), and a single lesion measuring less than 2 cm in diameter secondary to small vessel disease would all potentially lead to changes in patient management. In addition, the perfusion-diffusion mismatch pattern may also assist in determining stroke etiology;[88] however, as this pattern is quite dynamic, it is difficult to assess this association.

SUMMARY

Diffusion and perfusion MR imaging have proven to be highly useful in the clinical description and understanding of hyperacute ischemic stroke. In this article, we have given a brief overview of the basic concepts of diffusion and perfusion images and described some of the current challenges and limitations of these techniques as applied to acute cerebral ischemia. Diffusion imaging is

becoming a clinical standard for the identification of the acute stroke lesion. Perfusion imaging is useful in determining the tissue experiencing hypoperfusion, and, as a result of this hypoperfusion, is at risk of infarction. The diffusion-perfusion mismatch hypothesis unites these two imaging strategies to define the tissue that is not salvageable and the tissue that is salvageable with thrombolysis. This hypothesis is applied extensively, including showing utility in two recent clinical trials,[16,17] in addition to secondary studies and planned pooled analyses using the same study databases. Diffusion and perfusion imaging are additionally useful in examining and exploring minor stroke and TIA. For example, diffusion imaging has shown that many TIA are likely more severe than previously thought, as TIA lesions can be detected with diffusion imaging in the hyperacute and follow-up stages. As such, diffusion and perfusion imaging will serve important roles in further understanding minor stroke and TIA progression and triaging these patients to appropriate treatments in the future. Further to understanding minor stroke and TIA, diffusion and perfusion imaging are useful in determining stroke etiology and it is expected these imaging techniques will play essential roles in better understanding stroke pathophysiology and evolution and in better defining "tissue windows" for ischemic stroke treatment beyond the diffusion-perfusion mismatch paradigm. Although this paradigm is showing great utility, with improved acquisition and processing techniques and better understanding of stroke evolution, diffusion and perfusion imaging can have even greater roles in the diagnosis and treatment of ischemic stroke.

REFERENCES

1. Doyle KP, Simon RP, Stenzel-Poore MP. Mechanisms of ischemic brain damage. Neuropharmacology 2008;55(3):310–8.
2. Davis SM, Donnan GA, Butcher KS, et al. Selection of thrombolytic therapy beyond 3 h using magnetic resonance imaging. Curr Opin Neurol 2005;18(1): 47–52.
3. Baron JC. Perfusion thresholds in human cerebral ischemia: historical perspective and therapeutic implications. Cerebrovasc Dis 2001;11(Suppl 1): 2–8.
4. Perthen JE, Calamante F, Gadian DG, et al. Is quantification of bolus tracking MRI reliable without deconvolution? Magn Reson Med 2002;47(1):61–7.
5. Lin W, Lee JM, Lee YZ, et al. Temporal relationship between apparent diffusion coefficient and absolute measurements of cerebral blood flow in acute stroke patients. Stroke 2003;34(1):64–70.
6. Haley EC Jr, Brott TG, Sheppard GL, et al. Pilot randomized trial of tissue plasminogen activator in acute ischemic stroke. The TPA Bridging Study Group. Stroke 1993;24(7):1000–4.
7. Heiss WD, Thiel A, Grond M, et al. Which targets are relevant for therapy of acute ischemic stroke? Stroke 1999;30(7):1486–9.
8. Schellinger PD, Fiebach JB, Hacke W. Imaging-based decision making in thrombolytic therapy for ischemic stroke: present status. Stroke 2003;34(2): 575–83.
9. Umemura A, Suzuka T, Yamada K. Quantitative measurement of cerebral blood flow by (99m)Tc-HMPAO SPECT in acute ischaemic stroke: usefulness in determining therapeutic options. J Neurol Neurosurg Psychiatry 2000;69(4):472–8.
10. Tissue plasminogen activator for acute ischemic stroke. The National Institute of Neurological Disorders and Stroke rt-PA Stroke Study Group. N Engl J Med 1995;333(24):1581–7.
11. Olivot JM, Mlynash M, Thijs VN, Relationships between infarct growth, clinical outcome, and early recanalization in diffusion and perfusion imaging for understanding stroke evolution (DEFUSE) 2008;39(8):2258–63
12. Furlan A, Higashida R, Wechsler L, et al. Intra-arterial prourokinase for acute ischemic stroke. The PROACT II study: a randomized controlled trial. Prolyse in acute cerebral thromboembolism. JAMA 1999;282(21):2003–11.
13. Dijkhuizen RM, Asahi M, Wu O, et al. Delayed rt-PA treatment in a rat embolic stroke model: diagnosis and prognosis of ischemic injury and hemorrhagic transformation with magnetic resonance imaging. J Cereb Blood Flow Metab 2001;21(8):964–71.
14. Dijkhuizen RM, Asahi M, Wu O, et al. Rapid breakdown of microvascular barriers and subsequent hemorrhagic transformation after delayed recombinant tissue plasminogen activator treatment in a rat embolic stroke model. Stroke 2002;33(8):2100–4.
15. Heidenreich JO, Hsu D, Wang G, et al. Magnetic resonance imaging results can affect therapy decisions in hyperacute stroke care. Acta Radiol 2008; 49(5):550–7.
16. Albers GW, Thijs VN, Wechsler L, et al. Magnetic resonance imaging profiles predict clinical response to early reperfusion: the diffusion and perfusion imaging evaluation for understanding stroke evolution (DEFUSE) study. Ann Neurol 2006;60(5): 508–17.
17. Davis SM, Donnan GA, Parsons MW, et al. Effects of alteplase beyond 3 h after stroke in the echoplanar imaging thrombolytic evaluation trial (EPITHET): a placebo-controlled randomised trial. Lancet Neurol 2008;7(4):299–309.
18. Schellinger PD. EPITHET: failed chance or new hope? Lancet Neurol 2008;7(4):286–7.
19. Schellinger PD, Jansen O, Fiebach JB, et al. Feasibility and practicality of MR imaging of stroke in the management of hyperacute cerebral ischemia. AJNR Am J Neuroradiol 2000;21(7): 1184–9.
20. Baron JC, von Kummer R, del Zoppo GJ. Treatment of acute ischemic stroke. Challenging the concept of a rigid and universal time window. Stroke 1995; 26(12):2219–21.
21. Gonzalez RG. Imaging-guided acute ischemic stroke therapy: from "time is brain" to "physiology is brain." AJNR Am J Neuroradiol 2006;27(4): 728–35.
22. Kakuda W, Lansberg MG, Thijs VN, et al. Optimal definition for PWI/DWI mismatch in acute ischemic stroke patients. J Cereb Blood Flow Metab 2008; 28(5):887–91.
23. Cercignani M, Horsfield MA. The physical basis of diffusion-weighted MRI. J Neurol Sci 2001; 186(Suppl 1):S11–4.
24. Stejskal E, Tanner J. Spin diffusion measurements: spin-echoes in the presence of a time-dependent field gradient. J Chem Phys 1965;42(1):288–92.
25. Moseley ME, Kucharczyk J, Mintorovitch J, et al. Diffusion-weighted MR imaging of acute stroke: correlation with T2-weighted and magnetic susceptibility-enhanced MR imaging in cats. AJNR Am J Neuroradiol 1990;11(3):423–9.

26. Moseley ME, Mintorovitch J, Cohen Y, et al. Early detection of ischemic injury: comparison of spectroscopy, diffusion-, T2-, and magnetic susceptibility-weighted MRI in cats. Acta Neurochir Suppl (Wien) 1990;51:207–9.

27. Mintorovitch J, Yang GY, Shimizu H, et al. Diffusion-weighted magnetic resonance imaging of acute focal cerebral ischemia: comparison of signal intensity with changes in brain water and Na+,K(+)-ATPase activity. J Cereb Blood Flow Metab 1994;14(2):332–6.

28. Sevick RJ, Kucharczyk J, Mintorovitch J, et al. Diffusion-weighted MR imaging and T2-weighted MR imaging in acute cerebral ischaemia: comparison and correlation with histopathology. Acta Neurochir Suppl (Wien) 1990;51:210–2.

29. Sevick RJ, Kanda F, Mintorovitch J, et al. Cytotoxic brain edema: assessment with diffusion-weighted MR imaging. Radiology 1992;185(3):687–90.

30. Gass A, Niendorf T, Hirsch JG. Acute and chronic changes of the apparent diffusion coefficient in neurological disorders—biophysical mechanisms and possible underlying histopathology. J Neurol Sci 2001;186(Suppl 1):S15–23.

31. Kidwell CS, Saver JL, Mattiello J, et al. Thrombolytic reversal of acute human cerebral ischemic injury shown by diffusion/perfusion magnetic resonance imaging. Ann Neurol 2000;47(4):462–9.

32. Pereira RS, Harris AD, Sevick RJ, et al. Effect of b value on contrast during diffusion-weighted magnetic resonance imaging assessment of acute ischemic stroke. J Magn Reson Imaging 2002;15(5):591–6.

33. Chen PE, Simon JE, Hill MD, et al. Acute ischemic stroke: accuracy of diffusion-weighted MR imaging—effects of b value and cerebrospinal fluid suppression. Radiology 2006;238(1):232–9.

34. Falconer JC, Narayana PA. Cerebrospinal fluid-suppressed high-resolution diffusion imaging of human brain. Magn Reson Med 1997;37(1):119–23.

35. Latour LL, Warach S. Cerebral spinal fluid contamination of the measurement of the apparent diffusion coefficient of water in acute stroke. Magn Reson Med 2002;48(3):478–86.

36. Simon JE, Czechowsky DK, Hill MD, et al. Fluid-attenuated inversion recovery preparation: not an improvement over conventional diffusion-weighted imaging at 3T in acute ischemic stroke. AJNR Am J Neuroradiol 2004;25(10):1653–8.

37. Bykowski JL, Latour LL, Warach S. More accurate identification of reversible ischemic injury in human stroke by cerebrospinal fluid suppressed diffusion-weighted imaging. Stroke 2004;35(5):1100–6.

38. Kane I, Carpenter T, Chappell F, et al. Comparison of 10 different magnetic resonance perfusion imaging processing methods in acute ischemic stroke: effect on lesion size, proportion of patients with diffusion/perfusion mismatch, clinical scores, and radiologic outcomes. Stroke 2007;38(12):3158–64.

39. Carroll TJ, Teneggi V, Jobin M, et al. Absolute quantification of cerebral blood flow with magnetic resonance, reproducibility of the method, and comparison with H2(15)O positron emission tomography. J Cereb Blood Flow Metab 2002;22(9):1149–56.

40. Ostergaard L, Weisskoff RM, Chesler DA, et al. High resolution measurement of cerebral blood flow using intravascular tracer bolus passages. Part I: mathematical approach and statistical analysis. Magn Reson Med 1996;36(5):715–25.

41. Chen JJ, Smith MR, Frayne R. The impact of partial-volume effects in dynamic susceptibility contrast magnetic resonance perfusion imaging. J Magn Reson Imaging 2005;22(3):390–9.

42. Calamante F, Gadian DG, Connelly A. Delay and dispersion effects in dynamic susceptibility contrast MRI: simulations using singular value decomposition. Magn Reson Med 2000;44(3):466–73.

43. Salluzzi M, Frayne R, Smith MR. Is correction necessary when clinically determining quantitative cerebral perfusion parameters from multi-slice dynamic susceptibility contrast MR studies? Phys Med Biol 2006;51(2):407–24.

44. Smith MR, Lu H, Trochet S, et al. Removing the effect of SVD algorithmic artifacts present in quantitative MR perfusion studies. Magn Reson Med 2004;51(3):631–4.

45. Schellinger PD, Thomalla G, Fiehler J, et al. MRI-based and CT-based thrombolytic therapy in acute stroke within and beyond established time windows: an analysis of 1210 patients. Stroke 2007;38(10):2640–5.

46. Lansberg MG, Thijs VN, Bammer R, et al. Risk factors of symptomatic intracerebral hemorrhage after tPA therapy for acute stroke. Stroke 2007;38(8):2275–8.

47. Singer OC, Humpich MC, Fiehler J, et al. Risk for symptomatic intracerebral hemorrhage after thrombolysis assessed by diffusion-weighted magnetic resonance imaging. Ann Neurol 2008;63(1):52–60.

48. Bristow MS, Simon JE, Brown RA, et al. MR perfusion and diffusion in acute ischemic stroke: human gray and white matter have different thresholds for infarction. J Cereb Blood Flow Metab 2005;25(10):1280–7.

49. Lansberg MG, Thijs VN, Hamilton S, et al. Evaluation of the clinical-diffusion and perfusion-diffusion mismatch models in DEFUSE. Stroke 2007;38(6):1826–30.

50. Rowley HA. Extending the time window for thrombolysis: evidence from acute stroke trials. Neuroimaging Clin N Am 2005;15(3):575–87, x.

51. Parsons MW, Barber PA, Chalk J, et al. Diffusion- and perfusion-weighted MRI response to thrombolysis in stroke. Ann Neurol 2002;51(1):28–37.

52. Butcher KS, Parsons M, MacGregor L, et al. Refining the perfusion-diffusion mismatch hypothesis. Stroke 2005;36(6):1153–9.

53. Sandercock P, Wardlaw J, Dennis M, et al. EPITHET—where next? Lancet Neurol 2008;7(7):570–1 [author reply 571–3].

54. Alexandrov AW. Methodologic challenges in the design and conduct of hyperacute stroke research. AACN Adv Crit Care 2008;19(2):186–201.

55. Higashida RT, Furlan AJ, Roberts H, et al. Trial design and reporting standards for intra-arterial cerebral thrombolysis or acute ischemic stroke. Stroke 2003;34(8):e109–37.

56. Harris AD, Kosior JC, Ryder RC, et al. MRI of ischemic stroke in canines: applications for monitoring intraarterial thrombolysis. J Magn Reson Imaging 2007;26(6):1421–8.

57. Messe SR, Kasner SE, Chalela JA, et al. CT-NIHSS mismatch does not correlate with MRI diffusion-perfusion mismatch. Stroke 2007;38(7):2079–84.

58. Menezes NM, Ay H, Wang Zhu M, et al. The real estate factor: quantifying the impact of infarct location on stroke severity. Stroke 2007;38(1):194–7.

59. Simon JE, Bristow MS, Lu H, et al. A novel method to derive separate gray and white matter cerebral blood flow measures from MR imaging of acute ischemic stroke patients. J Cereb Blood Flow Metab 2005;25(9):1236–43.

60. Fiebach JB, Schellinger PD, Jansen O, et al. CT and diffusion-weighted MR imaging in randomized order: diffusion-weighted imaging results in higher accuracy and lower interrater variability in the diagnosis of hyperacute ischemic stroke. Stroke 2002;33(9):2206–10.

61. Davis DP, Robertson T, Imbesi SG. Diffusion-weighted magnetic resonance imaging versus computed tomography in the diagnosis of acute ischemic stroke. J Emerg Med 2006;31(3):269–77.

62. Coutts SB, Hill MD, Simon JE, et al. Silent ischemia in minor stroke and TIA patients identified on MR imaging. Neurology 2005;65(4):513–7.

63. Ay H, Oliveira-Filho J, Buonanno FS, et al. 'Footprints' of transient ischemic attacks: a diffusion-weighted MRI study. Cerebrovasc Dis 2002;14(3–4):177–86.

64. Crisostomo RA, Garcia MM, Tong DC. Detection of diffusion-weighted MRI abnormalities in patients with transient ischemic attack: correlation with clinical characteristics. Stroke 2003;34(4):932–7.

65. Inatomi Y, Kimura K, Yonehara T, et al. DWI abnormalities and clinical characteristics in TIA patients. Neurology 2004;62(3):376–80.

66. Kidwell CS, Alger JR, Di Salle F, et al. Diffusion MRI in patients with transient ischemic attacks. Stroke 1999;30(6):1174–80.

67. Rovira A, Rovira-Gols A, Pedraza S, et al. Diffusion-weighted MR imaging in the acute phase of transient ischemic attacks. AJNR Am J Neuroradiol 2002;23(1):77–83.

68. Coutts SB, Simon JE, Eliasziw M, et al. Triaging transient ischemic attack and minor stroke patients using acute magnetic resonance imaging. Ann Neurol 2005;57(6):848–54.

69. Prins ND, van Dijk EJ, den Heijer T, et al. Cerebral white matter lesions and the risk of dementia. Arch Neurol 2004;61(10):1531–4.

70. Vermeer SE, Hollander M, van Dijk EJ, et al. Silent brain infarcts and white matter lesions increase stroke risk in the general population: the Rotterdam Scan Study. Stroke 2003;34(5):1126–9.

71. Vermeer SE, Longstreth WT Jr, Koudstaal PJ. Silent brain infarcts: a systematic review. Lancet Neurol 2007;6(7):611–9.

72. Vermeer SE, Prins ND, den Heijer T, et al. Silent brain infarcts and the risk of dementia and cognitive decline. N Engl J Med 2003;348(13):1215–22.

73. Boulanger JM, Coutts SB, Eliasziw M, et al. Diffusion-weighted imaging-negative patients with transient ischemic attack are at risk of recurrent transient events. Stroke 2007;38(8):2367–9.

74. Sylaja PN, Coutts SB, Subramaniam S, et al. Acute ischemic lesions of varying ages predict risk of ischemic events in stroke/TIA patients. Neurology 2007;68(6):415–9.

75. Ay H, Koroshetz WJ, Benner T, et al. Transient ischemic attack with infarction: a unique syndrome? Ann Neurol 2005;57(5):679–86.

76. Prabhakaran S, Chong JY, Sacco RL. Impact of abnormal diffusion-weighted imaging results on short-term outcome following transient ischemic attack. Arch Neurol 2007;64(8):1105–9.

77. Purroy F, Montaner J, Rovira A, et al. Higher risk of further vascular events among transient ischemic attack patients with diffusion-weighted imaging acute ischemic lesions. Stroke 2004;35(10):2313–9.

78. Redgrave JN, Coutts SB, Schulz UG, et al. Systematic review of associations between the presence of acute ischemic lesions on diffusion-weighted imaging and clinical predictors of early stroke risk after transient ischemic attack. Stroke 2007;38(5):1482–8.

79. Calanchini PR, Swanson PD, Gotshall RA, et al. Cooperative study of hospital frequency and character of transient ischemic attacks. IV. The reliability of diagnosis. JAMA 1977;238(19):2029–33.

80. Johnston SC, Sidney S, Bernstein AL, et al. A comparison of risk factors for recurrent TIA and stroke in patients diagnosed with TIA. Neurology 2003;60(2):280–5.

81. Rajajee V, Kidwell C, Starkman S, et al. Diagnosis of lacunar infarcts within 6 hours of onset by clinical and CT criteria versus MRI. J Neuroimaging 2008;18(1):66–72.

82. Oppenheim C, Lamy C, Touze E, et al. Do transient ischemic attacks with diffusion-weighted imaging abnormalities correspond to brain infarctions? AJNR Am J Neuroradiol 2006;27(8):1782–7.

83. Krol AL, Coutts SB, Simon JE, et al. Perfusion MRI abnormalities in speech or motor transient ischemic attack patients. Stroke 2005;36(11):2487–9.

84. Flossmann E, Redgrave JN, Briley D, et al. Reliability of clinical diagnosis of the symptomatic vascular territory in patients with recent transient ischemic attack or minor stroke. Stroke 2008;39(9):2457–60.

85. Coutts SB, Hill MD, Campos CR, et al. Recurrent events in transient ischemic attack and minor stroke: what events are happening and to which patients? Stroke 2008;39(9):2461–6.

86. Lee LJ, Kidwell CS, Alger J, et al. Impact on stroke subtype diagnosis of early diffusion-weighted magnetic resonance imaging and magnetic resonance angiography. Stroke 2000;31(5):1081–9.

87. Wessels T, Wessels C, Ellsiepen A, et al. Contribution of diffusion-weighted imaging in determination of stroke etiology. AJNR Am J Neuroradiol 2006;27(1):35–9.

88. Restrepo L, Jacobs MA, Barker PB, et al. Etiology of perfusion-diffusion magnetic resonance imaging mismatch patterns. J Neuroimaging 2005;15(3):254–60.

Arterial Spin-Labeled MR Perfusion Imaging: Clinical Applications

Jeffrey M. Pollock, MD[a,b,*], Huan Tan, MS[c], Robert A. Kraft, PhD[c], Christopher T. Whitlow, MD, PhD[a], Jonathan H. Burdette, MD[a], Joseph A. Maldjian, MD[a]

KEYWORDS

- Arterial spin-labeled MR imaging
- Perfusion • Applications • Stroke imaging
- Arterial spin labeling • Pulsed arterial spin labeling

Wake Forest University School of Medicine has implemented an automated processing pipeline capable of handling a substantial clinical volume of perfusion acquisitions. During the past 2 years, more than 10,000 clinical arterial spin-labeled (ASL) examinations have been performed. These cases have revealed many pathologic and physiologic processes readily identified with quantitative perfusion imaging.[1–11]

ASL perfusion MR imaging was conceived more than 15 years ago.[12–14] Since that time the technique has existed largely in the research realm because of the complex postprocessing requirements. Many research studies have demonstrated the potential clinical utility of the sequence, but until now a large-scale clinical implementation has not been achieved.[1–8] The perfusion sequence offers several benefits over traditional contrast bolus techniques. First, ASL requires no gadolinium-based contrast agent. Because of the fear of nephrogenic systemic fibrosis, the acquisition of perfusion data in a clinical population containing patients who have chronic renal failure has been problematic and has caused great consternation for radiologists developing study protocols.[15] ASL allows the acquisition of perfusion data without this concern. Acquiring perfusion data with bolus techniques has also been problematic in young children because of the need for intravenous access. Because contrast is not needed for the routine examination, ASL avoids the need for a needle stick in a sleeping baby.

The second major benefit of ASL, as compared with conventional bolus techniques, is that ASL can be quantitative.[16] Most of the available perfusion techniques are qualitative, showing relative changes in cerebral blood volume (CBV), cerebral blood flow (CBF), and mean transit time.[17] Quantification allows regional and global assessments of cerebral perfusion. It is inherently difficult to reveal global hypo- or hyperperfusion with relative perfusion techniques. Absolute quantification allows easy recognition of states such as hypercapnia or diffuse hypoxic/anoxic injury. Regional assessments of cerebral perfusion allow easy comparisons between pre- and posttreatment states in patients undergoing chemotherapy, endarterectomy, thrombolysis, or therapy for migraines or

This work was supported by the Human Brain Project and the National Institute of Biomedical Imaging and Bioengineering through Grants EB004673 and EB004673-02S2. This work also was supported in part by the Center for Biomolecular Imaging of Wake Forest University School of Medicine.

a Department of Radiology, Wake Forest University School of Medicine, Medical Center Boulevard, Winston--Salem, NC 27157, USA
b Department of Radiology, Oregon Health and Science University, 3181 S.W. Sam Jackson Park Road, Portland, OR 97239, USA
c Department of Biomedical Engineering, Wake Forest University, Medical Center Boulevard, Winston-Salem, NC 27157, USA
* Corresponding author.
E-mail address: jeffmpollock@gmail.com (J.M. Pollock).

Magn Reson Imaging Clin N Am 17 (2009) 315–338
doi:10.1016/j.mric.2009.01.008

seizures. A growing body of evidence also indicates that perfusion values can be correlated with the histologic grade of neoplasms.[18,19]

During the last 15 years, refinements in scanner technology and computer processing capabilities have allowed automation of the necessary postprocessing. During that time, teams of researchers worked to improve the robustness of the sequence, acquisition time, and resolution and to reduce the known technical failures and artifacts.[20,21] Individual vendors have developed various versions of ASL, which can vary significantly in the techniques employed.

TECHNICAL CONSIDERATIONS

Understanding and interpreting the clinical applications of ASL requires some basic knowledge of the technical parameters of the sequence. In general, ASL is based on "labeling" protons in the blood in the supplying vessels outside the imaging plane, waiting for a period of time known as the "postlabeling delay" (PLD) for the labeled blood to reach the parenchyma, and then imaging the parenchyma in the labeled and control (ie, unlabeled) state. The width and location of the labeling plane varies depending on the ASL implementation, as discussed in greater detail in later sections.

Subtraction of the labeled images from the control images eliminates the static tissue signal from the parenchyma. The remaining signal is a relative measure of the perfusion. The difference between the control and the labeled images yields a signal proportional to the local CBF and can be sensitized to specific tissue perfusion.[12] The signal difference usually is a fraction (1%–2%) of the tissue signal and depends on many parameters, such as flow rate, T1 of the blood and tissue, and transit time for blood to travel from the tagging region to the imaging plane. Multiple control and label images are acquired to ensure sufficient signal-to-noise ratio (SNR) for diagnostic review. An absolute quantitative perfusion map can be obtained using the General Kinetic Model developed by Buxton and colleagues.[22]

ASL images are acquired with MR imaging pulse sequences that have two distinct and independent components, a preparation component and an acquisition component. The preparation component labels the inflowing blood in different magnetic states for the control and labeled images. Once the blood has been labeled, the acquisition component acquires the data. The acquisition component typically uses a fast acquisition method such as spiral or echo planar imaging (EPI). The distinct and independent nature of the preparation and acquisition components

has allowed researchers to choose the combination best suited for their specific application.

Currently there are four types of ASL preparation components, pulsed ASL (PASL), continuous ASL (CASL), pseudocontinuous ASL (PCASL), and velocity-selective ASL (VS-ASL). These four ASL methods were developed to address the limitations and technical challenges encountered in the early implementations of ASL techniques and differ primarily in the technique that magnetically tags the inflowing blood.

PASL uses short (5- to 2-millisecond) radiofrequency (RF) pulses to invert a thick slab of spins in the tagging plane proximal to the imaging region.[23] Original PASL methods such as flow-sensitive alternating inversion recovery (FAIR),[24] proximal inversion with control for off-resonance effects,[25] and echo-planar imaging and signal targeting with alternating radio frequency[23] used a single inversion pulse during the preparation component to label the spins magnetically. These methods differ in the location of the labeling plane and the choice of the magnetically labeled state of the blood for the control and labeled images. These techniques were refined when adiabatic hyperbolic secant (AHS) RF pulses, which are insensitive to B1 field inhomogeneity, were used to improve inversion efficiency.[23,24] Further improvements in the slice profile of the labeling plane were achieved with Frequency Offset Correction Inversion AHS RF pulses.[26] Although PASL techniques have a higher inversion efficiency and lower RF power deposition than CASL, a limitation of PASL was the poorly defined distal edge of the labeling plane, which introduces a systematic bias to the CBF quantification. This limitation was overcome with quantitative imaging of perfusion using a single subtraction (QUIPPS) and QUIPPS II with thin-slice TI1 periodic saturation[17,26] techniques that apply a saturation pulse at a specified time after the inversion pulse to define sharply the labeling plane's distal edge, thereby eliminating the systematic bias.

CASL uses long and continuous RF pulses (1–2 seconds) along with a constant gradient field to induce a flow-driven adiabatic inversion in a narrow plane of spins, usually just below the imaging plane.[27,28] The spins within a physiologic range of velocities traveling perpendicular through the tagging region can be inverted by adjusting the amplitudes of the gradients and the RF pulse through a phenomenon known as flow-driven adiabatic inversion.[14] In CASL the spins are inverted continuously as they pass through the tagging plane, resulting in higher perfusion sensitivity than obtained with PASL. Although higher perfusion sensitivity is desirable, CASL has several drawbacks that have limited its widespread acceptance. The primary limitation of CASL is the need for continuous RF transmitting hardware, which is not commonly available on commercial clinical scanners. Unless special precautions are taken, the long RF pulses used in CASL deposit large amounts of RF energy into the patient; this can exceed the Food and Drug Administration guidelines for RF power deposition, also known as the "specific absorption rate" (SAR).[29] Magnetization transfer (MT) effects also are a drawback of CASL, requiring a second inversion to accomplish the control state. Higher RF power deposition and MT effects associated with CASL can be overcome by using a separate small RF surface coil for labeling the blood as it flows through the carotid arteries.[9,30,31] The need for additional hardware restricts this solution to a small number of research sites. Another disadvantage of CASL is that the average inversion efficiency of CASL is lower (80%–95%) than that of PASL (95%).[30,31] The closer inversion to the imaging plane minimizes the loss of perfusion signal caused by T1 relaxation, however, and compensates for the lower inversion efficiency.

PCASL was introduced to match the inversion efficiency of CASL while reducing the RF power deposition. First developed by Garcia and colleagues,[32] PCASL uses a train of discrete RF pulses in conjunction with a synchronous gradient field to mimic the flow-driven adiabatic inversion seen in CASL without the need for special hardware. This technique provides a better balance between tagging efficiency and SNR, as well as reducing MT effects and RF power deposition compared with CASL methods. Depending on the implementation, PCASL is susceptible to B0 inhomogeneity and eddy currents.[30]

PASL, CASL, and pCASL invert the inflowing blood at a specific location. VS-ASL saturates the blood that is moving at a faster velocity than the specified cutoff value to achieve perfusion contrast. In theory, this technique results in a smaller and more uniform transit delay for the delivery of blood to the target tissue and allows quantitative measurements of CBF under slow and collateral flow conditions (eg, in patients who have experienced stroke).[33] Disadvantages of VS-ASL include lower SNR and difficulty in determining the optimal cutoff velocity. Inappropriate values of cutoff velocity result in incorrect local perfusion information and produce image artifacts. **Table 1** summarizes the advantages and disadvantages of each method.

Once the blood has been labeled in the preparation component of the ASL sequence, the acquisition component acquires the images. ASL images have been acquired conventionally with EPI in the Cartesian trajectory because of the fast acquisition speed and simple reconstruction. Because of relaxation, echo time (TE) plays an important role in perfusion sensitivity. A spiral trajectory can be used to achieve optimal TE to improve SNR further. In addition, suppression of the static tissue signal is an effective way to improve signal stability and reduce imaging noise.[32,34,35] There are many implementations of ASL techniques; the interested reader may refer to recent ASL reviews for detailed explanations.[29,36,37]

Regardless of the method used, one of the most significant factors in the appearance of the perfusion image is the presence or absence of additional crusher gradients during the acquisition component (**Table 2**). Ideally, all the signal imparted to the protons would be deposited in the tissues by the time the parenchyma is imaged; frequently, however, residual tagged signal remains within the vasculature. Including the vascular signal would give artificially high measurements when trying to quantify perfusion. By applying bipolar gradients

Table 1
Advantages and disadvantages of different ASL methods

ASL Types	Advantages	Disadvantages
PASL	Higher tagging efficiency Lower SAR Improved transit time effects	Lower SNR Increased transit delay
CASL	Higher SNR than PASL Shorter transit delay	Lower tagging efficiency Continuous RF transmit hardware required Higher SAR Magnetization transfer effects
PCASL	Higher SNR than PASL Higher tagging efficiency than CASL Improved transit time effects	Higher SAR Limited clinical availability
VS-ASL	Ability to measure low flow	Lower SNR

Table 2
The effects of bipolar crusher gradients on clinical ASL imaging

With/Without Crusher Gradient	Benefits	Limitations	AVM	Very Slow Flow	Stroke Imaging	Physiologic Imaging
Crusher gradient applied	Allows quantitative perfusion imaging	Decreased overall available signal	Allows quantification of the steal phenomena	CBF map will resemble transit time map	Perfusion will be underestimated.	Global perfusion changes can be assessed
No crusher gradient	Increased available signal	Perfusion imaging is qualitative	Allows visualization of the A-V shunting	High signal will be in the affected territory	Perfusion will be overestimated	Relative regional perfusion changes can be assessed

before imaging the parenchyma, it is possible to suppress the moving signal that is within the vasculature. The benefit of crusher gradients is that they allow quantification by suppressing the intravascular signal. Because ASL has inherently low SNR, however, removing any signal from the image, even if it is in the vessel, can lower the apparent quality of the perfusion image.[1] The presence or absence of crusher gradients also significantly impacts the appearance of vascular pathologies, such as slow-flow states associated with infarction, or high-flow states associated with arteriovenous malformations (AVM) (Fig. 1).[38]

In ASL, the usual procedure of placing a tag, delaying for tissue deposition, and then imaging introduces significant importance to the length

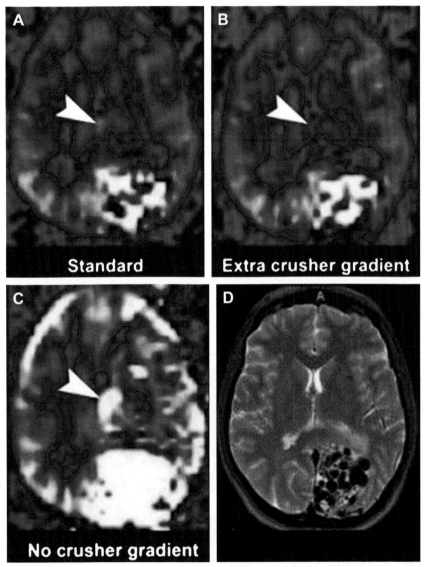

Fig. 1. The effect of bipolar gradients on PASL. (A) Standard bipolar gradients, (B) additional gradient directions, and (C) no bipolar gradients were used in a patient who had a large left occipital arteriovenous malformation (AVM). (D) Large flow voids are seen on the T2 image. The absence of bipolar gradients results in visualization of the intravascular signal, resulting in a brighter image. Without intravascular suppression (C), the entire AVM lesion, including the draining veins (*arrowhead*), is seen. With standard intravascular signal suppression (A), the intensity of the AVM's signal and that of the draining veins (*arrowhead*) are reduced significantly. With additional gradients (B), the AVM signal intensity is reduced further, and the signal in the draining vein is eliminated (*arrowhead*).

of the PLD in the sequence. The PLD, known as the inversion time in the PASL sequence, significantly affects the CBF perfusion map, especially when bipolar crusher gradients are used. With a very short PLD, in which the blood has not had sufficient time to reach the parenchyma, the perfusion signal is low. A shorter PLD allows a shorter acquisition time, but the perfusion image may not represent the cerebral perfusion accurately, because there has not been enough time for tissue exchange in the territories with slower flow. The moving intravascular signal then is crushed, resulting in an image that overestimates perfusion defects and shows watershed territories as having significantly diminished perfusion.[1] At longer PLD, there is more time for the tag to be deposited in the tissue, leading to a more accurate global assessment of cerebral perfusion. Images in general appear more homogenous. Drawbacks of longer delays include longer acquisition time and less available signal at the time of imaging because of T1 relaxation. Unfortunately, there is no perfect mean between the two extremes.

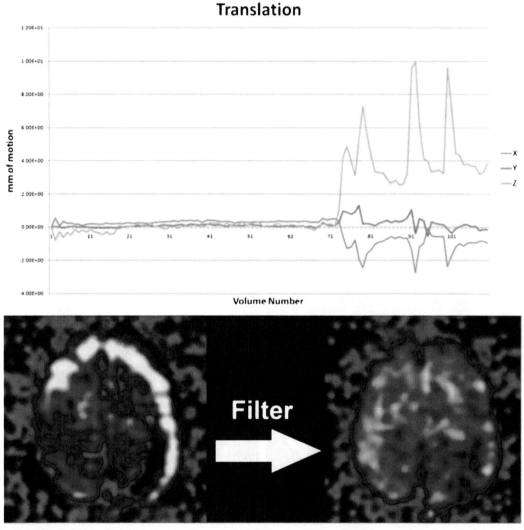

Fig. 2. Motion during the ASL examination can result in significant signal loss and a characteristic ring of increased signal because ASL is based on subtraction of one from the other of the control and labeled image pairs. PASL filtering can reduce these artifacts significantly by discarding image pairs with significant motion. (*Top*) The graph shows translational motion during the examination, which had four large spikes towards the end of the examination. (*Bottom left*) This motion manifests on imaging as the ring of high signal intensity at the periphery of the cerebral cortex. (*Bottom right*) Filtering discards the image pairs associated with the motion spikes, resulting in an image without artifact.

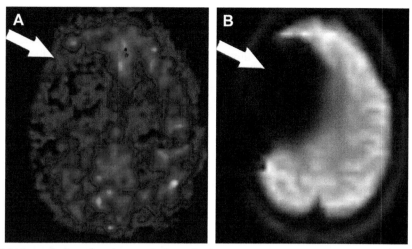

Fig. 3. (*A*) CBF PASL perfusion map shows a large right frontal region of hypoperfusion (*arrow*). This apparent perfusion defect is an artifact secondary to the craniotomy clips. (*B*) The susceptibility artifact (*arrow*) is demonstrated on the baseline magnetization echoplanar image.

The optimal PLD depends on the age and health of the patient. Imagers must find the balance that satisfies the imaging needs based on the clinical population. Regardless of the PLD selected, one should become familiar with the normal age-related appearance of the pulse sequence before declaring a perfusion pattern to be pathologic.[1]

Quantification Versus Qualification

The subtraction of the control and labeled image pairs yields signal differences that reflect the

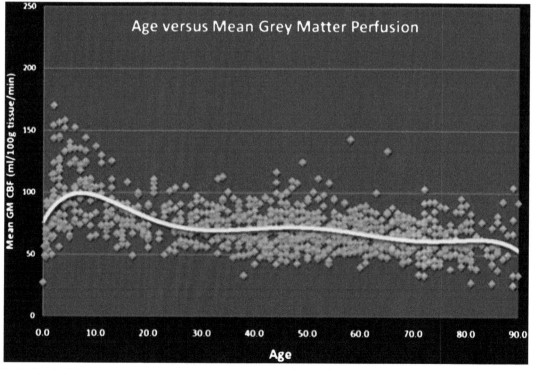

Fig. 4. Graph plots age in years versus mean gray matter perfusion for 959 normal patients imaged with PASL. Perfusion values peak in the 5- to 15-year-old range and then decrease quickly to age 30 years, after which a slow progressive decline is observed.

relative perfusion of the parenchyma. These relative perfusion maps are easily attainable but still reflect the choice of inversion time (delay), slice thickness, and presence of bipolar crusher gradients. To quantify cerebral perfusion, the following equation[13] must be solved:

$$CBF = \frac{\Delta M(TI_2)}{2M_{0,blood}\alpha TI_1 q_p\left(T_{1,tissue},T_{1,blood},TI_2\right)}e^{\left(\frac{TI_2}{T_{1,blood}}\right)}$$

where CBF is the cerebral blood flow, $\Delta M(TI_2)$ is the mean difference in the signal intensity between the labeled and control images, $M_{0,blood}$ is the equilibrium magnetization of blood, α is the tagging efficiency, TI_1 is the time duration of the tagging bolus, TI_2 is the inversion time of each slice, $T_{1,blood}$ is the longitudinal relaxation time of blood, and q_p is a correction factor that accounts for the difference between the T1 of blood and the T1 of brain tissue.[20] Several variables, such as the T1 of tissue, are measured directly and then introduced into the equation. Other variables used in the equation represent standard values taken from the published literature. Ideally, all the variables would be obtained de novo in each patient, but doing so is not possible in some cases and is not practical in others. These assumptions can introduce errors into the quantification. Most

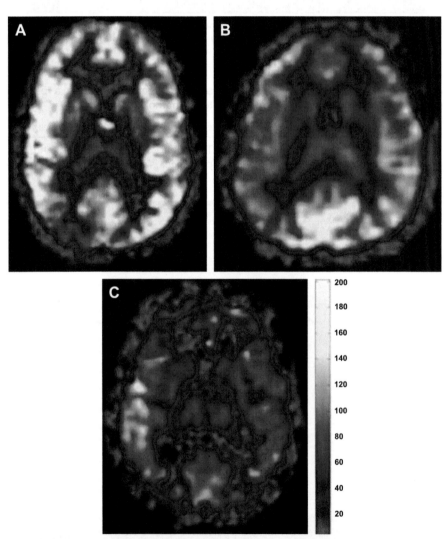

Fig. 5. (A) Normal physiologic pediatric hyperperfusion in a 10-year-old patient. Mean GM CBF = 94 mL/100 g tissue/minute. (B) Normal PASL cerebral perfusion in a 40-year-old patient. Mean GM CBF = 70 mL/100 g tissue/minute. (C) Normal cerebral perfusion in an 80-year-old patient. Note the areas of apparent hypoperfusion in the anterior and posterior watershed territories. Such areas are encountered frequently and reflect the increasingly slow transit times in the elderly. Mean GM CBF = 49 mL/100 g tissue/minute.

important are the T1 values of blood and tissue. The T1 of blood increases as hematocrit increases.[39–41] If standard published values for the T1 of blood are used in solving the equation for a severely anemic patient, quantification errors of 10% to 15% can result.[5,39,41] Fortunately, the T1 of tissue can be measured using Look-Locker techniques, but doing so adds time and complexity: the T1 data must be computed on a voxelwise basis, and then those T1 values are used to calculate CBF values. Understanding the influence and variables in the CBF quantification equation yields more accurate interpretations of the quantified CBF values.[42]

ARTIFACTS

A few frequently encountered artifacts in the clinical population must be addressed before the clinical applications of ASL are discussd.[1] Familiarity with these artifacts facilitates interpretation and allows the radiologist to be proactive in problem solving. Unlike graduate students who often volunteer to be subjects for MR sequence testing, clinical patients frequently move during scanning. Even the most subtle head or respiratory motion can impact the quality of the ASL image significantly, given the subtraction technique that is employed. At the Wake Forest University School

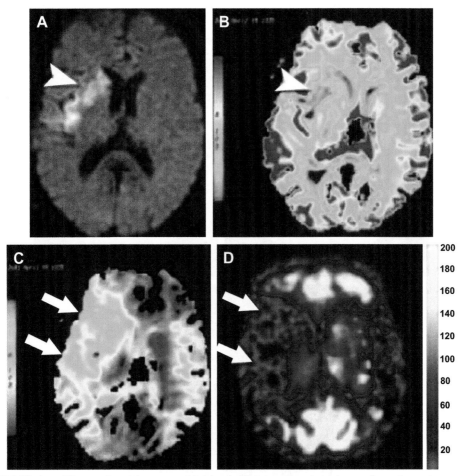

Fig. 6. (A) Diffusion, (B) negative enhancement integral, (C) mean time to enhance from dynamic susceptibility contrast perfusion imaging, and (D) PASL perfusion imaging in a patient who has a proximal right middle cerebral artery occlusion. (A) Diffusion restriction is seen the right basal ganglia and insular cortex (arrowhead). (B) The diffusion restriction corresponds to decreases in blood volume (blue areas, arrowhead) seen on the negative enhancement integral. (C) The mean time to enhance shows a much larger region of at-risk tissue (green area, arrows,) surrounding the core infarct. (D) PASL shows a similar region of hypoperfusion (arrows) corresponding to the defect on the mean time to enhance map. PASL perfusion imaging cannot distinguish small perfusion differences below 20 mL/100 g/minute, so infarction resembles at-risk tissue. In these low-flow situations, the PASL perfusion defect is comparable to the mean time to enhance rather than reflecting true CBF.

of Medicine, a filter has been developed that detects and discards bad subtraction pairs related to large movements or transient hardware gradient malfunctions.[43] This filter has improved the quality of scans markedly, but it is significantly more difficult to identify motion-corrupted data when a patient moves throughout the scan continuously. Vendors probably will employ similar techniques to filter the data and apply motion correction in future iterations of ASL. Despite these efforts, motion is the single most commonly seen artifact in the clinical population (Fig. 2).

Another commonly seen artifact is susceptibility. The ASL sequence frequently uses EPI because of the need for rapid acquisition. The disadvantage of EPI is the prevalence of susceptibility artifacts around surgical hardware, craniotomy sites, hemorrhages, calcifications, and the paranasal sinuses. The susceptibility effects create artifactual defects in the perfusion imaging that can be easily misinterpreted as pathology (Fig. 3). For example, the susceptibility associated with the paranasal sinus limits the utility of ASL in the medial temporal lobes and skull base.[1]

CLINICAL APPLICATIONS

To interpret pathology on ASL, the radiologist must have an understanding of normal ASL images. If quantitative techniques are used with the sequence, marked age-dependent variability is seen. Pediatric patients in the 5- to 15-year-old range have some of the highest perfusion

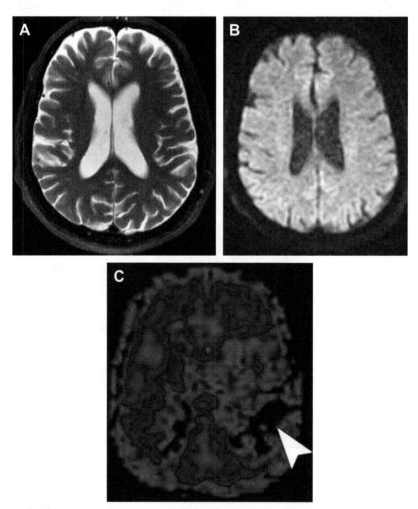

Fig. 7. Tissue at risk. This 70-year-old man presented with transient ischemic attacks involving the right-sided extremities. (A) T2 and (B) diffusion were normal except for mild diffuse cerebral atrophy. (C) PASL CBF map revealed significant hypoperfusion in the left frontal and parietal hemisphere. The patient had a follow-up CT angiography showing a high-grade stenosis of the left internal carotid artery that was corrected surgically without further clinical sequelae.

values for gray matter.[44–46] After approximately age 30 years, there is a gradual decline in gray mater perfusion (**Fig. 4**). Furthermore, if bipolar crusher gradients are used in elderly patients, the anterior and posterior watershed territories frequently appear more hypoperfused because of the prolonged transit times in these regions (**Fig. 5A–C**). If one alters the sequence to prolong the inversion time, the apparent hypoperfusion caused by transit time delay can be improved.

Cerebral Infarction

One of the most frequent applications of any perfusion technique is the evaluation of cerebral infarction. In comparison with bolus techniques, standard ASL provides only CBF.[47] Cerebral infarction typically has been defined as a CBF below which neuronal metabolism ceases. In clinical practice, however, measurement of the blood volume and transit time with perfusion imaging has supplanted the CBF concept. This change is a practical consequence of the current techniques, because accurate CBF data are notoriously difficult to obtain from bolus perfusion studies. Transit time typically depicts the tissue at risk, whereas volume shows the area of infarction. The difference between these two values defines the presence or absence of the penumbra.[48] Currently, ASL measures only CBF, although some promising techniques for generating transit time data are on the horizon.[49,50] The lack of blood volume or transit time parameters changes the interpretation of perfusion data generated by ASL.[2] The authors' unpublished experience with concomitant ASL

and dynamic susceptibility contrast perfusion imaging in patients who have suffered stroke is that the ASL CBF defect most closely corresponds to the transit time defect (**Fig. 6**). When vascular territories are affected by a significant stenosis or occlusion so that perfusion decreases below 15–20 mL/100 g tissue/minute, the associated diminution in ASL signal makes it difficult to resolve CBF values accurately. This limitation unfortunately is near the threshold of resolution for distinguishing a penumbra from an infarct. Thus, in the setting of an infarct, the ASL CBF map should be interpreted as showing the tissue at risk if bipolar crusher gradients are used. Traditional diffusion sequences can be used to demonstrate the area of infarction, with the difference between the diffusion abnormality and the ASL-imaged CBF defect representing the penumbra. Future applications of ASL using dynamic acquisitions at multiple inversion times may be able to generate arrival time parameters in addition to CBF.[51]

One significant benefit of incorporating perfusion into all cerebral imaging protocols is the detection of significant perfusion defects before they manifest clinically as infarctions. Large perfusion defects that cannot be explained as artifactual should warrant further investigations with MR or CT angiography. The authors have identified several patients, imaged for a variety of indications, demonstrating normal clinical imaging but a large perfusion defect on ASL imaging. In many of these patients, follow-up MR, CT, or conventional angiography demonstrated high-grade proximal stenotic lesions amenable to treatment to prevent future ischemic events (**Fig. 7**).

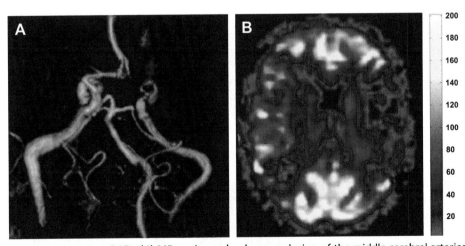

Fig. 8. Moya-moya pattern on PASL. (*A*) MR angiography shows occlusion of the middle cerebral arteries bilaterally and also suggests the presence of extensive small vessel collaterals in the basal ganglia. (*B*) PASL CBF map shows bilateral hypoperfusion in the territories of the middle cerebral arteries. The perfusion reflects the marked transit time delay caused by the suppression of the intravascular signal. The perfusion in the affected territories is underestimated.

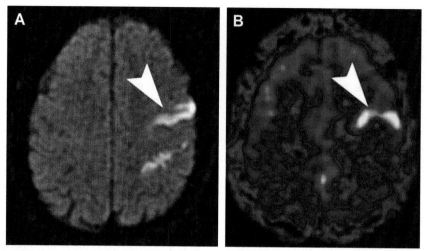

Fig. 9. Diffusion (*A*) shows a linear area of high signal (*arrowhead*) corresponding to a linear area of hyperperfusion (*arrowhead*) on PASL with a bipolar crusher gradient employed (*B*). This pattern of hyperperfusion can be seen when there has been lysis of the thrombus and local autoregulatory dysfunction. A similar appearance can be seen if bipolar crusher gradients are not used, and there is slow flow in the region of infarction.

Perfusion Patters in Stroke with Arterial Spin Labeling

Three different patterns of cerebral perfusion associated with cerebral infarction[2] can be seen based primarily on the use of bipolar crusher gradients to suppress intravascular signal. In patients who have very slow flow but not complete occlusion, the ASL tag may be suppressed in the vessels at the time of crusher gradient application before deposition in tissue. Any prolonged transit time delay results in a CBF perfusion defect corresponding to that delay. The resulting CBF map corresponds very closely to a transit time map (see **Fig. 6**).

The extreme case of slow transit time exists with a Moya-Moya pattern of cerebral perfusion. Moya-Moya is associated with prolonged stenosis resulting in marked development of collateral vessels. Transit time is increased significantly in the small perforating vessels of the basal ganglia and in leptomeningeal collaterals. This increased transit time manifests as large areas devoid of CBF when ASL is used with crusher gradients, because much of the tag remains in the intravascular compartment

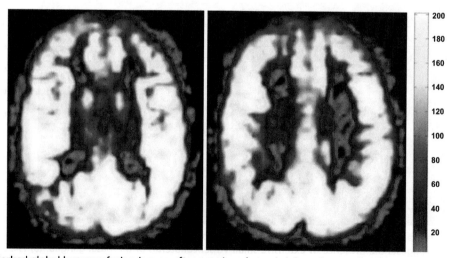

Fig. 10. Marked global hyperperfusion is seen after anoxic or hypoxic injury. Conventional sequences (not shown) revealed characteristic diffusion restriction in the basal ganglia and cortex. Mean GM CBF = 190 mL/100 g/minute.

and subsequently is suppressed. Although these patients frequently have multiple infarctions, the regions devoid of CBF frequently appear normal on conventional sequences. This discordant finding between perfusion and conventional images should not be misinterpreted as true lack of CBF (Fig. 8).

The second pattern is encountered when crusher gradients are not used, and there is very slow flow. In this setting, the intravascular signal is not suppressed, and the vessels are visualized. On the CBF map, this nonsuppressed, very slow flow has the appearance of linear areas of high signal along the cortical margins and affected vessels. This pattern reflects an overestimation of CBF; depending on the degree of stenosis, the resulting map more closely corresponds to a mix between CBV and transit time.[52]

The third pattern encountered with cerebral infarction is hyperperfusion. Occasionally thrombotic or embolic infarctions autolyse or lyse with intravenous or intra-arterial thrombolytic administration. If blood flow is restored to the area of ischemia, the local autoregulatory vasoconstrictive mechanisms may not be able to compensate, resulting in localized vasodilatation. This pattern manifests on ASL as regional areas of hyperperfusion corresponding to the regions of diffusion abnormality (Fig. 9).[2]

The extreme form of this hyperperfusion in the setting of stroke is seen with anoxic or hypoxic ischemic injury. In a retrospective case series using quantitative ASL CBF maps, anoxic patients demonstrated significant global hyperperfusion compared with the control group (Fig. 10).[2,6] A global loss of autoregulation likely resulted in diffuse vasodilatation and hyperperfusion in those cases. Not all cases of global hyperperfusion are secondary to anoxic injury, however. Global hyperperfusion also can be seen in other

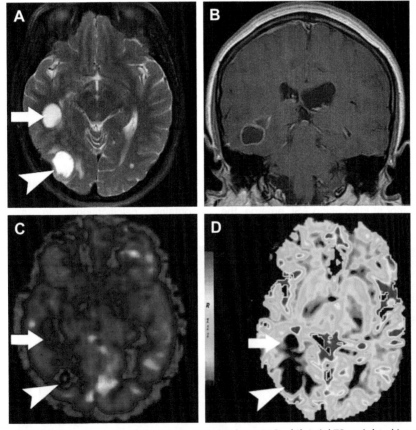

Fig. 11. Hypoperfused cystic non-small cell carcinoma metastasis on PASL. (A) Axial T2-weighted image shows two large hyperintense cystic lesions (arrow and arrowhead) with minimal surrounding vasogenic edema. (B) Postcontrast coronal image shows smooth ring enhancement of the more anterior lesion. (C) PASL CBF map shows both lesions (arrow and arrowhead) to be significantly hypoperfused relative to gray matter. The more anterior lesion (arrow) is centered within the white matter and is less distinct on PASL. (D) Negative enhancement integral from a dynamic susceptibility contrast perfusion study shows decreased blood volume in both the cystic masses (arrow and arrowhead).

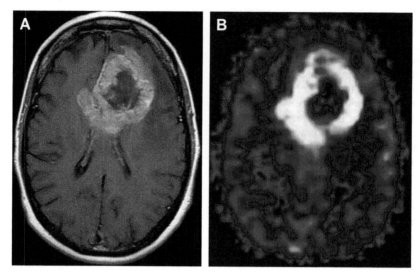

Fig. 12. (A) Glioblastoma multiforme. A large irregular ring-enhancing mass is seen in the left frontal lobe on the postcontrast image. (B) The PASL CBF map shows marked hyperperfusion corresponding to the ring-enhancing portion of the tumor and central hypoperfusion corresponding to the central necrotic areas.

circumstances, including in normal pediatric patients and in patients who have hypercapnia.

Tumor Evaluation

ASL perfusion maps frequently are used to evaluate an intra- or extra-axial neoplastic process. A growing body of research has shown that tumor grade frequently correlates with various perfusion parameters.[19,53,54,55] Most of the studies have reported CBV measurements based on contrast bolus techniques. The ASL CBF perfusion data in a tumor are affected by both transit time and blood volume. As tumor studies using ASL emerge, the

relationship between CBF and tumor grade will be defined better.

Hypoperfusion

Hypoperfused tumors on ASL frequently are cystic or are a lower histologic grade (Fig. 11).[53] There are, however, several factors other than histologic grade that can affect the ASL signal, and several questions must be considered before concluding that a tumor is hypoperfused and, therefore, of low histologic grade. First, it must be determined if the tumor has hemorrhaged, if it is cystic, or if it contains calcifications. In any of these

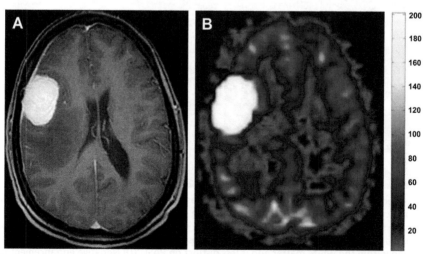

Fig. 13. (A) Meningioma. Axial postcontrast image shows a dural-based mass with avid homogenous enhancement and associated enhancing dural tail. (B) PASL CBF map shows dramatic characteristic hyperperfusion.

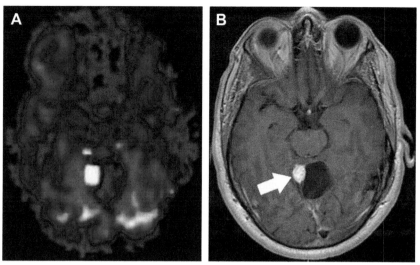

Fig. 14. Hemangioblastoma. (*A*) PASL CBF map shows an intensely hyperperfused posterior fossa nodule adjacent to a hypoperfused cyst. (*B*) Postcontrast T-1 imaging shows the intensely enhancing mural nodule and cyst (*arrow*).

circumstances, the ASL signal may be artificially low. If the patient already has had surgery, and metallic craniotomy clips were used, large artificial perfusion defects may mask an underlying recurrent or primary neoplasm. Finally high-grade neoplasms frequently are heterogeneous and may have central necrosis. CBF in these necrotic regions is characteristically low, but the rim of the mass typically is hyperperfused or similar to gray matter. Therefore, when measuring the mean perfusion of the tumor with ASL, it is very important to know which portion of the tumor was evaluated.

Hyperperfusion

Recent studies have shown that for most PASL imaging applications with malignant neoplasms, the higher the perfusion of the mass, the higher the histologic grade (**Fig. 12**).[19,53,54,55] Not all hyperperfused masses are high grade, however. Meningiomas are among the hyperperfused lesions most frequently encountered in clinical practice (**Fig. 13**). The hypervascularity of these lesions is known to correlate with the typical prolonged angiographic blush during contrast administration. The enhancing mural nodule of

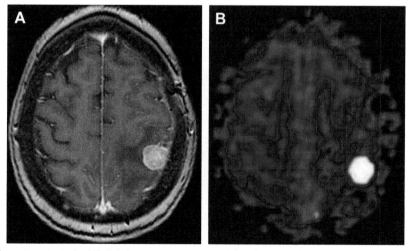

Fig. 15. Solid breast metastasis. (*A*) Axial postcontrast T1-weighted image shows a solid enhancing focus in the posterior left frontal lobe with surrounding vasogenic edema. (*B*) PASL CBF map shows an intensely hyperperfused focus.

neoplasms, such as hemangioblastomas, are some of the most highly perfused lesions the authors have encountered (**Fig. 14**). Metastatic lesions that are solid tend to be hyperperfused (**Fig. 15**); neoplasms that are cystic tend to be hypoperfused (see **Fig. 11**). As future studies are performed on different tumor subtypes and grades, it is likely that guidelines will emerge that can help differentiate between these lesions. Hyperperfusion has relatively high positive predictive value in diagnosing a neoplasm, and the absence of hyperperfusion may have significant negative predictive value for excluding the presence of a neoplasm. When trying to distinguish malignant high-grade tumors from infection or abscess, the perfusion characteristics of the lesion frequently are complementary to conventional sequences. If a lesion appears highly malignant, but the perfusion appears low, then the lesion may contain some intrinsic component, such as blood or calcium, that causes artifactual hypoperfusion. Alternatively, if no such confounding technical factors are identified, the nature of the lesion might need to be reconsidered.

Infectious Etiologies

Occasionally the imaging appearance of CNS infection can be confused with a neoplastic process. In the authors' experience with PASL, most infections demonstrate hypoperfusion (**Fig. 16**), but infectious conditions also can present with hyperperfusion. Cortical

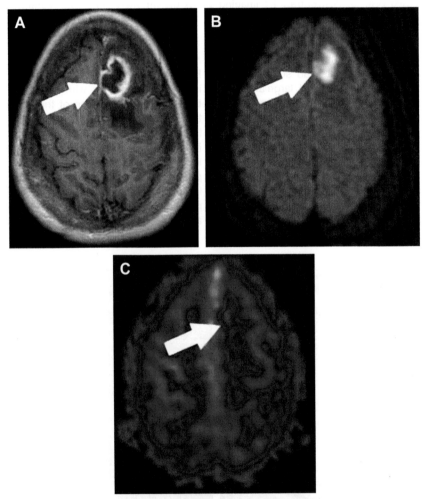

Fig. 16. Pyogenic cerebral abscess. (*A*) Postcontrast axial T1-weighted image shows irregular thick ring enhancement with surrounding edema (*arrow*). (*B*) The center of the lesion shows homogenous restricted diffusion (*arrow*). (*C*) PASL CBF map shows hypoperfusion corresponding to the center of the lesion (*arrow*). No hyperperfusion corresponding to the enhancing rim can be identified.

hyperperfusion, for example, can be seen adjacent to epidural abscesses and with conditions such as herpes encephalitis. Even when there is adjacent cerebritis, the abscess itself usually remains hypoperfused (**Fig. 17**).

Physiologic Quantification

One of the benefits of using quantitative ASL in a clinical population is that physiologic processes that affect global cerebral perfusion can be detected readily. Qualitative perfusion measurements can show relative perfusion differences quite reliably, but if the process is global or symmetric, it may become difficult, if not impossible, to detect. One of the main driving forces behind cerebral perfusion is CO_2. The autoregulatory mechanisms of the central nervous system are exquisitely sensitive to both hypercapnia and hypocapnia.[56,57,58] Hypercapnia produces cerebrovascular vasodilatation that increases in a linear fashion up to partial pressure of CO_2 values of 75 mm Hg. It has been shown that hypercapnia can produce global central nervous system hyperperfusion without concomitant findings on conventional MR imaging sequences (**Fig. 18**).[5] Similarly, hypocapnia secondary to hyperventilation can result in vasoconstriction

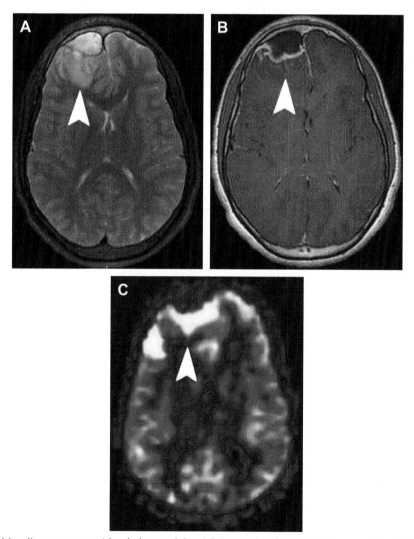

Fig. 17. Cerebritis adjacent to an epidural abscess. (*A*) Axial T2-weighted image shows an epidural fluid collection and adjacent edema (*arrowhead*) in the right frontal lobe. (*B*) Postcontrast imaging shows a rim enhancing epidural fluid collection, faint enhancement in the adjacent parenchyma (*arrowhead*), and enhancement of the right frontal subarachnoid spaces. (*C*) PASL CBF map demonstrates marked hyperperfusion of the edematous cortex (*arrowhead*).

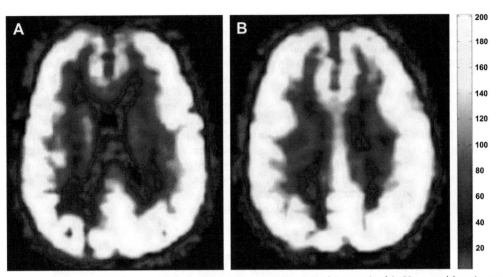

Fig. 18. Hypercapnia. (A, B) Global hyperperfusion (mean GM CBF = 168.4) is seen in this 60-year-old patient with normal conventional imaging findings but marked hypercapnia. This patient had a subsequent arterial blood gas PCO$_2$ measurement of 76.6 mm Hg (normal range 35–45 mm Hg).

and subsequent hypoperfusion.[5,59,60,61,62] Indeed, hypocapnia can result in global hypoperfusion that is severe enough to decrease the amount of usable ASL signal markedly, resulting in uninterpretable perfusion data in an otherwise clinically normal-appearing patient. These changes in physiologic perfusion may manifest while imaging ventilator-dependent, emphysematous, or claustrophobic patients.

Pediatric Patients

The pediatric patient population is one of the optimal groups for clinical ASL because reliable perfusion imaging can be obtained without the use of ionizing radiation or power injection of intravenous contrast materials. The sequence can be repeated safely for the reacquisition of data if an error should occur. Pediatric patients have intrinsically higher CBF that can be detected and quantified using ASL. Therefore, the same normative global perfusion values cannot be used in adult and pediatric populations. The authors' data show three discrete patterns of cerebral perfusion in pediatric patients. There is a rapid increase in cerebral perfusion between birth and age 3 years. Cerebral perfusion then plateaus between age 4 and 11 years; rates of CBF in most children in this age group are greater than 90 mL/100 g/minute. Cerebral perfusion decreases rapidly after age 11 years, so that rates of CBF in most adolescents and young adults (age 12–30 years) are less than 90 mL/100 g/ minute (see Fig. 4). From age 30 to 90 years, there is a very slow decline in mean CBF.[11]

Imaging very young pediatric patients presents a few problems for the ASL sequence. Because of the small size of the head and neck in a newborn, if the tag is applied well below the imaging plane, some of the tagged blood actually may be in the aortic arch and go to the arms and body rather than the brain. This situation results in a loss of signal and apparent cerebral hypoperfusion. In very young patients, the sequence should be modified to compensate for the patient's small size.[44,45]

Regional Causes of Hyperperfusion

Seizure

Epileptic foci have been studied extensively using nuclear medicine perfusion techniques. These methods require an ictal injection of a radiotracer, with a subsequent interictal injection. Such techniques capture a snapshot of cerebral perfusion at the time of tracer injection. Although the authors do not have a dedicated protocol for seizure imaging with ASL, they have captured several patients incidentally in the immediate postictal state. These ASL perfusion scans unambiguously demonstrated regional hyperperfusion corresponding to the abnormal cortical focus localized via clinical presentation and electroencephalogram monitoring (Fig. 19). ASL has been most successful in demonstrating supratentorial, extratemporal seizure foci.[63] Mesial temporal sclerosis has been difficult to image because of the susceptibility caused by the proximity to the skull base and sphenoid sinus.[64] Unlike nuclear medicine studies, ASL studies can be repeated within short time intervals. This property may lend itself to nearly real-time dynamic imaging of the cerebral perfusion during the immediate postictal state.

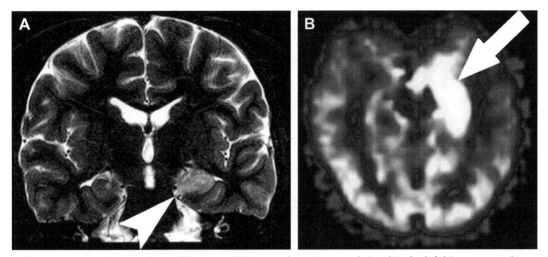

Fig.19. Hyperperfused seizure focus. (*A*) Coronal T2 image shows increased signal in the left hippocampus (*arrowhead*). (*B*) PASL CBF map reveals marked hyperperfusion in the medial left temporal lobe corresponding to the increased signal within the left hippocampus in this patient who had a recent left temporal lobe seizure.

Most patients who have clinical seizure are imaged in the interictal state. The seizure foci in these patients, unless they have a form of subclinical epileptic activity, shows hypoperfusion in the involved cortex (**Fig. 20**).[2,63] In the rare instance of postictal imaging, hyperperfusion has been shown with ASL studies up to 1 hour after seizure onset.[4]

Posterior reversible encephalopathy syndrome
A significant number of studies have sought to elucidate the pathogenesis of the posterior reversible encephalopathy syndrome (PRES). Various theories, from vasoconstriction to vasodilation, have been proposed, but no one theory can account for

the disparities in the clinical imaging and perfusion data.[65,66,67] PRES on ASL also can have a variety of appearances. The authors have found that patients who are imaged acutely show hyperperfusion in the occipital and frontal hemispheres, and patients who are imaged in the subacute phase show hypoperfusion in the occipital and frontal hemispheres (**Fig. 21**).[10] The variability and apparent discrepancies among studies investigating perfusion changes related to PRES may be secondary to the time course of the disease.

Migraine
Migraine headaches occasionally are imaged during the acute phase because the aura

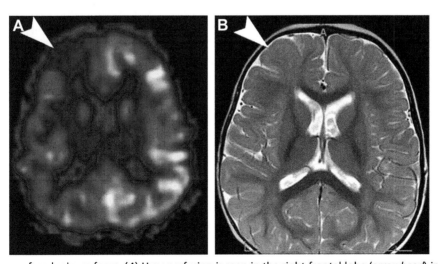

Fig. 20. Hypoperfused seizure focus. (*A*) Hypoperfusion is seen in the right frontal lobe (*arrowhead*) in this interictal pediatric patient. A second look at (*B*) the axial T2 image from the conventional sequences revealed a very subtle migrational anomaly with thickening in the right frontal cortex (*arrowhead*).

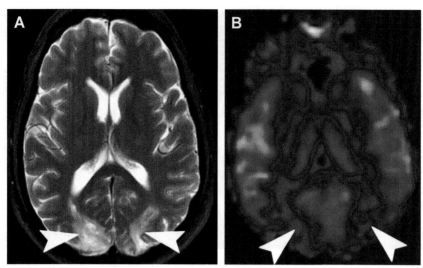

Fig. 21. Posterior reversible encephalopathy syndrome (PRES) on PASL. (*A*) Axial T2-weighted image shows increased symmetric bilateral signal in the occipital hemispheres (*arrowheads*). (*B*) PASL CBF map reveals significant hypoperfusion in the corresponding vascular territories (*arrowheads*). PRES seems to have a time-dependent appearance. Patients imaged acutely tend to have hyperperfusion in the affected territories, whereas patients imaged in the subacute phase are hypoperfused.

symptoms can mimic cerebral infarction. If the patient who has migraine happens to be imaged while having aura symptoms, ASL shows hypoperfusion in the cortex thought to correspond to those symptoms. More commonly the patients present to medical attention during the aura phase only to develop a headache later, near the time of imaging. If patients who have migraine are imaged during the headache phase, hyperperfusion is seen in the cortex and is thought to correspond to the prior aura symptoms (**Fig. 22**).[68,69,70,71] Conventional sequences usually are normal, but they may show some subtle cortical edema.[8]

Immunocompromised Patients

One occasional diagnostic dilemma in the immunocompromised patient is differentiating toxoplasmosis from lymphoma. In the authors' clinical experience with ASL to date, all cases of toxoplasmosis have been hypoperfused (**Fig. 23**), and the cases of lymphoma have been hyperperfused (**Fig. 24**). This simple distinction has proven reliable thus far, but a larger study is needed to confirm this hypothesis.

FUTURE DEVELOPMENTS

Even though ASL is being introduced into routine clinical imaging by several MR imaging vendors, the perfusion sequence remains a work in progress. Potentially the greatest barrier to the clinical acceptance of ASL is the lack of consistency in methodology and results. The number of options

available may seem daunting. The sequence will continue to be optimized in future iterations and will evolve as advances are made in the technology and scanners. Some techniques on the

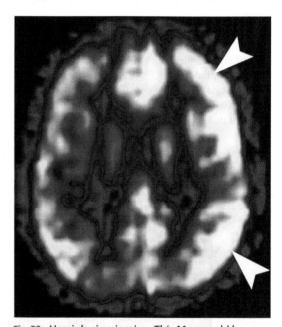

Fig. 22. Hemiplegic migraine. This 11-year-old boy presented with right hemiplegia followed by a severe migraine headache. All conventional sequences were normal. PASL showed marked hyperperfusion in the left cerebral cortex. Hyperperfusion of the symptomatic cortex is seen in patients imaged during the migraine headache. Hypoperfusion is seen if the patient is imaged during the aura phase.

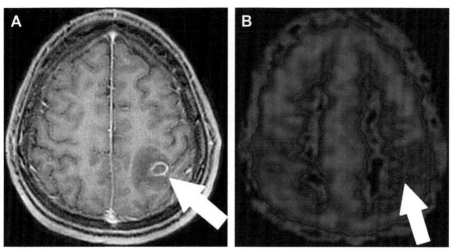

Fig. 23. Toxoplasmosis on PASL. (*A*) Axial postcontrast T1 image shows a ring-enhancing mass with surrounding edema in this immunocompromised patient (*arrow*). (*B*) PASL CBF map shows that the lesion is hypoperfused relative to gray matter. This hypoperfused pattern has been seen consistently in all toxoplasmosis cases to date and may be useful in distinguishing toxoplasmosis from lymphoma.

horizon that may be introduced into the sequence include propeller imaging, artifact reduction, territorial mapping,[72,73] and T1 mapping.

Extracranial Perfusion

The ASL methodology is ideal for imaging the cerebral circulation. There is little susceptibility in the cerebral hemispheres, and the brain does not move very much. As the ASL acquisition is extended inferiorly, increasing susceptibility artifacts at the skull base and near the paranasal sinuses are encountered. The authors frequently have imaged the orbits as part of the standard brain protocol,

with mixed degrees of success. Occasionally very vascular masses and infectious processes have shown hyperperfusion on ASL. The significance of the hyperperfusion in this setting is uncertain at this point, but as the susceptibility artifacts are reduced in the future, the ASL technique may be increasingly successful in imaging the skull base and extracranial soft tissues (**Fig. 25**).[9]

TRANSIT TIMES

Commonly used ASL techniques provide only CBF. Much of the literature on stroke, penumbra,

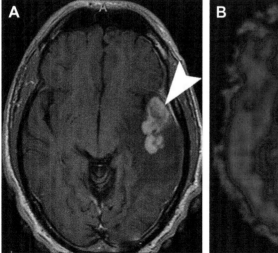
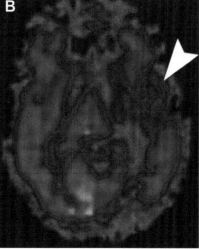

Fig. 24. Lymphoma on PASL. (*A*) Axial postcontrast images shows a solid enhancing mass (*arrowhead*) in the left temporal lobe with surrounding vasogenic edema in this immunocompromised patient. (*B*) PASL CBF map shows the mass (*arrowhead*) to have perfusion similar to the adjacent gray matter in this case of lymphoma.

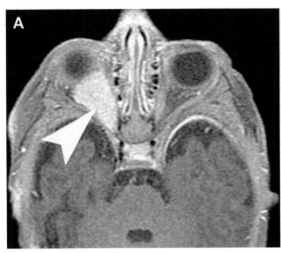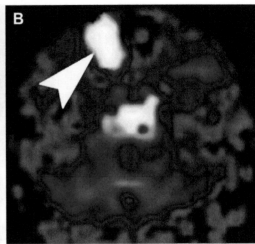

Fig. 25. PASL imaging of the orbit. (A) Axial postcontrast imaging of orbits in an infant shows an avidly enhancing right retrobulbar mass (*arrowhead*) consistent with an infantile or capillary hemangioma. (B) PASL CBF map reveals significant hyperperfusion in the mass (*arrowhead*). PASL imaging of the orbit is technically challenging because of the susceptibility artifacts from the paranasal sinuses and skull base. In infants, the relative lack of pneumatization may allow more successful imaging of orbital masses.

and tumors relies on transit time and blood volume parameters. In the future, multiphase dynamic ASL with multiple inversion times will be available. From this single multiphase acquisition, curves of voxelwise signal intensity versus time can be generated that can yield information about time to peak and tag arrival time. Although not a true transit time, these dedicated timing parameter maps will be a great addition to clinical perfusion imaging.[50]

SUMMARY

ASL has broad clinical applications in a routine neuroradiology practice. General understanding of the technique and the options used by the vendor are essential for accurate interpretation.

REFERENCES

1. Deibler AR, Pollock JM, Kraft RA, et al. Arterial spin-labeling in routine clinical practice, part 1: technique and artifacts. AJNR Am J Neuroradiol 2008;29: 1228–34.
2. Deibler AR, Pollock JM, Kraft RA, et al. Arterial spin-labeling in routine clinical practice, part 2: hypoperfusion patterns. AJNR Am J Neuroradiol 2008;29: 1235–41.
3. Maldjian JA, Laurienti PJ, Burdette JH, et al. Clinical implementation of spin-tag perfusion magnetic resonance imaging. J Comput Assist Tomogr 2008;32:403–6.
4. Pollock JM, Deibler AR, West TG, et al. Arterial spin-labeled magnetic resonance imaging in hyperperfused seizure focus: a case report. J Comput Assist Tomogr 2008;32:291–2.
5. Pollock JM, Deibler AR, Whitlow CT, et al. Manifestations of hyper and hypocapnia on arterial spin labeled MRI perfusion imaging. AJNR Am J Neuroradiol 2009;30(2):378–85.
6. Pollock JM, Whitlow CT, Deibler AR, et al. Anoxic injury-associated cerebral hyperperfusion identified with arterial spin-labeled MR imaging. AJNR Am J Neuroradiol 2008;29:1302–7.
7. Deibler AR, Pollock JM, Kraft RA, et al. Arterial spin-labeling in routine clinical practice, part 3: hyperperfusion patterns. AJNR Am J Neuroradiol 2008;29: 1428–35.
8. Pollock JM, Deibler AR, Burdette JH, et al. Migraine associated cerebral hyperperfusion with arterial spin-labeled MR imaging. AJNR Am J Neuroradiol 2008;29:1494–7.
9. Pollock JM, Kraft RA, Tan H, et al. Arterial spin labeled perfusion imaging of the orbit: initial experience. Presented at the American Society of Head and Neck Radiology 42th Annual Meeting. Toronto, Canada, 2008.
10. Whitlow CT, Pollock JM, Kraft RA, et al. Evolving temporal changes in cerebral blood flow associated with posterior reversible encephalopathy syndrome: a magnetic resonance arterial spin labeling investigation. Presented at the American Society of Functional Neuroradiology. Orlando, Florida, 2008.
11. Whitlow CT, Pollock JM, Mussat-Whitlow B, et al. Changes in global rates of cerebral perfusion associated with normal development as measured with MR arterial spin labeling. Presented at the American

Society of Neuroradiology 46th Annual Meeting. New Orleans, Louisiana, 2008.

12. Detre JA, Zhang W, Roberts DA, et al. Tissue specific perfusion imaging using arterial spin labeling. NMR Biomed 1994;7:75–82.

13. Alsop DC, Detre JA. Multisection cerebral blood flow MR imaging with continuous arterial spin labeling. Radiology 1998;208:410–6.

14. Williams DS, Detre JA, Leigh JS, et al. Magnetic resonance imaging of perfusion using spin inversion of arterial water. Proc Natl Acad Sci U S A 1992;89:212–6.

15. Sadowski EA, Bennett LK, Chan MR, et al. Nephrogenic systemic fibrosis: risk factors and incidence estimation. Radiology 2007;243:148–57.

16. Yang Y, Frank JA, Hou L, et al. Multislice imaging of quantitative cerebral perfusion with pulsed arterial spin labeling. Magn Reson Med 1998;39:825–32.

17. Wintermark M, Sesay M, Barbier E, et al. Comparative overview of brain perfusion imaging techniques. Stroke 2005;36:e83–99.

18. Chawla S, Wang S, Wolf RL, et al. Arterial spin-labeling and MR spectroscopy in the differentiation of gliomas. AJNR Am J Neuroradiol 2007;28:1683–9.

19. Noguchi T, Yoshiura T, Hiwatashi A, et al. Perfusion imaging of brain tumors using arterial spin-labeling: correlation with histopathologic vascular density. AJNR Am J Neuroradiol 2008;29:688–93.

20. Luh WM, Wong EC, Bandettini PA, et al. QUIPSS II with thin-slice TI1 periodic saturation: a method for improving accuracy of quantitative perfusion imaging using pulsed arterial spin labeling. Magn Reson Med 1999;41:1246–54.

21. Gunther M, Bock M, Schad LR. Arterial spin labeling in combination with a look-locker sampling strategy: inflow turbo-sampling EPI-FAIR (ITS-FAIR). Magn Reson Med 2001;46:974–84.

22. Buxton RB, Frank LR, Wong EC, et al. A general kinetic model for quantitative perfusion imaging with arterial spin labeling. Magn Reson Med 1998; 40:383–96.

23. Edelman RR, Siewert B, Darby DG, et al. Qualitative mapping of cerebral blood flow and functional localization with echo-planar MR imaging and signal targeting with alternating radio frequency. Radiology 1994;192:513–20.

24. Kim SG, Tsekos NV. Perfusion imaging by a flow-sensitive alternating inversion recovery (FAIR) technique: application to functional brain imaging. Magn Reson Med 1997;37:425–35.

25. Wong EC, Buxton RB, Frank LR. Implementation of quantitative perfusion imaging techniques for functional brain mapping using pulsed arterial spin labeling. NMR Biomed 1997;10:237–49.

26. Yongbi MN, Yang Y, Frank JA, et al. Multislice perfusion imaging in human brain using the C-FOCI inversion pulse: comparison with hyperbolic secant. Magn Reson Med 1999;42:1098–105.

27. Detre JA, Leigh JS, Williams DS, et al. Perfusion imaging. Magn Reson Med 1992;23:37–45.

28. Detre JA, Alsop DC. Perfusion magnetic resonance imaging with continuous arterial spin labeling: methods and clinical applications in the central nervous system. Eur J Radiol 1999;30:115–24.

29. Liu TT, Brown GG. Measurement of cerebral perfusion with arterial spin labeling: part 1. Methods. J Int Neuropsychol Soc 2007;13:517–25.

30. Wu WC, Fernandez-Seara M, Detre JA, et al. A theoretical and experimental investigation of the tagging efficiency of pseudocontinuous arterial spin labeling. Magn Reson Med 2007;58:1020–7.

31. Petersen ET, Zimine I, Ho YC, et al. Non-invasive measurement of perfusion: a critical review of arterial spin labelling techniques. Br J Radiol 2006;79: 688–701.

32. Garcia DM, Bazelaire CD, Alsop D. Pseudo-continuous flow driven adiabatic inversion for aterial spin labeling. Presented at the International Society for Magnetic Resonance in Medicine, May 2005.

33. Wong EC, Cronin M, Wu WC, et al. Velocity-selective arterial spin labeling. Magn Reson Med 2006;55: 1334–41.

34. St Lawrence KS, Frank JA, Bandettini PA, et al. Noise reduction in multi-slice arterial spin tagging imaging. Magn Reson Med 2005;53:735–8.

35. Ye FQ, Frank JA, Weinberger DR, et al. Noise reduction in 3D perfusion imaging by attenuating the static signal in arterial spin tagging (ASSIST). Magn Reson Med 2000;44:92–100.

36. Calamante F, Thomas DL, Pell GS, et al. Measuring cerebral blood flow using magnetic resonance imaging techniques. J Cereb Blood Flow Metab 1999;19:701–35.

37. Brown GG, Clark C, Liu TT. Measurement of cerebral perfusion with arterial spin labeling: part 2. Applications. J Int Neuropsychol Soc 2007;13:526–38.

38. Wolf RL, Wang J, Detre JA, et al. Arteriovenous shunt visualization in arteriovenous malformations with arterial spin-labeling MR imaging. AJNR Am J Neuroradiol 2008;29:681–7.

39. Lu H, Clingman C, Golay X, et al. Determining the longitudinal relaxation time (T1) of blood at 3.0 Tesla. Magn Reson Med 2004;52:679–82.

40. Silvennoinen MJ, Kettunen MI, Kauppinen RA. Effects of hematocrit and oxygen saturation level on blood spin-lattice relaxation. Magn Reson Med 2003;49:568–71.

41. Zhernovoi AI, Sharshina LM. [Effects of hematocrit on blood proton relaxation time]. Med Tekh 1997;33–4.

42. Buxton RB. Quantifying CBF with arterial spin labeling. J Magn Reson Imaging 2005;22:723–6.

43. Tan H Maldjian JA, Pollock JM, et al. A fast, effective filtering method for improving clinical pulsed arterial spin labeling MRI. J Magn Reson Imaging; in press.

44. Wang J, Licht DJ. Pediatric perfusion MR imaging using arterial spin labeling. Neuroimaging Clin N Am 2006;16:149–67.

45. Wang J, Licht DJ, Jahng GH, et al. Pediatric perfusion imaging using pulsed arterial spin labeling. J Magn Reson Imaging 2003;18:404–13.

46. Wang Z, Fernandez-Seara M, Alsop DC, et al. Assessment of functional development in normal infant brain using arterial spin labeled perfusion MRI. Neuroimage 2008;39:973–8.

47. Wolf RL, Alsop DC, McGarvey ML, et al. Susceptibility contrast and arterial spin labeled perfusion MRI in cerebrovascular disease. J Neuroimaging 2003;13:17–27.

48. Markus HS. Cerebral perfusion and stroke. J Neurol Neurosurg Psychiatr 2004;75:353–61.

49. Barbier EL, Silva AC, Kim SG, et al. Perfusion imaging using dynamic arterial spin labeling (DASL). Magn Reson Med 2001;45:1021–9.

50. Wang J, Alsop DC, Song HK, et al. Arterial transit time imaging with flow encoding arterial spin tagging (FEAST). Magn Reson Med 2003;50:599–607.

51. Hendrikse J, van Osch MJ, Rutgers DR, et al. Internal carotid artery occlusion assessed at pulsed arterial spin-labeling perfusion MR imaging at multiple delay times. Radiology 2004;233: 899–904.

52. Ye FQ, Mattay VS, Jezzard P, et al. Correction for vascular artifacts in cerebral blood flow values measured by using arterial spin tagging techniques. Magn Reson Med 1997;37:226–35.

53. Kim HS, Kim SY. A prospective study on the added value of pulsed arterial spin-labeling and apparent diffusion coefficients in the grading of gliomas. AJNR Am J Neuroradiol 2007;28:1693–9.

54. Warmuth C, Gunther M, Zimmer C. Quantification of blood flow in brain tumors: comparison of arterial spin labeling and dynamic susceptibility-weighted contrast-enhanced MR imaging. Radiology 2003; 228:523–32.

55. Wolf RL, Wang J, Wang S, et al. Grading of CNS neoplasms using continuous arterial spin labeled perfusion MR imaging at 3 Tesla. J Magn Reson Imaging 2005;22:475–82.

56. Noth U, Kotajima F, Deichmann R, et al. Mapping of the cerebral vascular response to hypoxia and hypercapnia using quantitative perfusion MRI at 3 T. NMR Biomed 2008;21(5):464–72.

57. Noth U, Meadows GE, Kotajima F, et al. Cerebral vascular response to hypercapnia: determination with perfusion MRI at 1.5 and 3.0 Tesla using a pulsed arterial spin labeling technique. J Magn Reson Imaging 2006;24:1229–35.

58. Raichle ME, Stone HL. Cerebral blood flow autoregulation and graded hypercapnia. Eur Neurol 1971;6:1–5.

59. Faraci FM, Breese KR, Heistad DD. Cerebral vasodilation during hypercapnia. Role of glibenclamide-sensitive potassium channels and nitric oxide. Stroke 1994;25:1679–83.

60. Floyd TF, Clark JM, Gelfand R, et al. Independent cerebral vasoconstrictive effects of hyperoxia and accompanying arterial hypocapnia at 1 ATA. J Appl Phys 2003;95:2453–61.

61. Raichle ME, Plum F. Hyperventilation and cerebral blood flow. Stroke 1972;3:566–75.

62. Raichle ME, Posner JB, Plum F. Cerebral blood flow during and after hyperventilation. Arch Neurol 1970; 23:394–403.

63. Wolf RL, Alsop DC, Levy-Reis I, et al. Detection of mesial temporal lobe hypoperfusion in patients with temporal lobe epilepsy by use of arterial spin labeled perfusion MR imaging. AJNR Am J Neuroradiol 2001;22:1334–41.

64. Engelhorn T, Doerfler A, Weise J, et al. Cerebral perfusion alterations during the acute phase of experimental generalized status epilepticus: prediction of survival by using perfusion-weighted MR imaging and histopathology. AJNR Am J Neuroradiol 2005;26:1563–70.

65. Bartynski WS. Posterior reversible encephalopathy syndrome, part 1: fundamental imaging and clinical features. AJNR Am J Neuroradiol 2008;29:1036–42.

66. Bartynski WS. Posterior reversible encephalopathy syndrome, part 2: controversies surrounding pathophysiology of vasogenic edema. AJNR Am J Neuroradiol 2008;29:1043–9.

67. Bartynski WS, Boardman JF, Zeigler ZR, et al. Posterior reversible encephalopathy syndrome in infection, sepsis, and shock. AJNR Am J Neuroradiol 2006;27:2179–90.

68. Friberg L, Olesen J, Lassen NA, et al. Cerebral oxygen extraction, oxygen consumption, and regional cerebral blood flow during the aura phase of migraine. Stroke 1994;25:974–9.

69. Goadsby PJ. Migraine pathophysiology. Headache 2005;45(Suppl 1):S14–24.

70. Hsu DA, Stafstrom CE, Rowley HA, et al. Hemiplegic migraine: hyperperfusion and abortive therapy with intravenous verapamil. Brain Dev 2008;30:86–90.

71. Jacob A, Mahavish K, Bowden A, et al. Imaging abnormalities in sporadic hemiplegic migraine on conventional MRI, diffusion and perfusion MRI and MRS. Cephalalgia 2006;26:1004–9.

72. Lim CC, Petersen ET, Ng I, et al. MR regional perfusion imaging: visualizing functional collateral circulation. AJNR Am J Neuroradiol 2007;28:447–8.

73. Golay X, Petersen ET, Hui F. Pulsed star labeling of arterial regions (PULSAR): a robust regional perfusion technique for high field imaging. Magn Reson Med 2005;53:15–21.

Dynamic Contrast-Enhanced MR Imaging of the Liver: Current Status and Future Directions

Richard Kinh Gian Do, MD, PhD, Henry Rusinek, PhD, Bachir Taouli, MD*

KEYWORDS

- Liver • MR imaging • Perfusion
- Dynamic contrast enhancement • Fibrosis
- Cirrhosis • Hepatocellular carcinoma • Metastases

MR imaging has an important role in the evaluation of diffuse and focal liver diseases, with new hardware and sequences being continuously developed to improve its diagnostic capabilities. Recently, dynamic contrast-enhanced MR imaging (DCE-MR imaging) has been applied to quantify perfusion changes in the liver parenchyma observed in hepatic fibrosis and cirrhosis, and to quantify the angiogenic activity in malignant focal liver lesions. The unique dual blood supply of the liver presents both challenges and opportunities for DCE-MR imaging. This article will focus on the recent developments, applications, potential clinical utility, and future directions of DCE-MR imaging of the liver.

Chronic viral hepatitis B and C, in addition to alcohol abuse and liver steatosis are major risk factors for the development of liver fibrosis, cirrhosis, and subsequent risk of end-stage liver disease and hepatocellular carcinoma (HCC).[1] HCC is the most common primary liver cancer and the third most common cause of cancer mortality worldwide.[2] Advances in imaging techniques allow for the early detection of HCC, which has implications in clinical management, including

eligibility for liver transplantation[3] and locoregional therapies, and for prognosis.[4,5]

The liver is a unique organ given its dual blood supply, with the majority (75%) of the blood normally provided by the portal vein and the remainder through the hepatic artery (25%). These inflowing vessels subdivide into branches organized by portal tracts; these further subdivide and transport blood to low pressure sinusoids. Highly fenestrated endothelial cells and the intervening extracellular space of Disse separate these sinusoids from hepatocytes. This organization allows free passage of low-molecular-weight compounds such as CT or MR contrast materials between the vascular compartment and the extracellular space of Disse. These characteristics are exploited by DCE-MR imaging to characterize diffuse and local liver diseases.[6] In liver fibrosis, a number of different pathophysiological processes occur including progressive loss of endothelial fenestration and deposition of collagen in the space of Disse.[7] These processes reduce the rate of blood flow and prolong its transit time. Furthermore, the decrease in portal blood flow is compensated by an increase in arterial blood flow, resulting in an

Financial support: RSNA Scholarship Grant # 0710, Bracco Diagnostics Research Grant.
Department of Radiology, New York University Langone Medical Center, 530 First Avenue, MRI, New York, NY 10016, USA
* Corresponding author.
E-mail address: bachir.taouli@nyumc.org (B. Taouli).

Magn Reson Imaging Clin N Am 17 (2009) 339–349
doi:10.1016/j.mric.2009.01.009

elevated arterial perfusion fraction (known as the arterial buffer response).[8,9] Changes in blood transit time of contrast agents and relative arterial to portal venous blood flow can be estimated using DCE-MR imaging.

HCC and liver metastases exhibit local alterations in microvascular anatomy, both demonstrating neoangiogenesis, promoted by vascular endothelial growth factor (VEGF),[10–13] which is a potent angiogenic factor, inducing hyperpermeability of tumor vessels. Antiangiogenic therapies have demonstrated promising results in liver metastases and HCC.[14–17] Recently, sorafenib, a multikinase and anti-VEGF inhibitor, has been shown to improve overall survival by 3 months and extend the time to radiologic progression in advanced HCC, using Response Criteria In Solid Tumors.[18] Characterizing the angiogenic properties of HCC and metastatic lesions is important for determining eligibility of patients for antiangiogenic therapy, and can be used to monitor response to antiangiogenic drugs. Furthermore, as antiangiogenic drugs may stabilize tumors without shrinking them, measurement of tumor size alone may not be sufficient to monitor treatment response. Physiologic imaging techniques such as DCE-MR imaging begins to play a critical role in the evaluation of novel antiangiogenic drugs.[19]

DYNAMIC CONTRAST-ENHANCED MR IMAGING

Regional perfusion can be assessed by following the uptake and washout of contrast agent with either MR imaging or CT. MR imaging has several advantages over CT, including the lack of ionizing radiation. Therefore, it has the ability to image whole organs repeatedly and dynamically with high temporal resolution, and the possibility of repeating the study multiple times after treatment. In addition, intravenous gadolinium contrast for MR imaging is also generally preferable to iodinated CT contrast—given the larger side-effect profile associated with the latter, including the risk of contrast induced nephropathy and allergic reactions.[20] However, with the recent recognition of nephrogenic systemic fibrosis,[21–23] gadolinium-based contrast agents should be avoided in patients with severe renal impairment. Furthermore, unlike the linear relationship between iodine concentration and Hounsfield units on CT, the relationship between gadolinium concentration and signal intensity (SI) is nonlinear with MR imaging, complicating quantitative perfusion measurements.

Dynamic Contrast-Enhanced MR Imaging Acquisition

DCE-MR imaging requires a balance between anatomic coverage, spatial resolution, and temporal resolution. With recent advances in MR imaging technique, including high performance gradients and parallel imaging, it is now possible to cover the entire liver with good spatial and temporal resolution. Imaging parameters used for quantitative DCE-MR imaging have progressed as MR scanner hardware and software continue to evolve. However, there is limited literature on the use of DCE-MR imaging in liver imaging.

The majority of prior DCE-MR imaging studies have relied on a two-dimensional (2D) acquisition limited to a single axial slice to preserve high spatial and temporal resolution.[24–26] The initial experimental work on DCE-MR imaging by Scharf and colleagues[24] in 1999 on pigs (at 1.0 T) demonstrated a good correlation between MR perfusion parameters and a reference thermal diffusion probe in the setting of partial portal vein occlusion. Materne and colleagues,[25] and Annet and colleagues[26] (from the same group), performed DCE-MR imaging at 1.5 T using a single axial slice at the level of the portal vein, using cardiac triggering, which enabled high temporal resolution. Jackson and colleagues[27] were the early proponents of 3D volumetric coverage to measure perfusion in primary and metastatic liver lesions. They achieved a 4.1-sec. temporal resolution using a 128 × 128 matrix when imaging a slab restricted in thickness to the lesion of interest. Recently, Abdullah and colleagues[28] used a 2D technique with eight sagittal 8 mm slices, achieving a temporal resolution of 1.7 second for each slice; using a 128 × 78 matrix.

At the authors' institution, we chose to perform whole liver perfusion imaging at 1.5-T (Magnetom Symphony, Avanto or Sonata; Siemens, Erlangen, Germany) or 3-T (Magnetom Trio) using a three-dimensional (3D) interpolated spoiled gradient-recalled echo sequence in the coronal plane, with whole liver coverage and a parallel imaging factor of two to three.[29] The coronal imaging plane is used to minimize inflow artifacts and facilitates the computation of accurate arterial input function.[30] Compared with 2D acquisition, 3D acquisition has the advantage of covering the entire liver, which is necessary when following patients with multiple liver metastases or HCCs, and in liver fibrosis and cirrhosis, where there is potential heterogeneous distribution. This is at the expense of lower temporal resolution.

At the authors' institution, patients are instructed to fast for 6 hours before the scan,

Table 1
Proposed parameters for the 3D-spoiled gradient echo sequence used for liver DCE-MR imaging acquisition (using a 32 multichannel 1.5 T system; Magnetom Avanto, Siemens Medical Solutions)

Parameter	Values
TR	1.7-3.2 msec
TE	0.8 msec
FOV	40 cm (right-left) × 40 cm (superior-inferior)
Matrix	121 × 192 (voxel size 3.3 × 2.1 × 3.0 mm)
Slice thickness	3.0 mm
Flip angle	9°
Number of averages	1
Parallel imaging acceleration factor	3
Number of time points	36–40
Acquisition time/volume	3–5 sec
Dose of Gd-DTPA	10 mL at 5 mL/sec with 20 mL of saline flush

Abbreviations: FOV, field of view; Gd-DTPA, gadopentetate dimeglumine; TE, time to echo; TR, repetition time.

given the potential changes in portal venous flow occurring in the postprandial state.[31] One to three volume acquisitions are performed before contrast administration. We use 10 mL of intravenous contrast material: gadopentetate dimeglumine (Magnevist; Berlex Laboratories, Wayne, NJ) followed by a 20 mL saline flush, at an injection rate of 3 to 5 mL/sec. Recently, we have used gadobenate dimeglumine (Multihance; Bracco Diagnostics, Princeton, NJ), which, because of its higher T1 relaxivity,[32] can potentially be used at a lower dose, especially when DCE-MR imaging is performed in combination with routine pre- and postcontrast imaging. Approximately 36 to 40 coronal slices are acquired every 3 to 5 seconds (depending on the magnet and liver size). Proposed sequence parameters are provided in Table 1. The images are acquired first during a breath-hold and then during quiet free breathing, for a total acquisition time of 3 to 5 minutes. With the recent availability of k-space echo-sharing techniques combined with high parallel imaging factor, we were able to improve the temporal resolution to less than 3 sec.[33–35]

Dynamic Contrast-Enhanced MR Imaging Processing

By placing regions of interest in the tissue of interest, SI versus time curves are obtained. Different DCE-MR imaging postprocessing techniques can be used to analyze the data. The methods can be divided into semiquantitative and quantitative techniques.

Semiquantitative methods

DCE-MR imaging can be processed semiquantitatively by the analysis of SI changes in organs or lesions of interest.[36] This is possible with T1-weighted images given the T1-shortening effects of gadolinium-based contrast media. Parameters such as initial upslope, time to peak, maximum SI, and washout rate can be measured and correlated with different clinical parameters. In addition, on a plot of SI versus time, the initial area (integral) under the time signal curve has been described in oncology and breast MR imaging.[37,38] Semiquantitative DCE-MR imaging methods have the advantage of being easy to implement, without the need for a pharmacokinetic model, conversion to tracer concentration, or input functions. Limitations are related to the variability of MR SI and numerous sources of bias, such as scanning protocols, amplifier gain, injection technique, and cardiac output, which could potentially

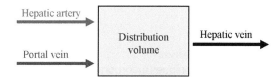

Fig. 1. Dual-input single compartment model applied for liver perfusion processing. Perfusion parameters in the liver are estimated using the dual-input single compartment model, reflecting the hepatic arterial and portal venous (dual) blood supply. The distribution volume is calculated as the ratio of the rates of inflow to the rate of outflow by way of the hepatic veins.

A

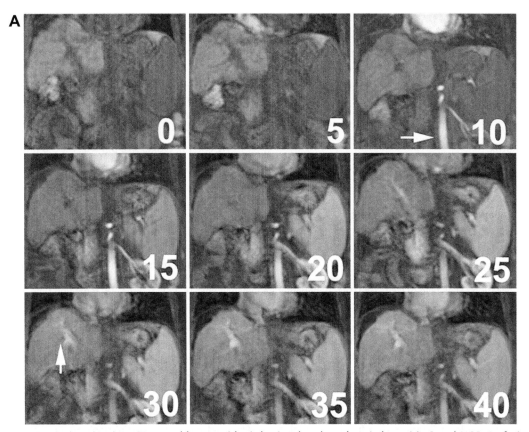

Fig. 2. DCE-MR imaging in a 65-year-old man with cirrhosis related to chronic hepatitis C and HCC. Perfusion parameters were determined from signal intensity versus time curves generated from DCE-MR imaging acquisition (using 5 sec temporal resolution). (*A*, *B*) First nine T1-weighted coronal images at two different levels at designated time intervals (sec) following administration of intravenous Gd-DTPA (*arrowhead*, HCC; *horizontal arrow*, aorta; *vertical arrow*, portal vein). (*C*) Signal intensity curves of the aorta (*red circle*), portal vein (*blue square*), liver (*black triangle*), and HCC (*green diamond*) are shown. Only the first 15 time points (out of 40) up to 70 sec are illustrated. (*D*) The small HCC in the dome demonstrates increased arterial perfusion and decreased portal perfusion compared with liver parenchyma, with no differences in MTT and DV (*Fa*, absolute arterial liver blood flow; *Fp*, absolute portal liver blood flow [ml/100 g/min]; *ART*, arterial fraction [%], *DV*, distribution volume [%]; *MTT*, mean transit time [sec]).

limit the reproducibility of semiquantitative parameters.[39,40] Nevertheless, the ease of use of these semiquantitative methods has generated important data of clinical interest, which will be discussed below.[41–43]

Quantitative methods

Quantitative techniques incorporate three steps in DCE-MR imaging quantification:

1. Calculation of tissue contrast agent concentrations from measured SI
2. Construction of arterial and portal vein input function
3. Fitting of tissue and input functions to a pharmacokinetic model.

In the liver, a dual input single compartment model can be used, which has been initially described with DCE-CT,[44,45] and has been validated with microspheres in rabbits. In addition, a modified two-compartmental Tofts model has been used to quantify perfusion parameters in liver metastases.[46–48]

For quantitative methods, regions of interest are placed in the main portal vein, proximal abdominal aorta (used as a surrogate for the hepatic artery), liver parenchyma, and lesions, if appropriate. van Laarhoven and colleagues[47] proposed the use of the spleen instead of the aorta as a vascular normalization function, showing improved reproducibility in 11 patients with colorectal metastases. This variability may be caused by vascular inflow effects on axial

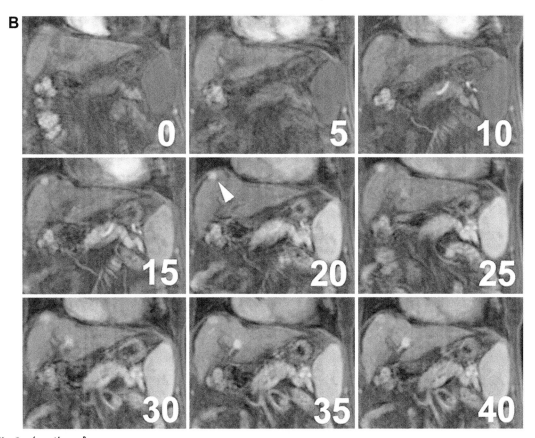

Fig. 2. (*continued*)

T1-weighted images, which could affect the arterial input function.[49]

Conversion of signal intensity to gadolinium concentration and calculation of dynamic contrast-enhanced MR imaging parameters

To simplify the perfusion quantification, a linear relationship between SI and gadolinium concentration [Gd] can be assumed for the range of expected concentrations in the liver (0.0–0.5 mM/L) and blood (0–5 mM/L), based on the authors' prior work on measurement of Gd-DTPA concentration in vivo and in vitro.[50] Therefore, the conversion was based on the approximation: $c = k\,(S\text{-}S_0)/S_0$,[51] in which S_0 is precontrast SI, S is postcontrast SI, and k the scaling constant (0.395 for liver and 0.201 for blood). These constants are based on earlier phantom and human calibration studies.[50] However, it is also possible to perform a potentially more accurate nonlinear conversion of SI to [Gd] using either analytic expressions[52] or calibration curves from phantom studies.

Nonlinear conversions may require measurement of precontrast T1 values in the liver. A segmented k-space version of the inversion recovery balanced steady-state free precession sequence can provide accurate T1 measurements in a single breath-hold.[50,53]

A dual-input single compartmental model (Fig. 1), which has been validated previously using radiolabeled microspheres in rabbits,[25] can be used to fit the resulting time-activity curves (Figs. 2 and 3). This model reflects the dual blood supply from the portal vein and hepatic artery received by the liver. The general equation for the dual-input kinetic model is:

$$C_L(t) = \int_0^t \left[k_{1a} C_a(t' - \delta) + k_{1p} C_p(t') \right] e^{-k_2(t-t')} dt',$$

where $C_a(t)$, $C_p(t)$ and $C_L(t)$ represent the concentrations of the contrast in the aorta (used as a surrogate for the hepatic artery), the portal vein and the liver respectively; δ represents the transit times from the aorta to the liver parenchyma, k_{1a} represents the aortic inflow rate constant, k_{1p} the portal venous inflow rate constant and k_2 the outflow rate constant. The distribution volume (*DV* in %) of Gd through the liver compartment is calculated as $DV = 100\,(k_{1a} + k_{1p})/k_2$, and mean transit time (*MTT* in sec) as $1/k_2$. MTT is the

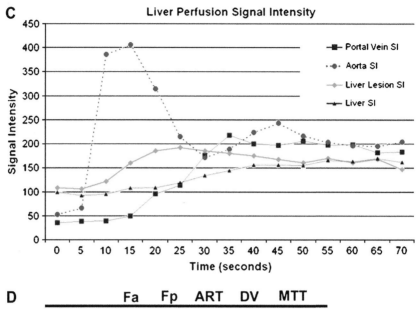

D	Fa	Fp	ART	DV	MTT
Liver	10.8	64.8	14%	19%	14.9
HCC	112	3.0	97%	21%	11.0

Fig. 2. (*continued*).

average time it takes a Gd molecule to traverse the liver from arterial-portal venous entry to the hepatic venous exit. The integration of these constants over the liver region or over the entire liver volume gives arterial F_a and portal F_p blood flow in ml/min. These values can be used to derive total liver blood flow ($F_a + F_p$), arterial fraction (ART, in %) = 100 x $F_a/(F_a + F_p)$, and portal venous fraction (PV, in %) = 100 - ART.

DYNAMIC CONTRAST-ENHANCED MR IMAGING APPLICATIONS IN THE LIVER

DCE-MR imaging is potentially useful for the diagnosis of advanced liver fibrosis and cirrhosis, and for the characterization of the angiogenic activity of HCC and liver metastases, and for monitoring antiangiogenic treatment response.

Diagnosis of Liver Fibrosis and Cirrhosis

Liver fibrosis and cirrhosis are associated with alterations in liver perfusion secondary to pathophysiologic alterations including endothelial defenestration and collagen deposition in the space of Disse. In a rabbit model of liver fibrosis, Van Beers and colleagues[54] demonstrated increased liver MTT using a low molecular contrast agent and decreased DV using a high molecular contrast agent that correlated with the collagen content in the liver. In a study of 46 patients with

cirrhosis, Annet and colleagues[26] demonstrated altered arterial, portal, and total liver perfusion, and increased MTT in cirrhotic livers compared with noncirrhotic livers, and found a correlation with severity of disease as assessed by the Child-Pugh classification and degree of portal hypertension. However, histologic evaluation of liver fibrosis was not available in their study.

The authors performed a prospective study assessing liver perfusion parameters, and demonstrated increased arterial flow, MTT and DV, and decreased portal venous flow in patients with advanced fibrosis and cirrhosis (n = 27).[29] DV, MTT, and F_a had the best sensitivity (76.9–84.6%) and specificity (71.4–78.5%) for the diagnosis of advanced fibrosis, as determined by histologic examination. The increased DV in patients with cirrhosis may be related to decreased hepatic outflow and increased interstitial volume. In comparison, the observed decrease in DV in a rabbit model of liver fibrosis described by Van Beers and colleagues[54] may be related to the use of a high molecular contrast agent. The increase in MTT may be explained by collagen deposition in the extracellular space of Disse restricting diffusion of small particles. This study was also the first to employ a 3D imaging technique that allows coverage of the entire liver for determination of parenchymal disease heterogeneity and coverage of individual lesions such as HCC.

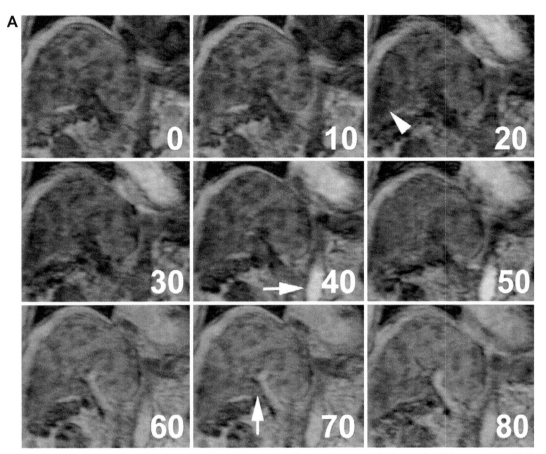

Fig. 3. DCE-MR imaging in a 78- year-old man with extensive liver metastases from small cell lung cancer. Perfusion parameters were determined from signal intensity versus time curves generated from DCE-MR imaging acquisition (using 5 sec temporal resolution). (A) Nine selected T1-weighted coronal images at the same level at designated time intervals (sec) following administration of intravenous Gd-DTPA (*arrowhead*, metastasis used for analysis; *horizontal arrow*, aorta; *vertical arrow*, portal vein). (B) Signal intensity curves of the aorta (*red circle*), portal vein (*blue square*), liver (*black triangle*), and liver metastasis (*green diamond*). Only the first 15 time points (out of 40) up to 70 sec are illustrated. (C) The metastasis in the right lobe is hypovascular with decreased arterial perfusion, portal perfusion, distribution volume, and increased mean transit time compared with liver parenchyma (*Fa*, absolute arterial liver blood flow; *Fp*, absolute portal liver blood flow [ml/100 g/min]; *ART*, arterial fraction [%]; *DV*, distribution volume [%]; *MTT*, mean transit time [sec]).

Assessment of Focal Liver Lesions

Semiquantitative and quantitative perfusion parameters have been used to characterize HCC and liver metastases, especially for monitoring treatment response to antiangiogenic drugs. Morgan and colleagues[46] demonstrated changes in tumor perfusion as early as two days following administration of a VEGF receptor tyrosine kinase inhibitor in a cohort of 26 patients with advanced colorectal liver metastases. Wang and colleagues[43] evaluated the enhancement characteristics of HCC treated with the antiangiogenic agent thalidomide, to distinguish patients who responded from those who progressed, with semiquantitative DCE-MR imaging. Based on 2D

T1-weighted spoiled gradient echo sequence, they measured SI of liver parenchyma and tumors to calculate peak enhancement in a first-pass study and maximal enhancement. In their study of seven patients, there were greater differences in these parameters in responders versus nonresponders, when comparing MR imaging obtained before and following (6–10 weeks) thalidomide administration. Measurement of the hepatic perfusion index (HPI) using semiquantitative DCE-MR imaging, to estimate the ratio of arterial hepatic perfusion to the total hepatic perfusion, has been implemented by two different groups.[41,42] In a cohort of 10 patients with metastatic liver disease, Miyazaki and colleagues[41] calculated HPI before and following treatment with the antiangiogenic

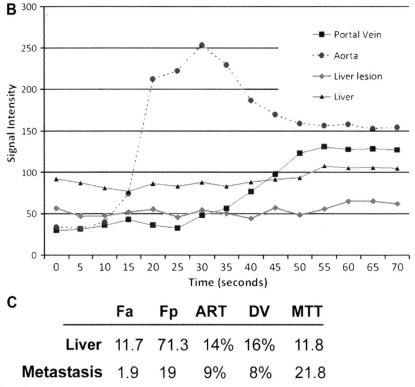

Fig. 3. *(continued)*.

compound BIBF1120. These authors found a decrease in mean HPI 28 days after treatment, even though lesions remained unchanged in size. Totman and colleagues[42] described an increase in overall HPI in patients with colorectal cancer metastases compared with normal controls, although there was a considerable overlap. Recently, Abdullah and colleagues[28] compared the perfusion characteristics of HCC (n = 13) and colorectal metastatic lesions (n = 13), with pathologic findings available for 35 of 50 lesions. Their results demonstrate increased total flow, including hepatic arterial and portal venous flow to HCC compared with colorectal metastases, and increased liver perfusion index for both.

The authors recently assessed DCE-MR imaging in patients who have HCC: 19 HCCs in 16 patients of which three were necrotic after transarterial chemoembolization (TACE) were initially studied. In this study, it was shown that F_a and ART were significantly higher and F_p lower in HCC compared with liver parenchyma, however there were no differences for MTT and DV. In addition, there were differences in F_a, ART, and PV between necrotic HCCs after TACE and untreated HCCs. These findings confirm the increased arterial supply of HCC lesions compared to cirrhotic liver, which is already elevated, and is consistent with prior results.[29] The authors were also able to demonstrate decreased arterial flow in necrotic HCC after TACE. Based on these data, the authors believe that DCE-MR imaging can be used as a noninvasive marker of HCC angiogenesis, and may be useful for predicting and monitoring response to targeted anti-angiogenic drugs currently in use against HCC.

DYNAMIC CONTRAST-ENHANCED MR IMAGING LIMITATIONS

In DCE-MR imaging, the selection of imaging parameters is important to optimize the competing demands of spatial resolution, anatomic coverage, and temporal resolution. This flexibility in parameter selection leads to institutional differences based on available MR imaging equipment and pulse sequence technology. Together with different pharmacokinetic models, the variability in methodology limits the comparison of DCE-MR imaging results from study to study. In addition, the intensive postprocessing required to obtain perfusion parameters is a nontrivial barrier to the widespread clinical use of DCE-MR imaging. Improvements and automation in image postprocessing will be an important step before DCE-MR imaging is implemented on a widespread and routine basis. Another limitation is related to respiratory misregistration, which can be partially corrected using registration algorithms. Navigator-based methods will have little role in DCE-MR imaging of the liver given the limited data sampling obtained, which limits information on early contrast uptake.

FUTURE DIRECTIONS

With improved hardware, parallel acquisition, and higher field magnets, DCE-MR imaging techniques will continue to improve in image quality, spatial resolution, and temporal resolution. DCE-MR imaging will likely be an important tool for drug trials assessing new antiangiogenic treatments, monitoring treatment response to antiangiogenic drugs, and may improve our sensitivity and specificity in the initial diagnosis of HCC and metastatic liver lesions. Differentiation between benign cirrhotic nodules and HCC could potentially be facilitated with DCE-MR imaging by providing a direct perfusion quantification of arterial versus portal inflow. Semiautomated software for perfusion quantification will fasten image processing, making DCE MR imaging a clinical reality. As more data are accumulated on the utility of DCE-MR imaging for the diagnosis and management of liver disease, it will become increasingly important to develop a consensus on standardized DCE-MR imaging protocols and methods of image analysis.

SUMMARY

DCE-MR imaging of the liver is an emerging tool for diagnosing focal and diffuse liver disease, with a potential role for staging of liver fibrosis and early detection of cirrhosis, before morphologic changes can be detected. DCE-MR imaging may also be useful for assessment of angiogenesis in HCC and liver metastases. A consensus on acquisition and processing methods will be needed.

REFERENCES

1. Afdhal NH, Nunes D. Evaluation of liver fibrosis: a concise review. Am J Gastroenterol 2004;99(6):1160–74.
2. El-Serag HB, Rudolph KL. Hepatocellular carcinoma: epidemiology and molecular carcinogenesis. Gastroenterology 2007;132(7):2557–76.
3. Mazzaferro V, Regalia E, Doci R, et al. Liver transplantation for the treatment of small hepatocellular carcinomas in patients with cirrhosis. N Engl J Med 1996;334(11):693–9.
4. Llovet JM, Real MI, Montana X, et al. Arterial embolisation or chemoembolisation versus symptomatic treatment in patients with unresectable hepatocellular carcinoma: a randomised controlled trial. Lancet 2002;359(9319):1734–9.
5. Llovet JM, Fuster J, Bruix J. The Barcelona approach: diagnosis, staging, and treatment of hepatocellular carcinoma. Liver Transpl 2004;10(2 Suppl 1):S115–20.
6. Pandharipande PV, Krinsky GA, Rusinek H, et al. Perfusion imaging of the liver: current challenges and future goals. Radiology 2005;234(3):661–73.
7. Martinez-Hernandez A. The hepatic extracellular matrix. II. Electron immunohistochemical studies in rats with CCl4-induced cirrhosis. Lab Invest 1985;53:166–86.
8. Richter S, Mucke I, Menger MD, et al. Impact of intrinsic blood flow regulation in cirrhosis: maintenance of hepatic arterial buffer response. Am J Physiol Gastrointest Liver Physiol 2000;279(2):G454–62.
9. Gulberg V, Haag K, Rossle M, et al. Hepatic arterial buffer response in patients with advanced cirrhosis. Hepatology 2002;35(3):630–4.
10. Terayama N, Terada T, Nakanuma Y. An immunohistochemical study of tumour vessels in metastatic liver cancers and the surrounding liver tissue. Histopathology 1996;29(1):37–43.
11. Park YN, Kim YB, Yang KM, et al. Increased expression of vascular endothelial growth factor and angiogenesis in the early stage of multistep hepatocarcinogenesis. Arch Pathol Lab Med 2000;124(7):1061–5.
12. Shimamura T, Saito S, Morita K, et al. Detection of vascular endothelial growth factor and its receptor expression in human hepatocellular carcinoma biopsy specimens. J Gastroenterol Hepatol 2000;15(6):640–6.
13. Takeda A, Stoeltzing O, Ahmad SA, et al. Role of angiogenesis in the development and growth of liver metastasis. Ann Surg Oncol 2002;9(7):610–6.
14. Abou-Alfa GK, Schwartz L, Ricci S, et al. Phase II study of sorafenib in patients with advanced hepatocellular carcinoma. J Clin Oncol 2006;24(26):4293–300.
15. Llovet J, Ricci S, Mazzaferro V, et al. Sorafenib improves survival in advanced Hepatocellular Carcinoma (HCC): results of a Phase III randomized placebo-controlled trial (SHARP trial). In: 2007 ASCO Annual Meeting Proceedings Part I. Journal of Clinical Oncology 2007;25(18S).
16. Alberts SR, Wagman LD. Chemotherapy for colorectal cancer liver metastases. Oncologist 2008;13(10):1063–73.
17. Siegel AB, Cohen EI, Ocean A, et al. Phase II trial evaluating the clinical and biologic effects of bevacizumab in unresectable hepatocellular carcinoma. J Clin Oncol 2008;26(18):2992–8.

18. Llovet JM, Ricci S, Mazzaferro V, et al. Sorafenib in advanced hepatocellular carcinoma. N Engl J Med 2008;359(4):378–90.

19. Provenzale JM. Imaging of angiogenesis: clinical techniques and novel imaging methods. AJR Am J Roentgenol 2007;188(1):11–23.

20. Weinreb JC. Which study when? Is gadolinium-enhanced MR imaging safer than iodine-enhanced CT? Radiology 2008;249(1):3–8.

21. Marckmann P, Skov L, Rossen K, et al. Nephrogenic systemic fibrosis: suspected causative role of gado-diamide used for contrast-enhanced magnetic resonance imaging. J Am Soc Nephrol 2006;17(9): 2359–62.

22. Kanal E, Barkovich AJ, Bell C, et al. ACR guidance document for safe MR practices: 2007. AJR Am J Roentgenol 2007;188(6):1447–74.

23. Thomsen HS, Marckmann P, Logager VB. Update on nephrogenic systemic fibrosis. Magn Reson Imaging Clin N Am 2008;16(4):551–60.

24. Scharf J, Zapletal C, Hess T, et al. Assessment of hepatic perfusion in pigs by pharmacokinetic analysis of dynamic MR images. J Magn Reson Imaging 1999;9(4):568–72.

25. Materne R, Smith AM, Peeters F, et al. Assessment of hepatic perfusion parameters with dynamic MRI. Magn Reson Med 2002;47(1):135–42.

26. Annet L, Materne R, Danse E, et al. Hepatic flow parameters measured with MR imaging and Doppler US: correlations with degree of cirrhosis and portal hypertension. Radiology 2003;229(2): 409–14.

27. Jackson A, Haroon H, Zhu XP, et al. Breath-hold perfusion and permeability mapping of hepatic malignancies using magnetic resonance imaging and a first-pass leakage profile model. NMR Biomed 2002;15(2):164–73.

28. Abdullah SS, Pialat JB, Wiart M, et al. Characterization of hepatocellular carcinoma and colorectal liver metastasis by means of perfusion MRI. J Magn Reson Imaging 2008;28(2):390–5.

29. Hagiwara M, Rusinek H, Lee VS, et al. Advanced liver fibrosis: diagnosis with 3D whole-liver perfusion MR imaging–initial experience. Radiology 2008; 246(3):926–34.

30. Ivancevic MK, Zimine I, Foxall D, et al. Inflow effect in first-pass cardiac and renal MRI. J Magn Reson Imaging 2003;18(3):372–6.

31. Burkart DJ, Johnson CD, Reading CC, et al. MR measurements of mesenteric venous flow: prospective evaluation in healthy volunteers and patients with suspected chronic mesenteric ischemia. Radiology 1995;194(3):801–6.

32. de Haen C, Cabrini M, Akhnana L, et al. Gadobenate dimeglumine 0.5 M solution for injection (Multi-Hance) pharmaceutical formulation and physicochemical properties of a new magnetic resonance imaging contrast medium. J Comput Assist Tomogr 1999;23(Suppl 1):S161–8.

33. Korosec FR, Frayne R, Grist TM, et al. Time-resolved contrast-enhanced 3D MR angiography. Magn Reson Med 1996;36(3):345–51.

34. Fink C, Ley S, Kroeker R, et al. Time-resolved contrast-enhanced three-dimensional magnetic resonance angiography of the chest: combination of parallel imaging with view sharing (TREAT). Invest Radiol 2005;40(1):40–8.

35. Song T, Laine AF, Chen Q, et al. Optimal k-space sampling for dynamic contrast-enhanced MR imaging with an application to MR renography. Magn Reson Med February 19, 2009 [Epub ahead of print].

36. Padhani AR. Dynamic contrast-enhanced MRI in clinical oncology: current status and future directions. J Magn Reson Imaging 2002;16(4):407–22.

37. Evelhoch JL. Key factors in the acquisition of contrast kinetic data for oncology. J Magn Reson Imaging 1999;10(3):254–9.

38. Kuhl CK, Mielcareck P, Klaschik S, et al. Dynamic breast MR imaging: are signal intensity time course data useful for differential diagnosis of enhancing lesions? Radiology 1999;211(1):101–10.

39. Tofts PS. Modeling tracer kinetics in dynamic Gd-DTPA MR imaging. J Magn Reson Imaging 1997;7(1):91–101.

40. Tofts PS, Brix G, Buckley DL, et al. Estimating kinetic parameters from dynamic contrast-enhanced T(1)-weighted MRI of a diffusable tracer: standardized quantities and symbols. J Magn Reson Imaging 1999;10(3):223–32.

41. Miyazaki K, Collins DJ, Walker-Samuel S, et al. Quantitative mapping of hepatic perfusion index using MR imaging: a potential reproducible tool for assessing tumour response to treatment with the antiangiogenic compound BIBF 1120, a potent triple angiokinase inhibitor. Eur Radiol 2008;18(7):1414–21.

42. Totman JJ, O'Gorman RL, Kane PA, et al. Comparison of the hepatic perfusion index measured with gadolinium-enhanced volumetric MRI in controls and in patients with colorectal cancer. Br J Radiol 2005;78(926):105–9.

43. Wang J, Chen LT, Tsang YM, et al. Dynamic contrast-enhanced MRI analysis of perfusion changes in advanced hepatocellular carcinoma treated with an antiangiogenic agent: a preliminary study. AJR Am J Roentgenol 2004;183(3):713–9.

44. Materne R, Van Beers BE, Smith AM, et al. Non-invasive quantification of liver perfusion with dynamic computed tomography and a dual-input one-compartmental model. Clin Sci (Lond) 2000;99(6): 517–25.

45. Van Beers BE, Leconte I, Materne R, et al. Hepatic perfusion parameters in chronic liver disease: dynamic CT measurements correlated with disease severity. AJR Am J Roentgenol 2001;176(3):667–73.

46. Morgan B, Thomas AL, Drevs J, et al. Dynamic contrast-enhanced magnetic resonance imaging as a biomarker for the pharmacological response of PTK787/ZK 222584, an inhibitor of the vascular endothelial growth factor receptor tyrosine kinases, in patients with advanced colorectal cancer and liver metastases: results from two phase I studies. J Clin Oncol 2003;21(21):3955–64.

47. van Laarhoven HW, Rijpkema M, Punt CJ, et al. Method for quantitation of dynamic MRI contrast agent uptake in colorectal liver metastases. J Magn Reson Imaging 2003;18(3):315–20.

48. Koh TS, Thng CH, Lee PS, et al. Hepatic metastases: in vivo assessment of perfusion parameters at dynamic contrast-enhanced MR imaging with dual-input two-compartment tracer kinetics model. Radiology 2008;249(1):307–20. Epub 2008 Aug 2011.

49. Peeters F, Annet L, Hermoye L, et al. Inflow correction of hepatic perfusion measurements using T1-weighted, fast gradient-echo, contrast-enhanced MRI. Magn Reson Med 2004;51(4):710–7.

50. Bokacheva L, Rusinek H, Chen Q, et al. Quantitative determination of Gd-DTPA concentration in T1-weighted MR renography studies. Magn Reson Med 2007;57(6):1012–8.

51. Jones RA, Easley K, Little SB, et al. Dynamic contrast-enhanced MR urography in the evaluation of pediatric hydronephrosis: part 1, functional assessment. AJR Am J Roentgenol 2005;185(6):1598–607.

52. Kim S, Quon H, Loevner LA, et al. Transcytolemmal water exchange in pharmacokinetic analysis of dynamic contrast-enhanced MRI data in squamous cell carcinoma of the head and neck. J Magn Reson Imaging 2007;26(6):1607–17.

53. Bokacheva L, Huang AJ, Chen Q, et al. Single breath-hold T1 measurement using low flip angle TrueFISP. Magn Reson Med 2006;55(5):1186–90.

54. Van Beers BE, Materne R, Annet L, et al. Capillarization of the sinusoids in liver fibrosis: noninvasive assessment with contrast-enhanced MRI in the rabbit. Magn Reson Med 2003;49(4):692–9.

Dynamic Contrast-Enhanced Breast MR Imaging

Marianne Moon, MD*, Daniel Cornfeld, MD, Jeffrey Weinreb, MD

KEYWORDS

- Breast • Breast cancer • Dynamic contrast-enhancement
- MR imaging

Breast cancer is the second most commonly diagnosed malignancy in women in the United States, with a one-in-eight lifetime risk.[1] American Cancer Society estimates reveal that in 2008, 182,460 women were diagnosed with breast cancer, and 40,480 will die of the disease.[2]

MR imaging of the breast is a highly sensitive, noninvasive technique for the detection of breast cancer.[3] In a large multicenter trial evaluating 995 breast lesions, the absence of enhancement on breast MR imaging had an 88% negative predictive value for any cancer, with a 94% negative predictive value for invasive breast cancer.[4]

In 2007, the American Cancer Society recommended annual screening with breast MR imaging for women with greater than 20% lifetime risk of breast cancer,[5] and it is among the fastest growing applications of MR imaging in the United States. MR imaging may be particularly valuable in patients with dense breasts where mammography may be limited. MR imaging is also useful for presurgical planning in newly diagnosed breast cancer;[6] to detect multifocal, multicentric,[7] and contralateral malignancy;[8,9] for evaluation of response to neoadjuvant chemotherapy; and for assessment of the postsurgical breast.

Of all MR imaging techniques used for assessment of breast cancer, dynamic contrast-enhanced MR imaging (DCE-MR imaging) is the most established and widely used. This article will discuss the basic principles of DCE-MR imaging of the breast, including technical parameters, image acquisition, and image interpretation. It will also discuss some more advanced techniques for performing DCE-MR imaging of the breast and investigate future applications.

PRINCIPLES OF DYNAMIC CONTRAST-ENHANCED MR IMAGING

Two major imaging features are used to interpret findings on breast MR imaging: appearance and enhancement pattern. Appearance is assessed on high-spatial-resolution T1 postcontrast, though T2-weighted images may also be useful. Prior studies have described morphologies of enhancing masses that predict benign and malignant etiologies.[10–12] Since this article is focused on DCE-MR imaging, the morphologies of benign and malignant findings are not discussed.

Enhancement characteristics are based on observing changes in signal intensity (SI) on precontrast and multiple postcontrast images. One recent study suggested that threshold enhancement based on precontrast images and a single postcontrast series acquired 2.5 minutes following the injection of intravenous contrast is sufficient for discriminating benign and malignant lesions.[13] However, common clinical practice is to obtain baseline precontrast images and a series of multiple postcontrast images for analysis. This is a practice already established in other parts of the body. For example, in liver imaging T1-weighted images are routinely acquired precontrast and in multiple postcontrast phases. In the liver, lesions are characterized based on

Department of Diagnostic Radiology, Yale New Haven Hospital, 333 Cedar Street, MRC-147, New Haven, CT 06520, USA

* Corresponding author.

E-mail address: marianne.moon@yale.edu (M. Moon).

Magn Reson Imaging Clin N Am 17 (2009) 351–362
doi:10.1016/j.mric.2009.01.010

how their enhancement qualitatively changes with time. The same principle applies in breast imaging, only the analysis can be qualitative or quantitative.

The principles of contrast enhancement are based on tumor angiogenesis. Angiogenesis is a key step in breast cancer growth, local invasion, and progression to metastasis.[14,15] Invasive breast cancers are highly metabolically active, with demand for oxygen and nutrients that outstrips the normal vascular supply. When breast cancers reach a diameter of approximately 3 mm (10^6 cells), they are no longer adequately nourished by diffusion and hypoxia ensues. Hypoxia induces expression of cytokines like vascular endothelial growth factor, leading to the rapid formation of a new abnormal vascular network that lacks a stabilizing matrix and is more prone to endothelial leakage. Studies have demonstrated the value of tumor microvessel density as a marker for angiogenesis and a prognostic indicator for breast cancer metastasis.[16,17] An increased blood supply combined with abnormal, leaky capillaries results in faster enhancement than the surrounding tissues. Increased diffusion of contrast in the opposite direction after the initial bolus of contrast results in lesions that de-enhance, or washout, more rapidly than the surrounding tissues.

For DCE-MR imaging, a small molecular weight gadolinium-based contrast agent (GBCA) is injected intravenously and circulates in the bloodstream before passing into the extravascular extracellular space. The gadolinium does not actually enter into the cancer cells. This occurs more rapidly and to a greater degree with the neovascularity present in cancers. Equilibration between the intravascular and extracellular spaces occurs minutes after injection. Detection of the differential uptake and washout of GBCA, and hence increased signal on T1-weighted images, by cancer versus normal breast tissue forms the basis for DCE-MR imaging of breast cancer.

The goal of a DCE-MR imaging protocol is to image rapidly enough to detect differential enhancement, but also at a high enough spatial resolution to enable characterization based on size, shape, margins, and internal features. Optimal assessment of breast cancer with DCE-MR imaging therefore requires rapid acquisition of high-spatial and high-temporal-resolution images. The temporal resolution required for DCE-MR imaging depends on the type of analysis that will be performed on the images. The most commonly used analysis of enhancement is qualitative. Initial enhancement is described as slow, medium, or rapid; and the enhancement pattern is described as progressive, plateau, or washout.

This conforms to the American College of Radiology's Breast Imaging Reporting and Data System MR imaging (MRI-BRIADS) lexicon[18] and will be discussed elsewhere in this issue.

TECHNICAL PARAMETERS FOR DYNAMIC CONTRAST-ENHANCED MR IMAGING OF THE BREAST
Spatial and Temporal Resolution

Historically, spatial resolution and temporal resolution represented competing goals. Previous limitations in the speed and sophistication of MR imaging systems necessitated prioritizing one at the expense of the other.

Early studies of very high-temporal-resolution scanning, covering only a few slices through a suspicious lesion, showed an increased specificity for diagnosing malignancy.[19] However, subsequent investigations of ultrafast scan techniques with acquisitions as fast as 1 second did not show any compelling advantage for detecting malignancies.[20] These ultrafast techniques are not currently widely used in routine clinical practice but will be discussed elsewhere this issue.

One recent study compared a high-temporal-resolution, low-spatial-resolution technique to a low-temporal-resolution, high-spatial-resolution technique for characterizing lesions seen on breast MR imaging.[21] Patients were scanned using both strategies within a 5-day period. The low-temporal-resolution, high-spatial-resolution technique involved acquiring images with a voxel size of 4.7 mm^3 (32 cm field of view, 256 × 256 matrix, 3 mm thick slices for 3 × 1.25 × 1.25 mm voxels) every 69 seconds. Images were acquired up to 8 minutes after injection of IV contrast (7 postcontrast volumes). The high-temporal-resolution, low-spatial-resolution technique involved acquiring images with a voxel size of 1.44 mm^3 (32 cm field of view, 400 × 512 matrix, 3 mm thick slices for 3 × 0.8 × 0.6 mm voxels) every 116 seconds. Images were acquired up to 10 minutes postcontrast injection (five postcontrast volumes). Both techniques were achievable on a commercial MR imaging unit. The authors concluded that the increased spatial resolution improved diagnostic confidence and accuracy and that no diagnostically relevant time course information was lost by scanning at the lower temporal resolution.

High-spatial-resolution images are required for detection of small lesions and for assessment of lesion morphology (ie, definition of shape, margins, and internal features of lesions). It is thought that a slice thickness less than or equal to 3 mm and an in-plane resolution of 1 mm or less is needed to detect clinically relevant lesions.

A malignant lesion typically will enhance maximally between 60 to 120 seconds after GBCA injection. Background normal fibroglandular tissue enhances progressively thereafter, resulting in decreasing tumor-to-background conspicuity over time. Most clinical protocols are therefore designed to image the breast at as high a spatial resolution as possible while keeping the temporal resolution for each data set below 2 minutes.

Elimination of Fat Signal

Contrast enhancement may lead to a lesion becoming isointense to fatty breast tissue on a T1-weighted image. Therefore, it is advantageous to suppress or remove background fat signal from the breast to facilitate lesion detection. Subtraction and fat suppression are two techniques that are used to minimize signal from fat.

Fat suppression minimizes or eliminates fat signal at the time of imaging. A number of techniques are used to achieve homogenous and effective fat suppression across the large field of view used for bilateral breast DCE-MR imaging. One technique employs a frequency-selective fat saturation pulse to the entire imaged volume. Since the precise frequency for fat varies with magnetic field strength, the effectiveness of this technique is highly dependent on a homogenous magnetic field, a condition which is not always present given the large field of view and inhomogeneous imaging region (the two breasts are at the edge of the field of view and there is air between then; this makes it difficult to achieve a homogenous magnetic field). A second technique uses a spectrally selective radio frequency pulse to partially invert the signal from fat and then images at an inversion time to null the signal from fat. More recently, three-dimensional techniques that separate fat from water based on 2-point or 3-point Dixon techniques without applying a fat suppression pulse have become available—providing rapid, effective, and uniform fat suppression.[22]

Subtraction is a postprocessing technique that subtracts a precontrast data set from a postcontrast data set on a pixel-by-pixel basis. Subtraction is not sensitive to magnetic field inhomogeneity and does not entail an increase in scanning time. However, signal-to-noise ratio (SNR) is low on the subtracted images, and patient motion between the pre- and postcontrast scans can lead to signal misregistration and spurious enhancement. Additional postprocessing with re-registration software may mitigate this problem, though source images should always be viewed to confirm apparent enhancement on subtraction images.

Fat-suppression and subtraction techniques are not mutually exclusive. Subtractions of fat suppressed images can improve conspicuity of enhancing structures. This is especially true if a lesion is high SI on the fat suppressed images or if there is inhomogeneous fat suppression. At the authors' institution, we routinely perform our DCE sequences with fat suppression. Additional subtraction images are also created automatically on the scanner.

Magnetic Field Strength

Although DCE-MR imaging can be performed at magnetic field strengths below 1.5 T, evaluation may be limited by low SNR, and there is scant published data to support its use. Compared with DCE-MR imaging of the breast at 1.5 T, at 3.0 T there is greater SNR. As a result, there should be increased lesion enhancement for the same dose GBCA, though this can be offset by increased T1 relaxation times at 3 T. There may also be greater susceptibility artifacts and dielectric effects, which might compromise uniform enhancement throughout the breast.[23]

The major difference between field strengths is SNR. At 3 T the SNR is almost double that at 1.5 T (depending on the specific tissue and pulse sequence), and this increased SNR can be exploited to image at a higher spatial resolution. Sample DCE-MR imaging protocols at 1.5 T and 3 T are presented in **Table 1**. At Yale New Haven Hospital, the DCE-MR imaging examination involves one precontrast sequence followed by four postcontrast sequences. Imaging is performed out to 8 minutes postcontrast administration. These parameters are guidelines, and knowledgeable MR imaging technologists will modify them on a case-by-case basis. For example, to cover a large breast in less than 2 minutes it may be necessary to decrease the spatial resolution. Alternatively, in a patient with small breasts, it may be possible to increase the spatial resolution and still keep the temporal resolution below 2 minutes.

Use of Gadolinium-Based Contrast Agents

Unlike computed tomography, where there is a linear relationship between iodine concentration and increased density or image enhancement, MR enhancement with GBCAs is complex and dependent on several factors, including T1-relaxivity, a measure of an agent's ability to promote T1-relaxation. There are a number of different commercially available GBCAs used for DCE-MR

Table 1
DCE-MR imaging protocol at 3 T and 1.5 T

	3 T	1.5 T
Plane	Axial	Sagittal
Field of view	32 cm	20 cm
Slice thickness	1 mm	2.2 mm
Matrix	320 × 320	224 × 224
Voxel size	1 × 1 × 1 mm (1 mm³)	2.2 × 0.9 × 0.9 mm (1.8 mm³)
Temporal resolution	90–120 seconds	90–120 seconds
Fat suppression	Nonselective IR prep	Nonselective IR prep
Imaging	1 precontrast 4 postcontrast	1 precontrast 4 postcontrast

Images are obtained once precontrast and four times postcontrast. The sequences are acquired using centric filling of k-space. There is a 15 second delay between injecting contrast and the start of the first postcontrast acquisition.
Abbreviation: IR, inversion recovery.

imaging in the United States, including gadopentetate dimeglumine (Magnevist), gadodiamide (Omniscan), gadoteridol (ProHance), and gadoversetamide (OptiMARK). Although they differ in structure and physiochemical properties, they display similar in vivo T1-relaxivity values of 4.3 to 5.0 L/mmol/sec. Another agent, gadobenate dimeglumine (MultiHance), demonstrates a greater T1-relaxivity of 9.7 L/mmol/sec,[24] which translates into more pronounced contrast-enhancement. Clinically, this may improve detection and delineation of cancers with DCE-MR imaging. However, it may also result in greater enhancement and conspicuity of benign tissues, possibly resulting in a greater number of false positive examinations. It may also result in changes in the pharmacokinetic thresholds that some have found useful to differentiate between benign and malignant tissues on DCE-MR imaging of the breast.

A prospective multicenter study showed a potential advantage for gadobenate dimeglumine for breast MR imaging. In this study, there was better lesion detection and higher sensitivity for detecting malignancy compared with gadopentetate dimeglumine administered at the same dose of 0.1 mmol/kg.[25] However, the validity of these results was questioned because of an unequal distribution of malignant, benign, solitary, and multifocal lesions between the four randomized parallel dose groups.

A separate, intraindividual study compared equal doses (0.1 mmol/kg) of gadobenate dimeglumine and gadopentetate dimeglumine for breast MR imaging at 1.5 T in 26 consecutive women suspected of having a breast tumor at mammography or sonography. The results showed a significant increase in sensitivity (94.7% versus 76.3%) and negative predictive value (80.0% versus 47.1%) with the gadobenate dimeglumine, particularly for

lesions less than 5 mm in size.[26] However, the specificity was 100% for both agents, a result which was inconsistent with other published studies of breast DCE-MR imaging, leading to questions about the validity of these results. The authors suggest that this may have been due to the limited total number of evaluated lesions, the high proportion of malignant lesions (38 of 46 lesions, 82.6%), and the low number of benign fibroadenomas (n = 3) in the overall lesion population.

Regardless of the specific GBCA, most radiologists who perform DCE-MR imaging of the breast in the United States employ a standard dose of 20 cc or 0.1 mmol/kg administered at a rate of 2 to 3 mL/sec, followed by saline flush. Some favor a higher contrast dose to increase lesion conspicuity, though there is little published data to support this approach.[27] An early study compared a dose of 0.1 mmol/kg with a dose of 0.16 mmol/kg at 1.0 T and found increased conspicuity of malignant lesions with the higher dose.[28] However, of the 152 studies in 132 patients, only 20 received both doses, and 10 received the higher dose because of uncertain diagnosis with the lower dose. These studies were also performed without the benefit of fat suppression or subtraction postprocessing, and no information about statistical significance or blinding was provided. Some have advocated the use of half-dose gadobenate dimeglumine as being equivalent to a single dose of other GBCAs, but there is little evidence to support this approach in the peer-reviewed literature.

Whichever GBCA and dose is administered, consistency of dose, saline flush, injection rate, timing, and imaging parameters are crucial for reliable interpretation and comparison of studies.

IMAGE INTERPRETATION

MR imaging findings should not be interpreted in isolation and should be correlated with mammographic and ultrasound findings, and medical history. When attempting to diagnose a cancer on DCE-MR imaging, the first step is to identify abnormally enhancing tissue and classify it into one of the following categories in the MRI-BIRADS lexicon: (1) a mass, (2) non-masslike enhancement, or (3) a focus. Details of these morphologic descriptors and their significance are discussed in other sources.[29] Once an enhancing finding is categorized, morphologic features described, and an assessment for bilateral symmetry performed, it may be further classified based on enhancement kinetics.

ENHANCEMENT KINETIC ANALYSIS: MASSES

Kinetics refers to the rate and intensity of lesion enhancement and de-enhancement over time. This may be performed by the reader by either visual assessment of the images obtained before and at various intervals after GBCA administration, or by tracking the SI in a manually selected region of interest (ROI) over the course of the dynamic series to produce a time-SI curve. This is called an ROI analysis.

Based on the MRI-BIRADS, analysis of enhancement kinetics is divided into two parts. The first part is the initial rate of enhancement based on comparison of the precontrast and first postcontrast data sets. The second part of the analysis is based on the shape of the time-SI curve. An example of a time-SI curve is shown in **Fig. 1**.

Initial Enhancement

Initial enhancement is divided into slow, medium, and rapid enhancement. These distinctions are somewhat arbitrary and, to our knowledge, there are no set definitions. Initial enhancement is quantified by calculating the percent enhancement $(SI_{post} - SI_{pre})/SI_{pre} \times 100$, where SI_{post} is the average SI within the ROI on the first postcontrast image and SI_{pre} is the average SI within the ROI on the precontrast images. One large study investigated the role of initial enhancement in characterizing breast lesions.[13] They evaluated 154 consecutive lesions in 125 consecutive patients who underwent an MR imaging-guided breast biopsy. Lesions were divided into groups based on initial percent enhancement thresholds of less than 50%, 50% to 100%, and greater than 100%. While there was no difference in the amount of enhancement between benign and malignant

A

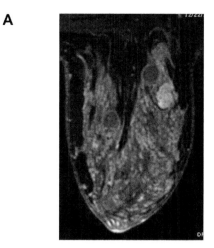

B

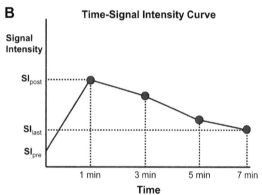

Fig. 1. Time-SI curve. (A) Axial post contrast image of the right breast. There is an enhancing mass in the lateral breast. A region of interest has been drawn around the mass (white oval). The average SI within this oval is calculated on the precontrast and each of the four postcontrast images and plotted in a time-SI curve as shown in (B). (B) Time-SI curve created from an ROI analysis of the mass depicted in (A). The percent enhancement is defined as the ratio $(SI_{post} - SI_{pre})/SI_{pre} \times 100$. This is a measure of how much the mass initially enhances. SI_{pre} is the SI of the mass on the precontrast image. SI_{post} is the SI of the mass on the first postcontrast image. SI_{last} is the SI of the mass on the last postcontrast image.

lesions, using a percent enhancement of greater than 100% as a marker for malignancy increased specificity and would have reduced the false-positive biopsy rate by 23%.

Shape of the Time-Signal Intensity Curve

The shape of the time-SI curve is described in one of three ways: persistent, plateau, and washout. A persistent curve is one where the SI continues to increase with time (ie, the lesion continues to enhance on each subsequent postcontrast data set). A plateau curve is a curve where the SI levels off after an initial enhancement. A washout curve is a curve where the SI initially increases after GBCA administration but then decreases on the subsequent postcontrast images. These curves are depicted in **Fig. 2**.

Many cancers, especially invasive ones, enhance rapidly and intensely, reaching an enhancement peak within the first 2 minutes after contrast injection and then de-enhancing. This is thought to be related to increased microvessel density and arteriovenous anastomoses leading to rapid inflow and outflow of contrast material,[30] but the precise pathophysiologic correlate is unknown. Benign tissues tend to demonstrate persistent kinetics, with enhancement continuing to increase after the initial phase, albeit often at a slower rate.

As for initial enhancement, there are no strict criteria for classifying these curves. A methodology used by one commercial vendor uses the following definition. If the SI at the last time point is greater than the SI at the first postcontrast time point by more than 10% the pattern is persistent. If the SI on the last image is within ± 10% of the SI on the first postcontrast image the pattern is plateau. If the SI decreases by greater than 10% then the pattern is washout (See **Fig. 2**).

Table 2 summarizes the correlation between enhancement pattern and whether a mass is benign or malignant. All studies referenced found significant overlap in curve characteristics for benign and malignant lesions. The largest of these studies is by Schnall and colleagues.[4] In this series of 995 lesions in 854 breasts, a mass with a washout enhancement curve was five times more likely to be malignant than a mass with a persistent curve. However, 45% of all cancers had a persistent enhancement curve. Clearly, using the shape of the enhancement curve alone is not sufficient for diagnosing a mass as benign or malignant. The morphology of the lesion must also be considered.

Postprocessing

Various parameters derived from an ROI analysis can be color coded to visually depict enhancement characteristics and these can be overlaid onto the anatomic images. Computer aided diagnostic programs can automatically process the pre- and postcontrast images and identify pixels with slow, medium, or rapid enhancement; and pixels with persistent, plateau, or washout enhancement curves. For example, in **Fig. 3**, pixels with initial percent enhancement of greater than 100% are presented in color. Pixels with a persistent curve are colored blue, pixels with a plateau curve are colored yellow, and pixels with a washout curve are colored red. Viewing images in this manner can provide a quick overview of a case and can be useful for identifying masses that might have missed when looking at the anatomic images alone. These graphics overlays are easily created with commercial products in real time.

When viewing these images it is important to remember that there is considerable kinetic overlap between benign and malignant lesions. There are many cancers, particularly noninvasive types that may not enhance intensely or demonstrate washout or plateau kinetics. Conversely, there are also many benign entities, including fibroadenomas, fibrocystic changes, scars, sclerosing adenosis, lobular carcinoma in situ, focal fibrosis, and atypical ductal hyperplasia that demonstrate "malignant" curves.[31] Thus, enhancement kinetics should not be evaluated without consideration of lesion morphology.

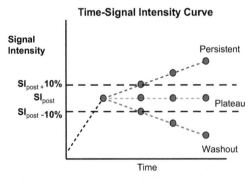

Time-Signal Intensity Curve

Signal Intensity

Persistent

SI_{post} +10%
SI_{post}
SI_{post} -10%

Plateau

Washout

Time

Fig. 2. Time-SI curve with different enhancement patterns. A persistent curve (*blue*), continues to increase, a plateau curve (*turquoise*) remains relatively flat, and a washout curve (*red*) decreases after an initial rise. In this example, a SI change of greater or less than 10% at the last time point differentiates between the different patterns. This distinction is arbitrary. These thresholds are determined at the physician's discretion, and may be a qualitative assessment.

ENHANCEMENT KINETIC ANALYSIS: NONMASSLIKE ENHANCEMENT AND FOCI

Kinetic analysis may be helpful in characterizing masses, but it seems to be less useful in the evaluation of nonmasslike enhancement. The differential diagnosis of nonmasslike enhancement includes a variety of benign entities as well as ductal carcinoma in situ and invasive lobular carcinoma, likely because cancers may be fed by existing fibroglandular capillaries and thus exhibit inconsistent angiogenic activity and variable enhancement kinetics.[32,33] The value of kinetic

Table 2
Sensitivity and specificity data of enhancement curve patterns

	Persistent	Plateau	Washout
Kuhl, et al.[30]	Sensitivity for malignancy 53% Specificity for malignancy 72%	Sensitivity for malignancy 42% Specificity for malignancy 75%	Sensitivity for malignancy 20% Specificity for malignancy 90%
Schnall et al.[4]	Pattern detected in 45% of cancers	—	Positive predictive value of 76% for identifying malignancy
Bluemke, et al.[36]	Present in 83% of benign lesions and 9% of malignant lesions	—	—

analysis for nonmasslike enhancement and foci is not well established.

DETECTION OF BREAST CANCER WITH DYNAMIC CONTRAST-ENHANCED MR IMAGING

DCE-MR imaging has been demonstrated to have a high sensitivity for invasive breast cancer, with published sensitivities between 89% and 100%,[31] consistently higher than mammography.[6,32,34] Very small cancers, cancers that display a diffuse growth pattern such as invasive lobular carcinoma, and cancers that exhibit "benign" morphology are particularly problematic with radiograph mammography. Breast fibroglandular tissue, more prominent in younger women, also limits mammography where sensitivity for breast cancer may be as low as 45% compared with 100% for predominantly fatty breasts. In one study comparing 177 breast lesions across multiple imaging modalities including MR imaging with a histologic reference standard, sensitivities of mammography and MR imaging were 81% versus 95% for invasive ductal carcinoma, 34% versus 96% for invasive lobular carcinoma, and 55% versus 89% for ductal carcinoma in situ.[35]

Though highly sensitive for breast carcinoma, DCE-MR imaging is only moderately specific. A multicenter study of 404 malignant lesions in 821 patients demonstrated a sensitivity of 88.1% and specificity of 67.7% for detecting malignancy.[36] Compared with radiograph mammography, DCE-MR imaging may be less specific, resulting in increased recalls and benign biopsies. Currently, DCE-MR imaging cannot be considered a replacement for radiograph mammography and breast ultrasound for most applications—but rather an adjunct.

PRACTICAL LIMITATIONS AND QUANTITATIVE ANALYSIS

There are several important limitations to consider when interpreting DCE-MR imaging. First, there are no universally accepted definitions for what constitutes slow, medium, or rapid enhancement. In the three published studies referenced in **Table 2**, curve characteristics were determined qualitatively. Independent readers characterized the curves based on their general shapes. Therefore, when using computer aided diagnostic analysis, it is important to remember that threshold parameters are set by the user based on experience (or vendor suggestions) and comfort level.

Secondly, no rigorous studies have been performed to measure the effect of DCE-MR imaging on decision making and eventual outcomes. For these reasons, DCE-MR imaging as described above is a qualitative analysis.

In response to these limitations, more quantitative analysis of DCE-MR imaging data can be performed. Various parameters derived from the time-SI curve—such as maximum slope of enhancement, time to peak enhancement, and degree or percent enhancement over baseline—can also be calculated, color coded, and displayed as an overlay on the anatomic images.

One sample parameter is called signal enhancement ratio (SER), which is defined as $(SI_{post} - SI_{pre})/(SI_{last} - SI_{pre})$. In a recent study,[37] 48 women were imaged before and after neoadjuvant chemotherapy for invasive breast cancer. Images were obtained before contrast, 2.5 minutes after

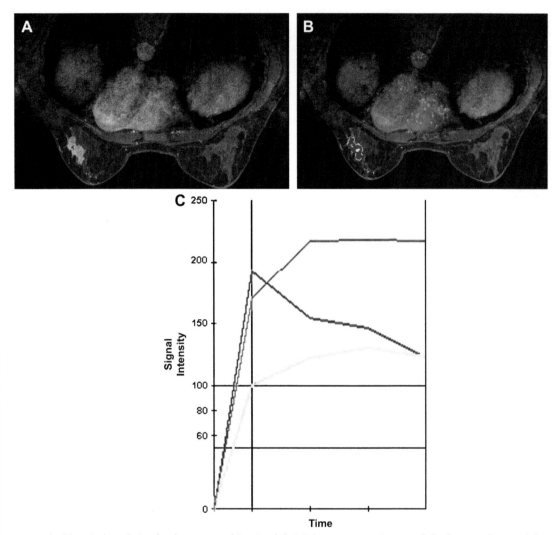

Fig. 3. Pixel-by-pixel analysis of enhancement kinetics. (A) Axial postcontrast image of the breasts shows a lobulated infiltrative ductal carcinoma in the left breast. (B) Fused image containing anatomic information and a pixel-by-pixel analysis of enhancement kinetics. Pixels with percent enhancement of greater than 100% are displayed in color. Pixels with a persistent enhancement curve are blue. Pixels with a plateau enhancement curve are yellow. Pixels with a washout curve are red. (C) Sample time-SI curves from three separate pixels in the mass seen in (A) and (B).

contrast, and at 7.5 minutes after contrast. Thus, the time enhancement curve had three points. SER was calculated before and after therapy and correlated with disease-free survival following surgery. Average tumor SER based on ROI analysis and the volume of tumor meeting threshold SER values (ie, the number of pixels within the tumor above a threshold SER value) were positively correlated with the risk of recurrence.

Studies like this are useful because they provide a more concrete framework for interpreting DCE-MR imaging images. However, quantitative analysis is limited when there are few points on the time-SI curve. For example, with only five data points spaced 2 minutes apart (precontrast and 4 postcontrast), the maximum slope of enhancement is effectively the same as the percent enhancement since all masses will maximally enhance on the first postcontrast image. Thus, there has been recent research on performing DCE-MR imaging with a much higher temporal resolution, resulting in many more data points on the time-SI curve.

HIGH-TEMPORAL-RESOLUTION DCE-MR IMAGING

Graphs of gadolinium concentration as a function of time can be constructed from a series of high-temporal-resolution images. This data can be fit to either heuristic[38,39] or pharmacologic[40,41] models of tumor perfusion. To optimally fit data points to a curve, there must be three to five data points over the most rapidly changing portion of the curve. For breast neoplasms, this requires a temporal resolution of 5 to 15 seconds. By contrast, the DCE-MR imaging described above uses a temporal resolution of 90 to 120 seconds. Current commercial pulse sequences will not allow imaging this fast at an acceptable spatial resolution, and most high-temporal DCE-MR imaging is performed in the research setting. However, several developmental sequences will allow for fast imaging[42] at adequate spatial resolution and in the future may be available for commercial use.

In the clinical setting, DCE-MR imaging as previously described is primarily used to screen breasts for malignancy. In the research setting, high-temporal-resolution DCE-MR imaging is used as a biomarker for measuring or predicting the response of breast tumors to therapy. Early studies have shown that perfusion parameters derived from pharmacologic models of the time-SI curve can predict which tumors will respond to anti-angiogenesis chemotherapy agents.[43] Similarly, early studies have suggested that perfusion parameters derived from these models can determine which tumors have responded to chemotherapy.[44] For example, **Fig. 4** shows the results of a DCE-MR imaging examination performed on a patient with breast cancer.

Limitations of high-temporal-resolution DCE-MR imaging include complex imaging techniques and postprocessing. Most of the required pulse sequences are not commercially available and postprocessing requires time and software. Fitting of the data to the heuristic or pharmacologic models requires specific software usually written by researchers within a research institution. Although at least one noncommercial software package is available to institutions wishing to perform these analyses,[45] analysis is time consuming and is impractical to perform in a clinical setting.

FUTURE DEVELOPMENTS

The technology underpinning DCE-MR imaging will continue to improve. As imaging becomes faster, higher-temporal-resolution DCE-MR imaging will become possible, and advances made in the research environment can be moved into the clinical setting. This may allow breast MR imaging to serve as a noninvasive diagnostic and prognostic tool. Other promising MR imaging techniques for breast cancer evaluation are undergoing investigation, including diffusion-weighted imaging,

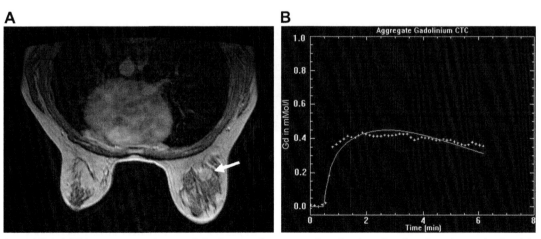

Fig. 4. (A) Axial T1 postcontrast image of the breasts shows an enhancing invasive ductal carcinoma in the right breast (*white arrow*). (B) Signal-time intensity curve taken from ROI analysis of the tumor using high-temporal-resolution DCE-MR imaging. The temporal resolution of the scan was 6 seconds. Notice how many more points are on the curve than in Fig. 3. (C) This is a table depicting the results of DCE-MR imaging at three different time points: before chemotherapy, after 2 weeks of chemotherapy, and after 6 months of chemotherapy. It also depicts a pixel histogram of a perfusion parameter called K^{trans}, which is a variable derived from a pharmacologic model that describes tumor vascularity. It is related to arterial input, macroscopic vessel density, microscopic vessel density, and capillary permeability. Higher values of K^{trans} indicate a more vascular tumor. Although the tumor size did not change during therapy, the appearance of the time-SI curves and the pixel-by-pixel distribution of K^{trans} did. Whether this pattern is predictive of long term response is currently under study.

C

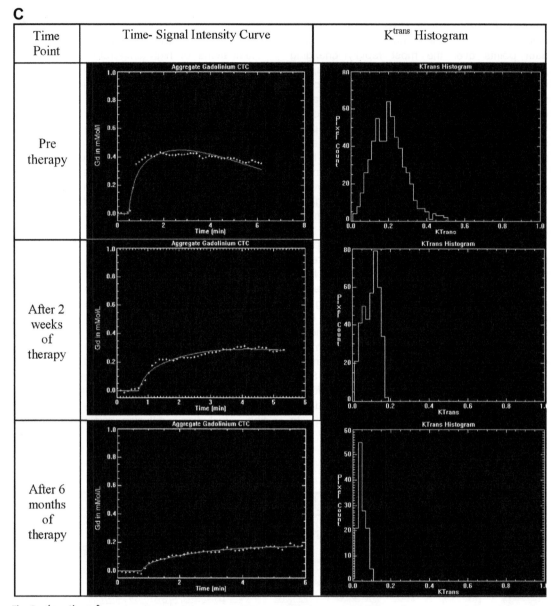

Time Point	Time- Signal Intensity Curve	K^{trans} Histogram
Pre therapy		
After 2 weeks of therapy		
After 6 months of therapy		

Fig. 4. (*continued*)

spectroscopy, blood oxygen level dependent imaging, targeted macromolecular contrast agents, and elastography.[46–48]

SUMMARY

Dynamic contrast-enhanced magnetic resonance imaging of the breast is a noninvasive technique that uses differential gadolinium-based contrast-enhancement patterns related to the increased endothelial leakage of malignant angiogenesis to detect breast cancer.

Clinical DCE-MR imaging of the breast has undergone considerable growth from a once investigational technique to an important clinical tool in widespread use. Progress in MR technology and refinement of MR imaging parameters now allow for concurrent acquisition of high-spatial-resolution and adequate-temporal-resolution images, which are necessary for accurate assessment of breast lesion morphology and qualitative kinetic analysis. More advanced DCE-MR imaging techniques involving higher-temporal-resolution images and rigorous quantitative analysis of the time-signal enhancement curves are currently an area of research.

DCE-MR imaging has been demonstrated to have a high sensitivity for breast cancer, though still only a moderate specificity for breast lesions, making it a useful adjunct though not a substitute for radiograph mammography, ultrasound, and high-spatial-resolution MR imaging. Applications in breast cancer diagnosis, treatment planning, and measurement of treatment response will continue to expand as DCE-MR imaging technique evolves.

REFERENCES

1. Ries LAG, Melbert D, Krapcho M, et al. SEER cancer statistics review, 1975–2005. National Cancer Institute. Bethesda, MD. Available at: http://seer.cancer.gov/csr/1975_2005/. Accessed August 2008.
2. American Cancer Society. Cancer facts & figures 2008. Atlanta (GA): American Cancer Society; 2008.
3. Peters NH, Rinkes IH, Suithoff NP, et al. Meta-analysis of MR imaging in the diagnosis of breast lesions. Radiology 2008;246:116–24.
4. Schnall MD, Blume J, Bluemke DA, et al. Diagnostic architectural and dynamic features at breast MR imaging: multicenter study. Radiology 2006;238:42–53.
5. Saslow D, Boetes C, Burke W, et al. American Cancer Society guidelines for breast screening with MRI as an adjunct to mammography. CA Cancer J Clin 2007;57:75–89.
6. Bedrosian I, Mick R, Orel SG, et al. Changes in the surgical management of patients with breast carcinoma based on preoperative magnetic resonance imaging. Cancer 2003;98:468–73.
7. Fischer U, Kopka L, Grabbe E. Breast carcinoma: effect of preoperative contrast-enhanced MR imaging on the therapeutic approach. Radiology 1999;213:881–8.
8. Liberman L, Morris EA, Kim CM, et al. MR imaging findings in the contralateral breast of women with recently diagnosed breast cancer. AJR Am J Roentgenol 2003;180:333–41.
9. Lehman CD, Gatsonis C, Kuhl CK, et al. MRI evaluation of the contralateral breast in women with recently diagnosed breast cancer. N Engl J Med 2007;356(13):1295–303.
10. Lee CH. Problem solving MR imaging of the breast. Radiol Clin North Am 2004;42:919–34.
11. Nunes LW, Schnall MD, Orel SG. Update of breast MR imaging architectural interpretation model. Radiology 2001;238:42–53.
12. Kuhl CK, Bieling HB, Gieseke J, et al. Healthy premenopausal breast parenchyma in dynamic contrast-enhanced MR imaging of the breast: normal contrast medium enhancement and cyclical-phase dependency. Radiology 1997;203:137–44.
13. Williams TC, Demartini WB, Partridge SC, et al. Breast MR imaging: computer-aided evaluation program for discriminating benign from malignant lesions. Radiology 2007;244:94–103.
14. Schneider BP, Miller KD. Angiogenesis of breast cancer. J Clin Oncol 2005;23:1782–90.
15. Folkman J, Watson K, Ingbr D, et al. Induction of angiogenesis during the transition from hyperplasia to neoplasia. Nature 1989;339:58–61.
16. Weidner N, Semple JP, Welch WR, et al. Tumor angiogenesis and metastasis-correlation in invasive breast carcinoma. N Engl J Med 1991;324(1):1–8. PMID: 1701519.
17. Uzzan B, Nicolas P, Cucherat M, et al. Microvessel density as a prognostic factor in women with breast cancer: a systematic review of the literature and meta-analysis. Cancer Res 2004;64(9):2941–55.
18. Erguvan-Dogan B, Whitman G, Kushwaha A, et al. BI-RADS-MRI: a primer. AJR Am J Roentgenol 2006;187:W152–60.
19. Boetes C, Barentsz JO, Mus RD, et al. MR characterization of suspicious breast lesions with a Gadolinium-enhanced tuboFLASH subtraction technique. Radiology 1994;193:777–81.
20. Schorn C, Fischer U, Luftner-Nagel S, et al. Diagnostic potential of ultrafast contrast-enhanced MRI of the breast in hypervascularized lesions: are there advantages in comparison with standard dynamic MRI? J Comput Assist Tomogr 1999;23(1):118–22.
21. Kuhl C, Schild H, Morakkabati N. Dynamic bilateral contrast enhanced MR imaging of the breast: trade off between spatial and temporal resolution. Radiology 2005;236:789–800.
22. Ma J. A single-point Dixon technique for fat-suppressed fast 3D gradient-echo imaging with a flexible echo time. J Magn Reson Imaging 2008;27(4):881–90.
23. Kuhl CK, Jost P, Morakkabati N, et al. Contrast enhanced MR imaging of the breast at 3.0T and 1.5T in the same patients: initial experience. Radiology 2006;239:666–76.
24. deHaen C, Cabrini M, Akhnana L, et al. Gadobenate dimeglumine 0.5 M solution for injection (MultiHance): pharmaceutical formulation and physicochemical properties of a new magnetic resonance imaging contrast medium. J Comput Assist Tomogr 1999;23(S1):S161–8.
25. Knopp MV, Bourne MW, Sardanelli F, et al. Gadobenate dimeglumine-enhanced MRI of the breast: analysis of dose response and comparison with gadopentetate dimeglumine. AJR Am J Roentgenol 2003;181(3):663–76.
26. Pediconi F, Catalano C, Occhiato R, et al. Breast lesion detection and characterization at contrast-enhanced MR mammography: gadobenate

dimeglumine versus gadopentetate dimeglumine. Radiology 2005;237:45–56.

27. Helbich TH. Contrast-enhanced magnetic resonance imaging of the breast. Eur J Radiol 2000;34:203–19.

28. Heywang-Kobrunner SH, Haustein H, Pohl C, et al. Contrast-enhanced MR imaging of the breast: comparison of two different doses of gadopentetate dimeglumine. Radiology 1994;191:639–46.

29. American College of Radiology. Breast imaging reporting and data system atlas (BI-RADS atlas). Reston (VA): American College of Radiology; 2003.

30. Kuhl CK, Mielcareck P, Klaschik S, et al. Dynamic breast MR imaging: are signal intensity time course data useful for differential diagnosis of enhancing lesions? Radiology 1999;211:101–10.

31. Rausch DR, Hendrick RE. How to optimize clinical breast MR imaging practices and techniques on your 1.5-T system. Radiographics 2006;26(5):1469–84.

32. Kuhl CK. Current status of breast MR imaging part 1: choice of technique, image interpretation, diagnostic accuracy, and transfer to clinical practice. Radiology 2007;244(2):356–78.

33. Jansen SA, Fan X, Karczmar GS, et al. Differentiation between benign and malignant breast lesions detected by bilateral dynamic contrast-enhanced MRI: a sensitivity and specificity study. Magn Reson Med 2008;59:747–54.

34. Harms SE, Flamig DP, Hesley KL, et al. MR imaging of the breast with rotating delivery of excitation off resonance: clinical experience with pathologic correlation. Radiology 1993;187(2):493–501.

35. Berg WA, Gutierrez L, NessAvier MS, et al. Diagnostic accuracy of mammography, clinical examination, US, and MR imaging in pre-operative assessment of breast cancer. Radiology 2004;233:830–49.

36. Bluemke A, Gatsonis CA, Chen MH, et al. Magnetic resonance imaging of the breast prior to biopsy. JAMA 2004;292(22):2735–42.

37. Li K, Partfidge S, Joe B, et al. Invasive breast cancer: predicting disease recurrence by using high-spatial-resolution signal enhancement ratio imaging. Radiology 2008;248:79–87.

38. Huisman H, Engelbrecht M, Barentsz J. Accurate estimation of pharmacokinetic contrast-enhanced dynamic MRI parameters of the prostate. J Magn Reson Imaging 2001;13:607–14.

39. Moate P, Dougherty L, Schnall M, et al. A modified logistic model to describe gadolinium kinetics in breast tumors. Magn Reson Imaging 2004;22:467–73.

40. Tofts P. Modeling tracer kinetics in dynamic Gd-DTPA MR imaging. J Magn Reson Imaging 1997;7:91–101.

41. Tofts P, Brix G, Buckley D, et al. Estimating kinetic parameters from dynamic contrast-enhanced T1-weighted MRI of a diffusible tracer: standardized quantities and symbols. J Magn Reson Imaging 1999;10:223–32.

42. Dougherty L, Isaac G, Rosen M, et al. High frame-rate simultaneous bilateral breast DCE-MRI. Magn Reson Med 2007;57:220–5.

43. Thukral A, Thomasson D, Chow C, et al. Inflammatory breast cancer: dynamic contrast-enhanced MR in patients receiving bevacizumab—initial experience. Radiology 2007;244:727–35.

44. Yankeelov T, Lepage M, Chakravarthy A, et al. Integration of quantitative DCE-MRI and ADC mapping to monitor treatment response in human breast cancer: initial results. Magn Reson Imaging 2007;25:1–13.

45. d'Arcy J, Collins D, Padhani A, et al. Informatics in radiology (infoRAD): magnetic resonance imaging workbench: analysis and visualization of dynamic contrast-enhanced MR imaging data. Radiographics 2006;26:621–32.

46. Sinha S, Sinha U. Recent advances in breast MRI and MRS. NMR Biomed 2009;22(1);3–16.

47. Garra BS, Cespedes EI, Ophir J, et al. Elastography of breast lesions: initial clinical results. Radiology 1997;202:79–86.

48. Bartella L, Huang W. Proton (1H) MR spectroscopy of the breast. Radiographics 2007;27:S241–52.

Dynamic Contrast-Enhanced MR Imaging in the Evaluation of Patients with Prostate Cancer

Colm J. McMahon, MB[a],*, B. Nicolas Bloch, MD[a],
Robert E. Lenkinski, PhD[b], Neil M. Rofsky, MD[a]

KEYWORDS

- Prostatic neoplasm • MR imaging • Contrast media
- Neoplasm staging • Kinetics • Gadolinium-DTPA

The diagnosis and management of prostate cancer requires a multimodality and multidisciplinary approach, including urologists, radiation oncologists, pathologists, and radiologists. There are many factors to be considered in determining the optimal treatment pathway for patients with prostate cancer. The role of imaging, particularly MR imaging, in this clinical setting is evolving. Advances in dynamic contrast-enhanced (DCE) MR imaging may lead to a more central role of MR imaging in caring for these patients. This article focuses on DCE MR imaging in the assessment of patients with prostate cancer, with reference to the clinical dilemmas encountered in imaging and managing this disease.

PROSTATE CANCER—CLINICAL PERSPECTIVE AND THE ROLE OF IMAGING

Adenocarcinoma of the prostate gland is the most frequently diagnosed cancer in men, with over 186,000 new cases diagnosed in the United States in 2008.[1] Adjusted for age, the incidence rate is 163 per 100,000 men per year.[2] The number of deaths in the United States from prostate cancer in 2008 is estimated to be over 28,000.[1]

In clinical practice, a patient is suspected of having prostate cancer based on one or more clinical data points: an abnormal digital rectal examination (DRE), an abnormal prostate-specific antigen (PSA) or less commonly, hesitancy, urgency, or hematuria/hematospermia. Clearly, the DRE and PSA have facilitated earlier detection of disease; however, it must be recognized that each suffers from a limited sensitivity and specificity.[3–6] Furthermore, when the PSA is high enough to suggest cancer it cannot localize the tumor, if a tumor is present at all.

Treatment options for prostate cancer include surgery (radical prostatectomy), external beam radiotherapy, brachytherapy, cryotherapy, androgen deprivation therapy, and watchful waiting. There is substantial evidence that patients with low-risk prostate cancer can be successfully managed conservatively. In a study of 767 men treated conservatively or with androgen deprivation therapy alone, subjects with low-grade prostate cancers had a minimal risk of dying from prostate cancer.[7] For example, in subjects with prostate cancer having a Gleason grade of 2–4; there were 6 deaths per 1000 person-years. For subjects with prostate cancer having a Gleason

This article was supported in part by NIH grant R01CA116465.

[a] Department of Radiology, Beth Israel Deaconess Medical Center, 330 Brookline Avenue, Boston, MA 02215, USA

[b] MRI Research Division, Ansin 2nd Floor, Beth Israel Deaconess Medical Center, 330 Brookline Avenue, Boston, MA 02215, USA

* Corresponding author.

E-mail address: cmcmahon@bidmc.harvard.edu (C.J. McMahon).

Magn Reson Imaging Clin N Am 17 (2009) 363–383
doi:10.1016/j.mric.2009.01.013

grade of 8–10, however, there were 121 deaths per 1000 person-years.[7] Given the variable natural history of this disease, side effects of treatment are an important factor in considering therapy for prostate cancer.

Radical prostatectomy carries risks of urinary incontinence, urethral stricture, impotence, and the morbidity associated with general anesthesia.[8] External beam radiotherapy can result in acute cystitis, proctitis, and enteritis. Cryotherapy is associated with risks of impotence, incontinence, urethral sloughing, urinary fistula or stricture, and bladder neck obstruction. Hormonal therapy includes luteinizing hormone-releasing hormone agonists, side effects of which include impotence, hot flashes, depression and loss of libido.

Given the usual age of diagnosis of prostate cancer (median age is 68 years[1]), comorbidity and overall life expectancy need to be considered in addition to the stage and grade of disease in determining an appropriate management plan for a given patient. For these reasons, radical prostatectomy is generally only considered in patients with disease confined to the prostate gland, and when the patient has a life expectancy of 10 years or more.[9] The determination of the status of prostate cancer disease status is of critical importance in stratifying patients into their appropriate treatment algorithms.

When there is a suspicion of prostate cancer, a patient is frequently referred to transrectal ultrasound-guided biopsy. Considering the limited ability of ultrasound to provide a reliable biopsy target,[10] and that each biopsy specimen represents only 1/10,000 of the gland, the false negative rate of 11–25% overall seems remarkably low, yet remains a substantial challenge for patient management.[11,12] In this context, the detection of prostate cancer in patients with a negative biopsy represents a key goal of imaging.

With a positive biopsy, certain predictive information can be derived: the percentage of a core that is positive, the number of cores that are positive, and the Gleason grade, all of which scale with the aggressiveness of the patient's disease.[13,14] The results of the DRE, PSA, and Gleason score have been combined into nomograms, popularized as the Partin tables, to suggest probabilities of disease aggressiveness, stage, and, ultimately, prognosis.[15] Whereas this information can guide patients and their physicians toward a treatment approach, it too has pitfalls and much remains unknown about the particular individual's cancer.[16–18] This circumstance leaves the patient with a variety of options and a range of potential responses and side effects, often creating confusion and anxiety.

Thus, additional details about a particular man's own cancer are vital to improve the physician–patient dialog and to optimize their care and management. Imaging holds promise to provide more in-depth information about a given individual's cancer, such as the designation of a dominant focus, a determination of multifocality, a determination of singular and aggregate disease volume, and a more comprehensive assessment of the disease vascularity, its metabolism, stage, and grade. Research and development in MR imaging over time have achieved slow and steady gains toward realizing such promises.

The current role of MR imaging in prostate cancer is to facilitate treatment planning and to assess response to therapy. This is largely accomplished by localizing and staging biopsy-proven cancer, and by facilitating a diagnosis when the cancer is occult. A determination of the aggressiveness of a patient's tumor represents an additional challenge that is being addressed with MR techniques.[19,20]

The requirements of imaging differ depending on the clinical goal. If detection is the key goal, then high-resolution, broad coverage of the gland and seminal vesicles is necessary. High-resolution imaging has become increasingly important since the era of PSA screening, an era associated with a down-staging of disease[21] and detection of smaller volume of disease.[22]

The interest in developing watchful waiting strategies for serially following a relevant tumor focus and for pursuing response to therapy evaluations is increasing,[23] now that attention is being directed toward the assessment of limited disease burden and dominant focal cancers, with the recognition that indolent cancers are probably being over-treated,[4] That has implications for focused, limited anatomic coverage assessments. In those scenarios, the use of limited through-plane coverage and high temporal resolution DCE MR imaging may be attractive, offering quantitative, kinetic parameters to follow over time. Rigorous test/re-test evaluations are necessary to establish confidence before relying upon such an approach.

Ideally, effective detection needs to be accompanied by accurate and comprehensive tissue characterization, including a determination of tumor volume and aggressiveness. Considering the demands for anatomic coverage and the array of techniques that can be applied in a given imaging session, a judicious selection of strategies is essential for yielding an optimized result within a feasible time frame.

PROSTATE MR IMAGING
Noncontrast MR Imaging

Traditionally, prostate MR imaging has relied predominantly on T2-weighted (T2w) imaging for the diagnosis, localization, and staging of prostate cancer. An endorectal coil offers higher signal-to-noise in the region of the prostate gland. On T2w imaging, the normal peripheral gland is high in signal intensity, and most prostate cancers are seen as focal areas of low signal intensity within this anatomic location.[24]

While low signal intensity relative to the background tissue on T2w imaging is the MR appearance of many cancers, that finding has limited sensitivity and specificity. Mucinous adenocarcinoma demonstrates high signal intensity on T2w imaging[25] and therefore may be obscured in the normal high signal background of the peripheral zone, where most tumors occur. Sensitivity can also be limited by peripheral zones that display diffusely low signal intensity (sometimes due to chronic prostatitis), which blunts the expected contrast of tumor within the peripheral zone. Finally, in terms of sensitivity, the low and heterogeneous signal that typifies the central gland, particularly in benign prostatic hypertrophy, can also obscure the low signal intensity of tumors located in that portion of the gland. Specificity on T2w imaging can be limited by the presence of prostatitis, hemorrhage, fibrosis, inflammation, and posttreatment changes, all capable of yielding focal and diffuse low signal intensity.

A critical determinant of prostate cancer operability is the presence or absence of extracapsular extension. In an assessment for extracapsular extension on T2w imaging, the following factors are typically considered: (a) broad (>12 mm) tumor contact with the prostate capsule, (b) smooth capsular bulge, (c) irregular capsular bulge, (d) obliteration of the rectoprostatic angle, and (e) asymmetry of the neurovascular bundle.

Beyersdorff and colleagues[26] demonstrated that invasion of the neurovascular bundle, direct periprostatic invasion and loss of the rectoprostatic angle were specific (83%–100%), but not sensitive (0%–20%) for the diagnosis of extracapsular extension of prostate cancer. In the same study, extended contiguity with the capsule and bulge were sensitive (80%–100%), but less specific (23%–39%). In a study by Yu and colleagues,[27] the highest specificity findings for extracapsular extension were loss of the rectoprostatic angle and asymmetry of the neurovascular bundle. The finding of irregular capsular bulge was of intermediate sensitivity and specificity.

The results of prostate cancer staging using noncontrast morphologic imaging alone have been modest. The ranges of reported sensitivity and specificity of unenhanced MR for prostate cancer detection are broad, from 35%–89% and from 56%–90%, respectively.[28–35] For detection of extracapsular extension, the ranges of reported sensitivity and specificity of T2w MR are from 23%–95% and from 49%–100%, respectively.[27,29,32,34–37]

These variable and modest results have limited the widespread implementation of prostate MR in prostate cancer staging. In an evidence-based review of the available literature and cost–benefit analysis performed in 2000, one expert panel's opinion was against the use of prostate MR for staging purposes.[38] However, in the same review, a cost–benefit analysis found that staging with MR was a more cost-effective approach than surgical staging. More recently, early experience with 3T MR using an endorectal coil has shown improved staging accuracy, with a sensitivity and specificity up to 88% and 96%, respectively.[39,40] The apparent improvement in accuracy using 3T MR is likely due to improved signal-to-noise ratio and the higher resolution imaging that this higher field facilitates.

Contrast-Enhanced MR Imaging of the Prostate

The limitations of morphologic imaging of prostate cancer prompted investigators to assess a potential role for gadolinium-enhanced imaging in the staging of prostate cancer. The early use of contrast-enhanced MR involved an initial precontrast T1-weighted (T1w) sequence followed by a single postcontrast phase with interpretation made by comparing the pre- and postcontrast images.

Using this technique, Mirowitz and colleagues[41] found that the depiction of prostate tumors on T1w images was improved, but that lesion characterization was not significantly improved over T2w images. In the same study, it was also found that the demonstration of seminal vesicle architecture and of seminal vesicle tumor invasion was improved, with better depiction of seminal vesicle tumor invasion on contrast-enhanced T1w images over T2-weighting in 23% of cases.[41] Enhancement within the lumen of the seminal vesicles was seen in patients with tumor invasion.

Dynamic Contrast-Enhanced MR Imaging: Rationale

The enhancement of prostate cancer on T1w images following gadolinium contrast medium is dependent on a number of factors, including the microcirculatory environment of the tumor, which differs from the surrounding normal tissue because of tumor neovascularization. DCE MR imaging involves a multiphasic pre- and postcontrast evaluation of the prostate to glean information about the local microcirculatory environment and, hence, tissue type. In this way, the neovascularization of prostate tumors can form an important substrate of imaging for cancer staging and detection, and also for the evaluation of the response to therapy with antiangiogenic agents and other therapies.[42]

ANGIOGENESIS AND PROSTATE CANCER

As in other cancers, angiogenesis plays a critical role in the biology of prostate cancer. In general, angiogenesis consists of the recruitment of new blood vessels to support the growth of tumor cells.[43] In addition to the direct perfusion of the tumor, the neoendothelium itself plays a role in the paracrine stimulation of tumor cells by several growth factors and matrix proteins.[43] Angiogenesis is a feature of tumor development that is required to permit tumor growth above a small size (0.2 to 2 mm diameter[42]) and allows the development of metastases. Metastases themselves must also promote angiogenesis to remain viable.[43,44]

Microvessel density (MVD) is a quantifiable measure of neovascularity. It has been shown that MVD is higher in areas of the prostate containing carcinoma than in benign prostate tissue.[45,46] Furthermore, MVD has been found to be substantially higher in prostate cancers that metastasize and in those of higher Gleason grade.[47] The switch to angiogenic phenotype within the tumor is promoted by angiogenic factors.[43,44] In prostate cancer, important angiogenic factors are thought to include vascular endothelial growth factor (VEGF), matrix metalloproteinases, fibroblast growth factor-2, transforming growth factor-B, cyclooxygenase-2, and others.[48] These factors are now the target of clinical and preclinical trials assessing the potential for antiangiogenic agents in the therapy of prostate cancer.

The microcirculation of any tissue can be conceptualized as containing three compartments: the intracellular space, the extravascular extracellular space (EES), and the microvasculature itself.[49] Tumor microcirculation and its immediate environs have fundamental differences compared with normal tissue.[49] The tumor microvessels have increased permeability and lack the branching hierarchical substructure seen in normal circulation, which alter the local flow dynamics and blood volume.[50] Additional alterations can result from vascular compression by space occupying masses.[42] Furthermore, the relative lack of intratumoral lymphatics[51] in the tumor bed can lead to increased interstitial fluid and interstitial pressure, with resulting alterations in local microcirculatory

flow dynamics. These fundamental microcirculatory differences will affect the dynamic behavior of diffusible tracers such as the traditional, nontargeted gadolinium chelates. The analysis of DCE MR imaging therefore offers a potential approach to capture the effects of angiogenesis.

BASIC PRINCIPLES OF DYNAMIC CONTRAST-ENHANCED MR IMAGING

When a low-molecular-weight contrast agent (eg, gadopentetate dimeglumine, Gd-DTPA) is injected into a peripheral vein, it passes from the venous system, via the heart, into the arterial system. When contrast reaches the blood vessels of a tumor, it leaks into the EES during the initial first pass. Having reached the EES, the contrast agent can freely diffuse, and later, when the intravascular concentration diminishes because of excretion, it diffuses out of the EES into the intravascular space and washes out.[52]

The main determinants of the dynamics of this process are: (a) the blood flow, (b) microvessel permeability, and (c) microvessel surface area.[49] The dynamics of the movement of contrast into and out of the tumor EES can be quantified using pharmacokinetic analysis. There are three principal parameters that describe this dynamic process, as indicated with a recently standardized nomenclature,[53] namely, the transfer constant (K^{trans}), the EES fractional volume (v_e), and the rate constant (k_{ep}), outlined below.

Description of Pharmacokinetic Parameters

The transfer constant (K^{trans})
This parameter relates the fraction of contrast agent transferred from blood to the interstitial space as a function of the concentrations of contrast in the blood vessel and in the interstitium. It is determined by the flow rate per unit volume, the permeability and the surface area of the tissue capillaries. In high permeability circumstances, the transfer constant is primarily flow-limited. In low permeability states, permeability becomes the main determining factor of K^{trans}, such that K^{trans} is equal to the permeability surface area product (PS).[54] (Previously used symbols for K^{trans} include EF, FE, $CL_d/V_t{}^b$.)

The extravascular extracellular space fractional volume (v_e)
This refers to the volume of EES per unit volume of tissue. (Alternative names were the interstitial space or the leakage space.)

The rate constant (k_{ep})

This is the ratio of the transfer constant to the EES. It represents the efflux constant from the EES to blood plasma. (Alternative nomenclature: k_{21}, k_2).

There are a number of potential approaches to evaluating the above factors using DCE MR imaging.

Dynamic Contrast Enhancement: Approaches

Tumor DCE is generally implemented by using a T1w sequence that is repeated before, during, and for a time period after the intravenous injection of a gadolinium chelate. Common sequences used include fast low-angle shot and 2-D and 3-D fast-spoiled gradient echo sequences. The movement of a gadolinium chelate from the intravascular space into the EES causes T1-shortening in the tumor EES, leading to increased signal intensity on T1w images. The changes in signal intensity over time are an index of the local microcirculatory physiology and hence an indirect measure of the angiogenesis associated with it. Such changes can be analyzed quantitatively, semiquantitatively, and qualitatively.

Quantitative analysis

During the passage of contrast medium from the blood vessel to the EES and back to the vessel, the signal changes can be used to estimate the local concentration of contrast agent in vivo. When the concentration of the agent in a given pixel or region of interest is plotted against time, a concentration versus time curve is generated. This curve can be mathematically fitted to a number of pharmacokinetic models and from these the quantitative modeling parameters can be derived (K^{trans}, v_e, k_{ep}). Popular pharmacokinetic models that have been applied include those described by Tofts and Kermode,[55] Larsson and colleagues,[56] and Brix and colleagues.[57] The details of these three models are summarized in a review by Tofts.[58]

Each model assumes the existence of a specified number of defined compartments in which contrast agent resides at a uniform concentration. The Tofts and Kermode model,[55] as an example, is a four-compartment model with plasma, extracellular space, tissue leakage space, and the renal (or excretory) compartment. The core kinetic parameters are related to the rate of change concentration of contrast agent by the following equation:

$$dC_t/dt = K^{trans} \cdot C_p - k_{ep} \cdot C_t$$

Where C_p is the concentration of contrast agent in arterial plasma, C_t is the concentration of contrast agent in tissue, t is time, and the terms K^{trans} and

k_{ep} are as previously defined. This approach assumes that all patients have the same plasma–clearance curve.

The advantage of model-based quantitative techniques is that they provide a means for quantifying factors important in characterizing tumor microcirculation that is independent of the MR scanner used and the particular imaging protocol employed. Importantly, this facilitates cross-institutional comparisons of data. A number of assumptions built into each of these models must be considered, however, as they may not be true and thus may expose some liabilities.[58]

The pharmacokinetic models assume that contrast agent concentration in a given compartment is in uniformly distributed. It is also assumed that the intercompartmental flux is linearly proportional to the concentration in each compartment. The parameters are assumed not to have changed during the acquisition. It is also assumed that the relaxivity of the gadolinium contrast agent is directly proportional to its concentration. Furthermore, the method of curve-fitting used for a model-based analysis itself can have a substantial impact on the accuracy of the determination of enhancement parameters.[59]

Strictly speaking, accurate quantification of parameters in a pharmacokinetic model relies on exact determination of the arterial input function (AIF),[60] which needs to be determined for each patient and each measurement.[61] Such a determination is vulnerable to T2* effects, particularly at higher field strengths.[62] In practice, a population-averaged AIF is often used that lacks detail and precision, but does provide a convenient (though perhaps dubious) solution.

Theoretical considerations and concerns aside, there is growing evidence that quantitative DCE techniques may improve prostate cancer detection. van Dorsten and colleagues[63] demonstrated higher k_{ep} and K^{trans} in areas of prostate cancer compared with normal peripheral gland. Futterer and colleagues,[64] using qualitative techniques, found that DCE was significantly more accurate than T2w images in tumor localization. In this analysis, v_e had the highest accuracy for tumor localization, whereas washout has the highest specificity; in that study, the combination of multiple parameters into a mean pharmacokinetic score proved the most accurate parameter, outperforming T2w imaging. Similarly, Ocak and colleagues[65] showed sensitivity and specificity of DCE MR imaging for prostate cancer detection of 73% and 88%, respectively, compared with 94% and 37% for T2w imaging, with significantly higher K^{trans} and k_{ep} in tumors than in normal peripheral gland. On the other hand, Storaas and colleagues[66] found no benefit of DCE over T2w images alone in prostate cancer localization using T1w dynamic postcontrast, 3D echo planar imaging.

The correlation of histopathologic markers of angiogenesis (including MVD) with quantitative pharmacokinetic parameters determined by DCE has been assessed with conflicting results by a small number of authors. Schlemmer and colleagues[67] found a correlation between MVD and k_{ep} (termed k_{21} in that paper), but did not find a correlation between quantitative parameters and Gleason grade. Conversely, Kiessling and colleagues[68] did not find that quantitative DCE parameters correlated with MVD. While a statistically significant association between MVD and prostate cancer recurrence has been demonstrated,[69,70] this has not been a universal finding.[71] Likewise the relationship between MVD and prostate cancer grades is not uniform.[69–72]

Semiquantitative analysis

Semiquantitative parameters describe tissue enhancement using a number of descriptors derived from signal intensity–time curves, without reference to a pharmacokinetic model. Parameters considered by semiquantitative analysis include the onset time (time from injection to signal intensity increase in the tumor tissue), time to peak signal intensity, the initial and mean gradient of the signal intensity–time curve upsweep, maximum signal intensity, washout gradient, and the initial area under the gadolinium concentration or signal intensity curve over a fixed time period.

Semiquantitative methods have the advantage of being relatively simple to implement, and not subject to the assumptions of the model-based quantitative techniques. However, they are subject to variations in scanner factors, such as repetition time (TR), echo time (TE), flip angle, scaling factors, and gain factors. They do not assess the local concentration changes of contrast agent in the tumor, but rather the signal intensity in the region over time.

Despite these limitations, semiquantitative techniques can provide a useful alternative to the pharmacokinetic parameters derived from model-based quantitative techniques. In an analysis of the relationship between semiquantitative measures and quantitative measures, Jesberger and colleagues[73] found that G_{peak}, initial area under the curve and other parameters correlated with near-linearity with K^{trans}. Additionally, some authors have used both quantitative and semiquantitative analysis. Kiessling and colleagues,[68] for example, found no difference in discrimination of benign prostate tissue and cancer when quantitative parameters derived from a two-compartmental model

were compared with the area under the enhancement curve measurement.

In assessing the enhancement profile of prostate cancer semiquantitatively, several patterns are consistently found in the literature. Compared with normal peripheral gland, prostate cancer tends to reach maximal enhancement earlier and also reaches higher amplitude of enhancement as compared with benign tissue.[74–76]

In addition to higher peak enhancement, Padhani and colleagues[19] also showed an earlier onset of contrast enhancement in malignant regions. Engelbrecht and colleagues[77] introduced an additional factor: "relative peak enhancement," defined as peak enhancement in lesion minus average peak enhancement in the accompanying tissue, and found that this value had the highest discriminatory value between benign and malignant tissue. From a practical standpoint, Kim and colleagues[78] found a higher sensitivity and specificity of semiquantitative DCE (using wash-in rate as an indication of carcinoma) than T2w imaging (96% and 82% versus 65% and 60%, respectively). Other authors have also demonstrated the utility of semiquantitative DCE in the localization of prostate cancer.[74]

Qualitative analysis

Subjective visual assessment of contrast-enhanced images of the prostate to visualize carcinoma and to evaluate staging, without measurement of enhancement parameters or directly quantifying pharmacokinetic measurements, can be referred to as qualitative assessment.

The practical impact of using a qualitative assessment of DCE MR imaging data in clinical practice can be found in the detection and characterization of breast cancer.[79] In this approach, analysis of signal intensity yields three patterns of contrast enhancement – type 1 (progressive enhancement), type 2 (wash-in and plateau), and type 3 (wash-in and wash-out), assisting in the characterization of breast lesions.

In an early study of contrast-enhanced MR of the prostate by Brown and colleagues[80] using a scan time of 3 minutes, 48 seconds, an initial postcontrast series was followed by a more delayed postcontrast phase. In this study, visual evaluation of the early postcontrast phase depicted the prostate tumor with better definition than T2w images, and also improved the assessment of extracapsular extension. In that study, the delayed-phase postcontrast image was not considered helpful.

More recently, Girouin and colleagues[81] used simple visual criteria to detect prostate cancer.

The study did not employ an endorectal coil and only assessed the early postcontrast sequences for analysis. Using 'arterial' phase enhancement of peripheral gland nodules as a criterion for malignancy, DCE-MR imaging had a higher per sector localization than T2w, correctly depicting 78%–81% of tumors greater than 0.3 cm^3 compared with 50%–60% when T2w images were used. The specificity of DCE with this technique was lower than T2w and both T2 and DCE performed poorly in the detection of lesions less than 0.3 cm^3 in volume and tumors of lower Gleason grade.

Using an endorectal coil, Ogura and colleagues[82] described sensitivity and specificity for the detection of peripheral zone cancers of 81% and 79%, respectively, when T2w images are combined with DCE imaging (using visual criteria); the independent performance and contributions from T2w imaging and DCE were not reported.

Dynamic Contrast Enhancement: Temporal Versus Spatial Resolution

In order to accurately assess the enhancement kinetics of prostate cancer, many researchers use an approach with high temporal resolution, ranging from 1.25 to 16 seconds.[39,64–66,68,76,77,83–89] In these protocols, there is usually limited spatial resolution and/or incomplete coverage of the prostate gland, factors that can diminish the practical utility for assessing prostate cancer. Other researchers use a more moderate temporal resolution (22–30 seconds), more often covering the whole gland but still with only moderate spatial resolution.[75,78,81,82,90]

Recognizing that accurate depiction of regional variations in the distribution of contrast-enhancement time curves was important in the localization and accurate anatomic depiction of tumors in the breast, Degani and colleagues[91] proposed a higher spatial resolution implementation of DCE. With this approach, a lower temporal resolution is accepted and the analysis of kinetics depends on data from three carefully selected time points: a precontrast time point, an early postcontrast time point, and a delayed postcontrast time point. Using this three time point (3TP) method, an index of tumor microvascular heterogeneity can be depicted with a high spatial resolution.

This method also allows quantitative measurement including microvascular permeability (microcapillary surface area permeability product) and V_e. These quantitative parameters can be depicted with a high spatial resolution, potentially allowing better analysis of tumor location and stage. Recently, Bloch and colleagues[40] demonstrated

the efficacy of such a technique in staging of prostate cancer. In this study, whole-mount histopathologic analysis of the excised prostate gland was used as a gold standard. Using this high-resolution quantitative 3TP approach, the sensitivity and specificity of DCE MR imaging in the detection of extracapsular extension or seminal vesicle infiltration was 82%–91% and the specificity was 86%. The overall sensitivity for detection of extracapsular extension was improved by 25% when DCE images were reviewed in combination with T2w images versus T2w images alone.

When high spatial resolution is coupled with sparsely sampled temporal resolution, it is essential to obtain the component sequences of DCE MR imaging at the optimal time. In particular, the early postcontrast sequences should be timed to maximize the enhancement of carcinoma over background glandular tissue. This concept was explored by Rouviere and colleagues,[88] who used a high temporal resolution approach through one slice only, including an area of prostate gland containing carcinoma, as depicted on T2w imaging (and correlated results with histopathology). By restricting the acquisition to a single slice, high in-plane spatial resolution was achieved with a 30-second temporal resolution. In that study, based on the enhancement curves obtained from patients and simulation experiments, it was determined that a start delay of 36 seconds provided the optimal contrast of peripheral gland cancer versus benign glandular tissue.[88]

To probe the interplay between temporal resolution and signal-to-noise ratio, we performed a series of model simulations. We calculated the noise variance from sample DCE MR imaging studies performed at our institution using our standard protocol (Table 1)[40] at 3T, using an endorectal coil. We then performed a Monte Carlo simulation (n = 1000) with different random noise added with the same noise variance as experienced on our clinical examinations using the so called "Tofts Model." We did this with representative DCE signal intensity curves of a prostate cancer (K^{trans} = 1, V_e = 0.25). We then fit the signal from the simulations using nonlinear least squares fitting to the Tofts Model to give values of K^{trans} and V_e. We then constructed a histogram for each of these parameters derived from the fits.

Based on the derived histograms (Fig. 1), it can be seen that a greater accuracy of evaluation of Ve is possible than K^{trans} at the temporal and spatial resolution used at our institution. If all else remains equal and the simulation is repeated with the expected noise variance of an equivalent 1.5T examination, a wider standard deviation of

Table 1
Beth Israel Deaconess Medical Center MR imaging parameters at 3 Tesla

Sequence	T1w (SE or FSE)	T2w FSE	T2w FSE	High Spatial Resolution 3D GE
Imaging plane	Axial	Axial	Coronal	Axial
Coils	Combined torso- phased array and endorectal coil	Combined torso- phased array and endorectal coil	Combined torso- phased array and endorectal coil	Combined torso- phased array and endorectal coil
Anatomic coverage	Aortic bifurcation to pubic symphysis	Prostate and seminal vesicles	Prostate and seminal vesicles	Prostate and seminal vesicles
TE (msec)	12	165	165	2.1
TR (msec)	600–700	6375	7600	7.1
Slice thickness/ spacing (gap) (mm)	5/1	1.5–2/0	2/0	2–3/0; larger sections used for larger glands[a]
FOV	28–22 cm	12 cm	14 cm	12 cm
Frequency direction	Transverse	AP	AP or SI	AP
Matrix	256 × 192	320 × 224–192	320 × 224–192	256 × 224
NEX	2	4	4	2
Echo train length	—	22	22	—
Acquisition time	5 min	5–7 min	5–6 min	1 min, 32 sec each × 7 = 10 min, 44 sec total
Flip angle	90°	90°	90°	18°
Receiver bandwidth	50 kHz	31.25 kHz	31.25 kHz	20.83 kHz
Notes	Frequency: transverse to prevent endorectal coil motion artifact from obscuring pelvic nodes	Frequency: AP to prevent endorectal coil motion artifact from obscuring the prostate gland	Frequency: AP to prevent endorectal coil motion artifact from obscuring the prostate gland	Frequency: AP to prevent endorectal coil motion artifact from obscuring the prostate gland

[a] Constraint: maintain each DCE MR imaging 3D data-set with temporal resolution at ~ 90–95 sec for the parametric/kinetic analysis.
Courtesy of Beth Israel Deaconess Medical Center.

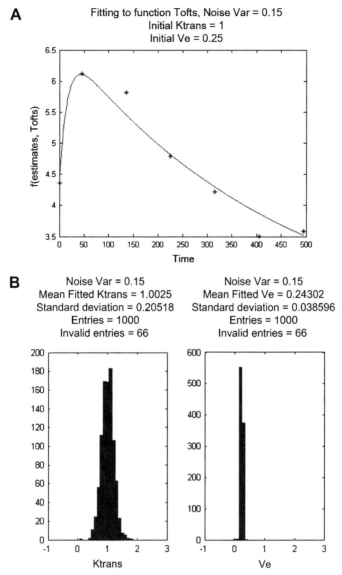

Fig. 1. (A) Concentration versus time curve of a typical prostate cancer with data points derived from simulation, based on the noise variance experienced on clinical DCE MR imaging using a temporal resolution of 90 seconds at 3T with an endorectal coil. (B). Histogram of the of K^{trans} and V_e derived from 1000 simulations of the results of clinical DCE MR imaging using a temporal resolution of 90 seconds at 3T with an endorectal coil.

measured K^{trans} is seen than at 3T because of lower signal-to-noise ratio (Fig. 2). If the simulation is repeated for the 3T protocol, but the temporal resolution is increased by a factor of two, the accuracy of determination of K^{trans} and V_e are not improved (Fig. 3) because the increase in temporal resolution results in decreased signal-to-noise ratio if the spatial resolution remains the same. This experiment demonstrates the inherent difficulty in determining an 'optimal' balance between spatial and temporal resolution.

Dynamic Contrast-Enhanced MR Imaging of the Prostate: What is the Gold Standard?

The efficacy assessment of any imaging technique relies on an appropriate gold standard. This is not without controversy when it comes to prostate cancer detection, grading, and staging. When prostate biopsy serves as a gold standard, sampling errors can substantially limit the utility. Histologic interpretations require pattern recognition; the small but significant interobserver variability in the assignment of Gleason grade to

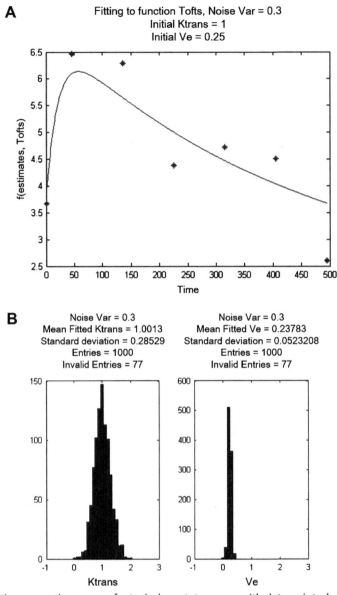

Fig. 2. (*A*) Concentration versus time curve of a typical prostate cancer with data points derived from simulation, based on the noise variance experienced on clinical DCE MR imaging using a temporal resolution of 90 seconds at 1.5T with an endorectal coil. (*B*) Histogram of the of K^{trans} and V_e derived from 1000 simulations of the results of clinical DCE MR imaging using a temporal resolution of 90 seconds at 1.5T with an endorectal coil.

prostate tumors by histopathologists is well recognized.[92]

The histologic determination of stage, including the presence or absence of extracapsular extension, is also associated with interobserver variability.[93] Scientific evaluation of DCE MR imaging as a surrogate marker for angiogenic status requires a gold standard, such as MVD. The evaluation of MVD at histology, however, depends on the use of vascular endothelium markers and immunohistochemical procedures. These technical approaches can vary significantly between

histology laboratories, which can also lead to variability in results.[94] Factors such as these should be borne in mind when assessing the technical efficacy of DCE MR imaging (as well as other imaging techniques) and when comparing results between centers.

IN SEARCH OF A BIOMARKER

The close connection between DCE MR imaging and angiogenesis, and the current consensus that more aggressive tumors exhibit greater

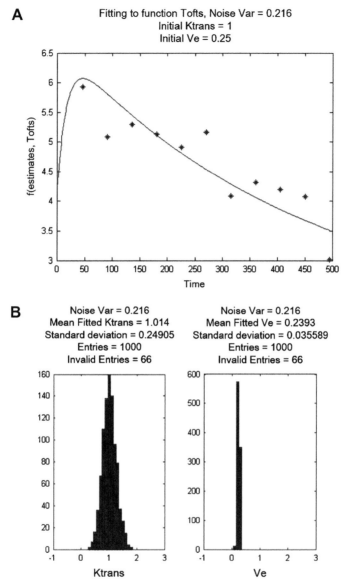

Fig. 3. (A) Concentration versus time curve of a typical prostate cancer with data points derived from simulation, based on the noise variance experienced on clinical DCE MR imaging using a temporal resolution of 45 seconds at 3T with an endorectal coil. (B) Histogram of the of K^{trans} and V_e derived from 1000 simulations of the results of clinical DCE MR imaging using a temporal resolution of 45 seconds at 3T with an endorectal coil.

angiogenesis, form the basis for suggesting that DCE MR imaging might serve as an "imaging" biomarker. As an example, a recent review by Rehman and Jayson[95] discusses the role of DCE MR imaging as a molecular imaging tool in assessing the efficacy of antiangiogenic agents, both in clinical and preclinical studies. More broadly, in his recent article, Oehr[96] reviews the use of noninvasive imaging modalities to probe genomics, proteomics, and metabolomics.

The induction of new blood vessels is a key event in the progression of a solid tumor as it grows beyond 1-2 mm in diameter and can no longer depend on simple passive diffusion to provide nutrients and clear toxic wastes (for a review see Folkman[97]). Both the outgrowth of new blood vessels from established vessels (angiogenesis) and the formation of new microvessels from circulating endothelial cells (vasculogenesis) can be co-opted by a cancer.[98]

Tumor-induced blood vessel formation has proven to be a complex pathologic event, and the early hopes for antiangiogenesis therapies have been tempered by the realization that cancers use multiple molecular pathways to induce and remodel a vascular network.

Assessments of angiogenic phenotypes using a variety of biomarkers are only beginning to be included into the clinical assessments of a patient's malignancy. There is great interest in developing, validating, and using noninvasive imaging technologies to replace these more invasive tests.

VEGF is one of the most intensively studied angiogenic factors in human cancers, and has generally been reported to be overexpressed in prostate cancer relative to benign prostate tissue. Thus, it is reasonable to expect that most if not all of the tumors that exhibit abnormal DCE MR imaging patterns would show overexpression of VEGF. However, it has been reported that the levels of VEGF overexpression in primary human prostate cancers are highly variable, both at the RNA and protein levels.[99–102] We have recently published the results of an analysis of gene expression patterns in low-VEGF, DCE MR imaging–positive prostate cancers to determine which pathways were involved in the angiogenesis of these tumors. Interestingly, one of the genes most highly overexpressed in low-VEGF cancers shown is neuropeptide Y (NPY).[103]

Although other groups have recognized NPY as one of many neuroendocrine markers that are overexpressed in a subset of prostate cancers, the ramifications of its overexpression has not yet been established.[104,105] The significance of NPY overexpression is that in model systems NPY produces microvessels that appear to be more mature and less permeable, or "leaky," than those induced by VEGF.[106,107] In principle, DCE MR imaging should be able to distinguish tumors with these more mature vessels from tumors with more leaky vessels. For example, using commonly employed pharmacokinetic analyses of DCE MR imaging results, eg, the Tofts Model,[53,58,108] the values of the parameter, K^{trans}, should be higher in tumors with leaky vessels. If this hypothesis were correct, there would be a noninvasive way to identify high VEGF expressing tumors from high NPY expressing tumors. DCE MR imaging could be used to identify patients who would respond to antiangiogenic therapy based on anti-VEGF approaches and also to monitor changes in response to therapy.

In summary, there is strong evidence to suggest that DCE MR imaging may emerge as an imaging biomarker. It may be used to estimate the degree of angiogenesis present in a given prostate cancer and the heterogeneity of this angiogenesis. Moreover, DCE MR imaging may be able to identify those patients with prostate cancers that show robust overexpression of VEGF and are likely to respond to anti-VEGF therapy.

BETH ISRAEL DEACONESS MEDICAL CENTER EXPERIENCE

Since 2004, at Beth Israel Deaconess Medical Center (BIDMC) we have combined the use of 3T clinical MR technology, T2w and high spatial resolution DCE MR imaging, and an endorectal coil.[109] This imaging strategy acquires higher-resolution images with smaller voxel sizes than has been possible with prior MR technology and more comprehensive tissue sampling compared with other presurgical assessments. This methodology makes it feasible to assess prostate tissue morphology and additional features of prostate cancer such as tissue kinetics and the vascular microenvironment, providing a non-invasive tool to: (1) detect extracapsular spread; (2) detect specific areas within the prostate that harbor cancer; and (3) direct biopsy and treatment specifically to diseased areas, resulting in a pretreatment evaluation that can assist in the rational selection of patients to undergo appropriate and definitive therapy for prostate cancer.

Currently, our patients are referred for MR of the prostate for four main reasons: (1) pretherapeutic staging in patients with biopsy-proven cancer, (2) detection of local recurrence in patients with rising PSA after definitive treatment (surgery, radiation therapy), (3) cancer detection in patients with rising PSA and repeat negative biopsies, and (4) pre- and postbrachytherapy planning studies (to designate a dominant nodule location before brachytherapy, to evaluate for seed distribution and dislocation after seed implantation, and to perform MR-based dosimetric studies). Preliminary data suggest that contrast-enhanced MR imaging has value for brachytherapy posttreatment evaluation and planning.[110]

Prostate MR Protocol

All patients, whether they are evaluated for pre- or posttherapeutic assessment, undergo the same standardized MR protocol at our institution.

Patient preparation

Patients are asked to refrain from ejaculation for 3 days preceding the examination to ensure optimal distension of the seminal vesicles. A sodium phosphate enema is administered on the day of the study to minimize fecal residue in the rectum. A 1 mg glucagon intramuscular injection is administered to reduce peristaltic motion of the rectum. The endorectal coil (Prostate eCoil, MEDRAD, Pittsburgh, PA) is inserted into the rectum and connected to a pelvic-phased array coil with a coupling device to combine the surface-phased array coil with the endorectal coil. A barium suspension is used to fill the endorectal coil balloon, with a typical volume of 80 cm^3. The volume injected into this balloon is adjusted for patient tolerance. The use of barium has been shown to reduce susceptibility effects when compared with air[111] and therefore should improve MR spectroscopy and diffusion-weighted imaging results.

MR imaging is performed on a 3.0 T MR imaging system (Genesis Signa LX Excite, GE Healthcare, Waukesha, WI). The coil position is verified with sagittal T2w localizer images and adjusted, if needed, so that the endorectal coil is optimally situated with respect to the prostate gland. The imaging parameters are summarized in Table 1.

T2-weighted acquisition
Transverse and coronal fast spin–echo T2w images are obtained from below the prostatic apex to above the seminal vesicles using the following parameters: repetition time msec/echo time msec (effective) 4,500–7600/165, 2.0–2.6 mm section thickness (depending on cranio–caudad size of the gland) and no intersection gap, 2–4 signal averages, 14-cm field of view (FOV), 320×192 matrix, and no phase wrap (100% phase oversampling). The frequency encoding direction is anterior–posterior. A unique attribute of this protocol is the use of thinner sections than have been the previous clinical routine. This results in 30%–50% more sampling of the gland compared with the traditional 3–4 mm section approach.

Axial spin–echo or fast spin–echo T1-weighted acquisition–nodal evaluation
T1w images from the aortic bifurcation to the symphysis pubis are obtained using TR/TE = 600–700/12msec, a slice thickness 4-6 mm, an interslice gap of 0–1 mm, a matrix of 256×192, 2 excitations, and a 20–32 cm FOV. Fat suppression is not employed. The frequency-encoding direction is left to right (to avoid motion-related artifacts from propagating into the pelvic nodes).

Three-dimensional T1-weighted gradient echo acquisition
Images are acquired before, during, and after contrast injection. DCE images are obtained after bolus injection of gadopentetate dimeglumine (Magnevist; Bayer Pharmaceuticals, Wayne, NJ) at a dose of 0.1 mmol per kilogram of body weight administered with a mechanical injection system (Spectris MR Injection System, MEDRAD, Pittsburgh, PA) at a flow rate of 4 mL/sec, immediately followed by 20 mL of normal saline at a flow rate of 4 mL/sec. The imaging parameters of the 3D gradient-recalled echo sequence are: TR/TE 7.1/2.1msec, flip angle 18°, FOV 14 cm, matrix 256×224, ST: 2.0–2.6 mm, 2 signal averages, no

phase wrap, which is obtained with a temporal resolution of 91–95 seconds. Two precontrast and five postcontrast sequential acquisitions are obtained. The first precontrast scan is used to ensure relevant anatomic coverage; the second is used as part of a continuous series of pre- and postacquisitions in which the instrument settings (gain and attenuation values) are identical. Contrast injection is initiated during the last 5–7 seconds of the 2nd precontrast acquisition.

Kinetic analyses of dynamic contrast-enhanced MR imaging
DCE images are processed at pixel resolution, using a 3TP model (noncommercial software courtesy of Hadassa Degani, PhD, Weizmann Insitute, Israel) to analyze the time evolution of contrast enhancement. The results are translated into a color-coded scheme as previously published.[40,91]

CLINICAL MR APPLICATIONS AT BETH ISRAEL DEACONESS MEDICAL CENTER
MR Staging and Detection of Extracapsular Disease at Beth Israel Deaconess Medical Center

A study that combined a T2w and DCE MR protocol revealed a mean sensitivity, specificity, positive predictive value, and negative predictive value for the detection of extracapsular extension of 86%, 95%, 90% and 93%, respectively.[40] The sensitivity for extracapsular extension was improved by more than 25% using the combined T2w/DCE MR imaging approach compared with T2w MR imaging alone. The sensitivity and specificity of DCE MR imaging alone in the detection of extracapsular extension or seminal vesicle infiltration was 82%–91% and the specificity was 86%. The combined approach had a mean overall staging accuracy of 95%, as determined by the area under the receiver operating characteristic curve. Staging results were significantly improved (P<.05) using the combined approach compared with T2w MR imaging alone. Fig. 4 shows an example of MR imaging at 3T performed for pre-therapeutic evaluation and staging.

Clinical MR Imaging for Local Recurrence of Prostate Cancer at Beth Israel Deaconess Medical Center

T2w MR imaging cannot readily distinguish between the low signal intensities of cancerous tissue versus fibrotic changes, post-radiation changes, and scar tissue after prostatectomy. DCE MR imaging, however, is able to differentiate between neoplasm and fibrotic or radiated tissue based on the enhancement features. Fig. 5 shows

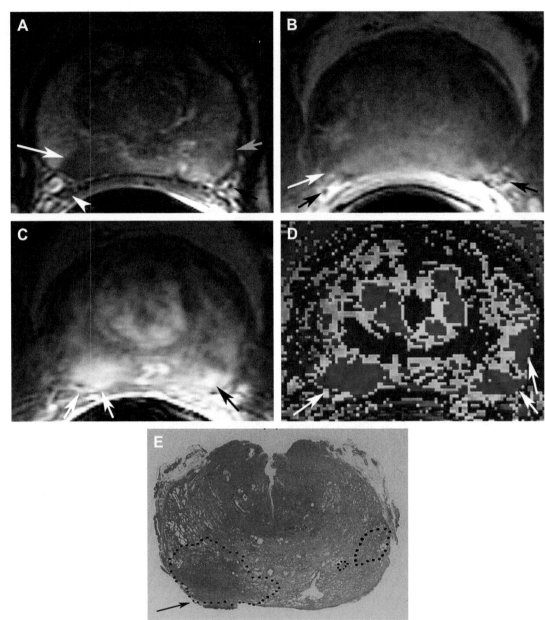

Fig. 4. T2w, DCE MR, and DCE MR-based color-coded images in correlation with whole mount histopathology of a 55-year-old patient with positive biopsy on the right, Gleason score 3 + 4 = 7. On biopsy no malignancy was identified on the left, resulting in a clinical stage of T2a. (*A*) Axial T2w FSE (5800/1600), 2.2 mm-thick image of the mid-third of the prostate. Note the large hypointense area in the right peripheral zone (*white arrow*). The tumor abuts the neurovascular bundle and the ill-defined capsule. The hypointense tissue extends beyond the capsule (*white arrowhead*). The black arrow marks the contralateral neurovascular bundle, which shows normal hyperintense signal, surrounding the hypointense nerves. The gray area marks a small area of slightly hypointense signal intensity in the left peripheral gland, suggesting a small tumor. The tumor was staged as T3a based on the T2w images. (*B*) DCE 3D gradient-echo (6.9/2.1) 2.6 mm-thick precontrast image. Note the irregular pseudocapsule (*white arrow*), and the visualization of the nerves within the neurovascular bundle (*black arrows*). (*C*) Corresponding DCE 3D gradient-echo (6.9/2.1) 2.6 mm-thick early postcontrast image. Note the larger bulging tumor (*white arrows*) and the smaller contralateral tumor showing early wash-in (*black arrow*). With poor delineation between the neurovascular bundle/pseudocapsule, the bilateral tumor was staged as T3a. (*D*) Corresponding color-coded DCE 3D gradient-echo (6.9/2.1) 2.6 mm-thick image showed cancer (geographic areas with confluent bright red pixelation) bilateral in the peripheral zone (*white arrows*). The combined analysis of T2w and DCE MR imaging yielded an MR imaging diagnosis of bilateral tumor, stage T3a. (*E*) Whole-mount histopathology proved cancer (*black dotted lines*) bilaterally involving the peripheral zone with extracapsular extension on the right into the neurovascular bundle (*black arrow*), and stage pT3a.

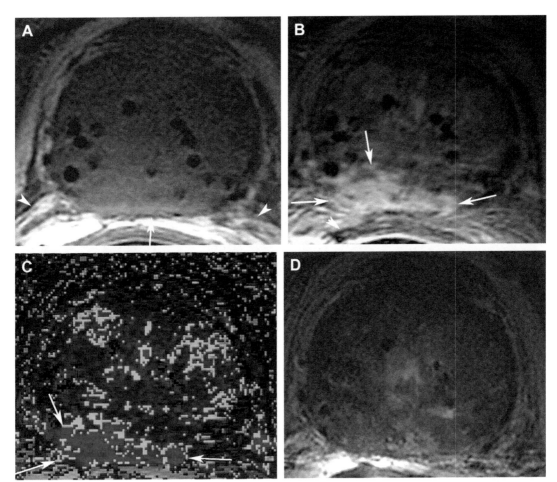

Fig. 5. (*A*) DCE 3D gradient-echo (6.9/2.1) 2.6 mm-thick precontrast image: Note the signal voids (seeds) and the clear depiction of prostate capsule (*white arrow*) and neurovascular bundles (*arrowheads*). (*B*) Corresponding DCE 3D gradient-echo (6.9/2.1) 2.6-mm-thick early postcontrast image. Note the tumor showing early wash-in (*white arrows*) on the background of relatively low perfusion of the radiated gland. The brachytherapy seeds are represented as focal signal voids. Note also the proximity of the tumor to the rectal wall (*white arrowhead*). (*C*) Corresponding color-coded DCE 3D gradient-echo (6.9/2.1) 2.6 mm-thick image showed cancer (geographic area with confluent bright red pixelation) in the right posterior peripheral zone (*white arrows*). (*D*) Axial T2w FSE (5800/160) 2.2 mm-thick image of the mid-third of the prostate. (Corresponding to Fig. 5 *A*, *B*). Note that the entire prostate gland shows low signal due to post- radiation changes and, therefore, the tumor cannot be delineated.

an example of high-resolution DCE MR imaging at 3T and detection of local recurrence after brachytherapy. The patient underwent brachytherapy seed implantation 3 years before the MR imaging, and was referred after PSA relapse. Note the local recurrence in a "cold spot" where there is a relative lack of seeds, in the posterior right peripheral zone. Note the seeds visualized as small signal voids (black) in postcontrast image (**Fig. 5**B) and the clear visualization of the cancer on the parametric map (**Fig. 5**C). The MR imaging diagnosis was confirmed by targeted biopsy.

Prostate Cancer Detection and Localization in Patients Who Have Repeat Negative Biopsies

In an ongoing prospective study we are currently investigating the value of high spatial resolution DCE MR imaging with high spatial resolution T2w endorectal coil MR imaging at 3T for detection and localization of prostate cancer in patients with repeat negative biopsies and rising PSA using histopathology of the subsequent biopsy as the reference standard. The preliminary results have shown that the MR-prompted biopsy detected prostate cancer in greater than 50% of patients, with the majority of tumors being located in the anterior gland, as predicted by MR imaging. These results are an improvement over previously reported results of randomly performed repeat biopsies or targeted sextant biopsies with emphasis on anterior and lateral tissue sampling.[112–114] The ability for MR imaging data to improve the positive biopsy yield in men after repeat negative biopsies holds an opportunity for earlier diagnoses and a reduction in the number of biopsy sessions. **Fig. 6** shows data from a 66-year-old patient with

2× repeat negative biopsies and a rising PSA (8.3 ng/mL) before the MR examination. A targeted ultrasound guided biopsy based on the MR imaging findings confirmed cancer in the anterior gland (Gleason score 7 [4 + 3 with a minor component of 5]). Consequently, the patient underwent prostatectomy providing imaging–histologic correlation.

Our 3T high spatial resolution T2w and DCE-MR imaging protocol is assisting clinicians in their efforts to more objectively and rationally select appropriate treatment for the individual patient with prostate cancer, based on improved pre- and

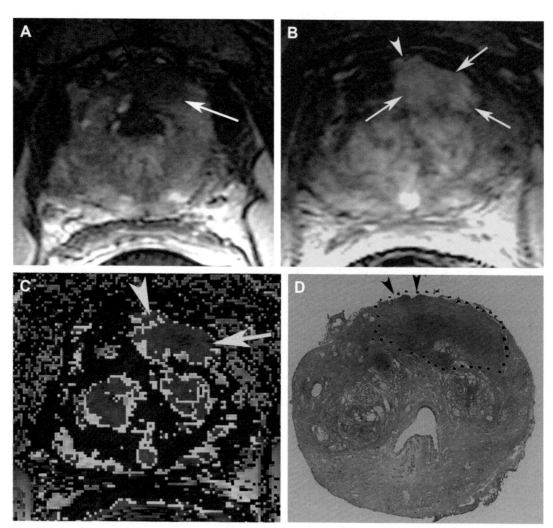

Fig. 6. (*A*) Axial T2w FSE (7050/156) 2.2 mm-thick image of the mid-third of the prostate. Note the subtle hypointense area in the anterior aspect of the gland (*white arrow*)—the cancer is not readily seen. The fibromuscular band cannot be delineated (*black arrow*). (*B*) Corresponding early postcontrast DCE 3D gradient-echo (6.9/2.1) 2.6 mm-thick image. Note readily the large anterior tumor as a geographic asymmetric area of early wash-in (*white arrows*), bulging and disrupting the fibromuscular band (*white arrow head*). (*C*) Corresponding color-coded DCE 3D gradient-echo (6.9/2.1) 2.6 mm-thick image. Note the large anterior tumor easily seen in bright red, extending through the fibromuscular band (*white arrowhead*). (*D*) Whole-mount histopathology proved cancer (*black dotted line*) in the anterior gland, with a final pathologic stage pT3a. with extracapsular extension right anteriorly (*arrowheads*) as reported by MR imaging.

posttherapeutic MR imaging studies, and is increasingly relied upon at our institution to detect and target cancer in patients with repeat negative biopsies and rising PSA levels. Further, we anticipate undertaking systematic studies that involve correlating the MR imaging features (phenotype) with underlying gene expression and protein expression profiles (genotype). Our preliminary results in this area have shown the potential of DCE MR imaging for establishing MR imaging parameters as validated biomarkers for human prostate cancer.[115]

SUMMARY

The diagnosis and treatment of prostate cancer requires a tumor-specific and patient-specific approach. There are many tumor factors that are of importance in optimally planning and monitoring therapy for each patient with prostate cancer. These include tumor stage, grade, aggressiveness, metastatic potential, and tumor volume.

Patients with low volume disease and patients with biopsy-occult tumor may present a particularly difficult clinical challenge. In this advancing field of patient care, DCE MR imaging of the prostate provides a functional window into the microcirculatory behavior of the prostate gland that can facilitate potential answers to critical, management-determining questions. Many different approaches to DCE MR imaging are feasible, all with inherent compromises.

The approach we illustrate in this article provides high spatial resolution with optimized timing of low temporal resolution acquisitions and we find that this provides improved performance in prostate cancer detection and staging. With the growing evidence–base for a positive contribution of DCE MR imaging to the evaluation of patients with prostate cancer, it seems likely that DCE MR imaging will become a routine part of clinical radiology practice.

REFERENCES

1. American Cancer Society. Cancer facts and figures 2008. Atlanta (GA): American Cancer Society; 2008.
2. National Cancer Institute. SEER cancer statistics review, 1975-2005. Available at: http://seer.cancer.gov/csr/1975_2005/. Accessed 2008.
3. Bock JL, Klee GG. How sensitive is a prostate-specific antigen measurement? How sensitive does it need to be? Arch Pathol Lab Med 2004; 128(3):341–3.
4. Hernandez J, Thompson IM. Prostate-specific antigen: a review of the validation of the most commonly used cancer biomarker. Cancer 2004; 101(5):894–904.
5. Schwartz MJ, Hwang DH, Hung AJ, et al. Negative influence of changing biopsy practice patterns on the predictive value of prostate-specific antigen for cancer detection on prostate biopsy. Cancer 2008;112(8):1718–25.
6. Gosselaar C, Kranse R, Roobol MJ, et al. The inter-observer variability of digital rectal examination in a large randomized trial for the screening of prostate cancer. Prostate 2008;68(9):985–93.
7. Albertsen PC, Hanley JA, Fine J. 20-year outcomes following conservative management of clinically localized prostate cancer. JAMA 2005;293(17): 2095–101.
8. National Cancer Institute. National Cancer Institute Physician Data Query (PDQ), 2008. Available at: http://www.cancer.gov/cancertopics/pdq/treatment/prostate.
9. Carlani M, Mancino S, Bonanno E, et al. Combined morphological, [1H]-MR spectroscopic and contrast-enhanced imaging of human prostate cancer with a 3-Tesla scanner: preliminary experience. Radiol Med 2008;113(5):670–88.
10. Gosselaar C, Roobol MJ, Roemeling S, et al. The value of an additional hypoechoic lesion-directed biopsy core for detecting prostate cancer. BJU Int 2008;101(6):685–90.
11. Cookson MS. Update on transrectal ultrasound-guided needle biopsy of the prostate. Mol Urol 2000;4(3):93–7 [discussion: 99].
12. Mettlin C, Lee F, Drago J, et al. The American Cancer Society National Prostate Cancer Detection Project. Findings on the detection of early prostate cancer in 2425 men. Cancer 1991; 67(12):2949–58.
13. San Francisco IF, Regan MM, Olumi AF, et al. Percent of cores positive for cancer is a better preoperative predictor of cancer recurrence after radical prostatectomy than prostate specific antigen. J Urol 2004;171(4):1492–9.
14. Sved PD, Gomez P, Manoharan M, et al. Limitations of biopsy Gleason grade: implications for counseling patients with biopsy Gleason score 6 prostate cancer. J Urol 2004;172(1):98–102.
15. Partin AW, Kattan MW, Subong EN, et al. Combination of prostate-specific antigen, clinical stage, and Gleason score to predict pathological stage of localized prostate cancer. A multi-institutional update. JAMA 1997;277(18):1445–51.
16. Steuber T, Karakiewicz PI, Augustin H, et al. Transition zone cancers undermine the predictive accuracy of Partin table stage predictions. J Urol 2005;173(3):737–41.
17. Aprikian AG. Risk stratification in clinically localized prostate cancer. Can J Urol 2002;9(Suppl 1): 18–20.

18. Zorn KC, Capitanio U, Jeldres C, et al. Multi-institutional external validation of seminal vesicle invasion nomograms: head-to-head comparison of Gallina nomogram versus 2007 Partin tables. Int J Radiat Oncol Biol Phys 2008, submitted for publication.

19. Padhani AR, Gapinski CJ, Macvicar DA, et al. Dynamic contrast enhanced MRI of prostate cancer: correlation with morphology and tumour stage, histological grade and PSA. Clin Radiol 2000;55(2):99–109.

20. Zakian KL, Sircar K, Hricak H, et al. Correlation of proton MR spectroscopic imaging with Gleason score based on step-section pathologic analysis after radical prostatectomy. Radiology 2005; 234(3):804–14.

21. Cooperberg MR, Lubeck DP, Meng MV, et al. The changing face of low-risk prostate cancer: trends in clinical presentation and primary management. J Clin Oncol 2004;22(11):2141–9.

22. Stamey TA, Caldwell M, McNeal JE, et al. The prostate specific antigen era in the United States is over for prostate cancer: what happened in the last 20 years? J Urol 2004;172(4 Pt 1):1297–301.

23. Eggener SE, Scardino PT, Carroll PR, et al. Focal therapy for localized prostate cancer: a critical appraisal of rationale and modalities. J Urol 2007; 178(6):2260–7.

24. Schiebler ML, Tomaszewski JE, Bezzi M, et al. Prostatic carcinoma and benign prostatic hyperplasia: correlation of high-resolution MR and histopathologic findings. Radiology 1989;172(1):131–7.

25. Outwater E, Schiebler ML, Tomaszewski JE, et al. Mucinous carcinomas involving the prostate: atypical findings at MR imaging. J Magn Reson Imaging 1992;2(5):597–600.

26. Beyersdorff D, Taymoorian K, Knosel T, et al. MRI of prostate cancer at 1.5 and 3.0 T: comparison of image quality in tumor detection and staging. AJR Am J Roentgenol 2005;185(5):1214–20.

27. Yu KK, Hricak H, Alagappan R, et al. Detection of extracapsular extension of prostate carcinoma with endorectal and phased-array coil MR imaging: multivariate feature analysis. Radiology 1997; 202(3):697–702.

28. Hricak H, Dooms GC, Jeffrey RB, et al. Prostatic carcinoma: staging by clinical assessment, CT, and MR imaging. Radiology 1987;162(2):331–6.

29. Quinn SF, Franzini DA, Demlow TA, et al. MR imaging of prostate cancer with an endorectal surface coil technique: correlation with whole-mount specimens. Radiology 1994;190(2):323–7.

30. Jager GJ, Ruijter ET, van de Kaa CA, et al. Local staging of prostate cancer with endorectal MR imaging: correlation with histopathology. AJR Am J Roentgenol 1996;166(4):845–52.

31. Tempany CM, Zhou X, Zerhouni EA, et al. Staging of prostate cancer: results of Radiology Diagnostic Oncology Group project comparison of three MR imaging techniques. Radiology 1994;192(1): 47–54.

32. Presti JC Jr, Hricak H, Narayan PA, et al. Local staging of prostatic carcinoma: comparison of transrectal sonography and endorectal MR imaging. AJR Am J Roentgenol 1996;166(1): 103–8.

33. Huch Boni RA, Boner JA, Debatin JF, et al. Optimization of prostate carcinoma staging: comparison of imaging and clinical methods. Clin Radiol 1995;50(9):593–600.

34. Bezzi M, Kressel HY, Allen KS, et al. Prostatic carcinoma: staging with MR imaging at 1.5 T. Radiology 1988;169(2):339–46.

35. Biondetti PR, Lee JK, Ling D, et al. Clinical stage B prostate carcinoma: staging with MR imaging. Radiology 1987;162(2):325–9.

36. Bartolozzi C, Menchi I, Lencioni R, et al. Local staging of prostate carcinoma with endorectal coil MRI: correlation with whole-mount radical prostatectomy specimens. Eur Radiol 1996;6(3):339–45.

37. Perrotti M, Kaufman RP Jr, Jennings TA, et al. Endo-rectal coil magnetic resonance imaging in clinically localized prostate cancer: is it accurate? J Urol 1996;156(1):106–9.

38. Jager GJ, Severens JL, Thornbury JR, et al. Prostate cancer staging: should MR imaging be used?–A decision analytic approach. Radiology 2000;215(2):445–51.

39. Futterer JJ, Engelbrecht MR, Huisman HJ, et al. Staging prostate cancer with dynamic contrast-enhanced endorectal MR imaging prior to radical prostatectomy: experienced versus less experienced readers. Radiology 2005;237(2): 541–9.

40. Bloch BN, Furman-Haran E, Helbich TH, et al. Prostate cancer: accurate determination of extracapsular extension with high-spatial-resolution dynamic contrast-enhanced and T2-weighted MR imaging–initial results. Radiology 2007;245(1):176–85.

41. Mirowitz SA, Brown JJ, Heiken JP. Evaluation of the prostate and prostatic carcinoma with gadolinium-enhanced endorectal coil MR imaging. Radiology 1993;186(1):153–7.

42. Folkman J, Beckner K. Angiogenesis imaging. Acad Radiol 2000;7(10):783–5.

43. Folkman J. Angiogenesis in cancer, vascular, rheumatoid and other disease. Nat Med 1995;1(1):27–31.

44. Li WW. Tumor angiogenesis: molecular pathology, therapeutic targeting, and imaging. Acad Radiol 2000;7(10):800–11.

45. Vartanian RK, Weidner N. Endothelial cell proliferation in prostatic carcinoma and prostatic hyperplasia: correlation with Gleason's score, microvessel density, and epithelial cell proliferation. Lab Invest 1995;73(6):844–50.

46. Strohmeyer D, Rossing C, Strauss F, et al. Tumor angiogenesis is associated with progression after radical prostatectomy in pT2/pT3 prostate cancer. Prostate 2000;42(1):26–33.

47. Weidner N, Moore DH 2nd, Ljung BM, et al. Correlation of bromodeoxyuridine (BRDU) labeling of breast carcinoma cells with mitotic figure content and tumor grade. Am J Surg Pathol 1993;17(10):987–94.

48. van Moorselaar RJ, Voest EE. Angiogenesis in prostate cancer: its role in disease progression and possible therapeutic approaches. Mol Cell Endocrinol 2002;197(1–2):239–50.

49. Taylor JS, Tofts PS, Port R, et al. MR imaging of tumor microcirculation: promise for the new millennium. J Magn Reson Imaging 1999;10(6):903–7.

50. Dewhirst MW, Tso CY, Oliver R, et al. Morphologic and hemodynamic comparison of tumor and healing normal tissue microvasculature. Int J Radiat Oncol Biol Phys 1989;17(1):91–9.

51. Leu AJ, Berk DA, Lymboussaki A, et al. Absence of functional lymphatics within a murine sarcoma: a molecular and functional evaluation. Cancer Res 2000;60(16):4324–7.

52. Alonzi R, Padhani AR, Allen C. Dynamic contrast enhanced MRI in prostate cancer. Eur J Radiol 2007;63(3):335–50.

53. Tofts PS, Brix G, Buckley DL, et al. Estimating kinetic parameters from dynamic contrast-enhanced T(1)-weighted MRI of a diffusible tracer: standardized quantities and symbols. J Magn Reson Imaging 1999;10(3):223–32.

54. Choyke PL, Dwyer AJ, Knopp MV. Functional tumor imaging with dynamic contrast-enhanced magnetic resonance imaging. J Magn Reson Imaging 2003;17(5):509–20.

55. Tofts PS, Kermode AG. Measurement of the blood-brain barrier permeability and leakage space using dynamic MR imaging. 1. Fundamental concepts. Magn Reson Med 1991;17(2):357–67.

56. Larsson HB, Stubgaard M, Frederiksen JL, et al. Quantitation of blood-brain barrier defect by magnetic resonance imaging and gadolinium-DTPA in patients with multiple sclerosis and brain tumors. Magn Reson Med 1990;16(1):117–31.

57. Brix G, Semmler W, Port R, et al. Pharmacokinetic parameters in CNS Gd-DTPA enhanced MR imaging. J Comput Assist Tomogr 1991;15(4):621–8.

58. Tofts PS. Modeling tracer kinetics in dynamic Gd-DTPA MR imaging. J Magn Reson Imaging 1997;7(1):91–101.

59. Huisman HJ, Engelbrecht MR, Barentsz JO. Accurate estimation of pharmacokinetic contrast-enhanced dynamic MRI parameters of the prostate. J Magn Reson Imaging 2001;13(4):607–14.

60. Kety S. Theory of blood-tissue exchange and its application to measurement of blood flow. Methods Med Res 1960;8:223–7.

61. Rijpkema M, Kaanders JH, Joosten FB, et al. Method for quantitative mapping of dynamic MRI contrast agent uptake in human tumors. J Magn Reson Imaging 2001;14(4):457–63.

62. de Bazelaire C, Rofsky NM, Duhamel G, et al. Combined T2* and T1 measurements for improved perfusion and permeability studies in high field using dynamic contrast enhancement. Eur Radiol 2006;16(9):2083–91.

63. van Dorsten FA, van der Graaf M, Engelbrecht MR, et al. Combined quantitative dynamic contrast-enhanced MR imaging and (1)H MR spectroscopic imaging of human prostate cancer. J Magn Reson Imaging 2004;20(2):279–87.

64. Futterer JJ, Heijmink SW, Scheenen TW, et al. Prostate cancer localization with dynamic contrast-enhanced MR imaging and proton MR spectroscopic imaging. Radiology 2006;241(2):449–58.

65. Ocak I, Bernardo M, Metzger G, et al. Dynamic contrast-enhanced MRI of prostate cancer at 3 T: a study of pharmacokinetic parameters. AJR Am J Roentgenol 2007;189(4):849.

66. Storaas T, Gjesdal KI, Svindland A, et al. Dynamic first pass 3D EPI of the prostate: accuracy in tumor location. Acta Radiol 2004;45(5):584–90.

67. Schlemmer HP, Merkle J, Grobholz R, et al. Can pre-operative contrast-enhanced dynamic MR imaging for prostate cancer predict microvessel density in prostatectomy specimens? Eur Radiol 2004;14(2):309–17.

68. Kiessling F, Lichy M, Grobholz R, et al. Simple models improve the discrimination of prostate cancers from the peripheral gland by T1-weighted dynamic MRI. Eur Radiol 2004;14(10):1793–801.

69. Bettencourt MC, Bauer JJ, Sesterhenn IA, et al. CD34 immunohistochemical assessment of angiogenesis as a prognostic marker for prostate cancer recurrence after radical prostatectomy. J Urol 1998;160(2):459–65.

70. Silberman MA, Partin AW, Veltri RW, et al. Tumor angiogenesis correlates with progression after radical prostatectomy but not with pathologic stage in Gleason sum 5 to 7 adenocarcinoma of the prostate. Cancer 1997;79(4):772–9.

71. Rubin MA, Buyyounouski M, Bagiella E, et al. Microvessel density in prostate cancer: lack of correlation with tumor grade, pathologic stage, and clinical outcome. Urology 1999;53(3):542–7.

72. Weidner N, Carroll PR, Flax J, et al. Tumor angiogenesis correlates with metastasis in invasive prostate carcinoma. Am J Pathol 1993;143(2):401–9.

73. Jesberger JA, Rafie N, Duerk JL, et al. Model-free parameters from dynamic contrast-enhanced-MRI: sensitivity to EES volume fraction and bolus timing. J Magn Reson Imaging 2006;24(3):586–94.

74. Tanaka N, Samma S, Joko M, et al. Diagnostic usefulness of endorectal magnetic resonance imaging with dynamic contrast-enhancement in patients with localized prostate cancer: mapping studies with biopsy specimens. Int J Urol 1999; 6(12):593–9.

75. Preziosi P, Orlacchio A, Di Giambattista G, et al. Enhancement patterns of prostate cancer in dynamic MRI. Eur Radiol 2003;13(5):925–30.

76. Noworolski SM, Henry RG, Vigneron DB, et al. Dynamic contrast-enhanced MRI in normal and abnormal prostate tissues as defined by biopsy, MRI, and 3D MRSI. Magn Reson Med 2005;53(2): 249–55.

77. Engelbrecht MR, Huisman HJ, Laheij RJ, et al. Discrimination of prostate cancer from normal peripheral zone and central gland tissue by using dynamic contrast-enhanced MR imaging. Radiology 2003;229(1):248–54.

78. Kim JK, Hong SS, Choi YJ, et al. Wash-in rate on the basis of dynamic contrast-enhanced MRI: usefulness for prostate cancer detection and localization. J Magn Reson Imaging 2005;22(5):639–46.

79. Kuhl CK, Mielcareck P, Klaschik S, et al. Dynamic breast MR imaging: are signal intensity time course data useful for differential diagnosis of enhancing lesions? Radiology 1999;211(1):101–10.

80. Brown G, Macvicar DA, Ayton V, et al. The role of intravenous contrast enhancement in magnetic resonance imaging of prostatic carcinoma. Clin Radiol 1995;50(9):601–6.

81. Girouin N, Mege-Lechevallier F, Tonina Senes A, et al. Prostate dynamic contrast-enhanced MRI with simple visual diagnostic criteria: is it reasonable? Eur Radiol 2007;17(6):1498–509.

82. Ogura K, Maekawa S, Okubo K, et al. Dynamic endorectal magnetic resonance imaging for local staging and detection of neurovascular bundle involvement of prostate cancer: correlation with histopathologic results. Urology 2001;57(4):721–6.

83. Jager GJ, Ruijter ET, van de Kaa CA, et al. Dynamic TurboFLASH subtraction technique for contrast-enhanced MR imaging of the prostate: correlation with histopathologic results. Radiology 1997; 203(3):645–52.

84. Namimoto T, Morishita S, Saitoh R, et al. The value of dynamic MR imaging for hypointensity lesions of the peripheral zone of the prostate. Comput Med Imaging Graph 1998;22(3):239–45.

85. Liney GP, Turnbull LW, Knowles AJ. In vivo magnetic resonance spectroscopy and dynamic contrast enhanced imaging of the prostate gland. NMR Biomed 1999;12(1):39–44.

86. Turnbull LW, Buckley DL, Turnbull LS, et al. Differentiation of prostatic carcinoma and benign prostatic hyperplasia: correlation between dynamic Gd-DTPA-enhanced MR imaging and histopathology. J Magn Reson Imaging 1999; 9(2):311–6.

87. Ito H, Kamoi K, Yokoyama K, et al. Visualization of prostate cancer using dynamic contrast-enhanced MRI: comparison with transrectal power Doppler ultrasound. Br J Radiol 2003;76(909):617–24.

88. Rouviere O, Raudrant A, Ecochard R, et al. Characterization of time-enhancement curves of benign and malignant prostate tissue at dynamic MR imaging. Eur Radiol 2003;13(5):931–42.

89. Buckley DL, Roberts C, Parker GJ, et al. Prostate cancer: evaluation of vascular characteristics with dynamic contrast-enhanced T1-weighted MR imaging–initial experience. Radiology 2004; 233(3):709–15.

90. Hara N, Okuizumi M, Koike H, et al. Dynamic contrast-enhanced magnetic resonance imaging (DCE-MRI) is a useful modality for the precise detection and staging of early prostate cancer. Prostate 2005;62(2):140–7.

91. Degani H, Gusis V, Weinstein D, et al. Mapping pathophysiological features of breast tumors by MRI at high spatial resolution. Nat Med 1997;3(7):780–2.

92. Montironi R, Mazzucchelli R, Scarpelli M, et al. Gleason grading of prostate cancer in needle biopsies or radical prostatectomy specimens: contemporary approach, current clinical significance and sources of pathology discrepancies. BJU Int 2005;95(8):1146–52.

93. Evans AJ, Henry PC, Van der Kwast TH, et al. Interobserver variability between expert urologic pathologists for extraprostatic extension and surgical margin status in radical prostatectomy specimens. Am J Surg Pathol 2008;32(10):1503–12.

94. Nico B, Benagiano V, Mangieri D, et al. Evaluation of microvascular density in tumors: pro and contra. Histol Histopathol 2008;23(5):601–7.

95. Rehman S, Jayson GC. Molecular imaging of anti-angiogenic agents. Oncologist 2005;10(2):92–103.

96. Oehr P. 'Omics'-based imaging in cancer detection and therapy. Per Med 2006;3(1):19–32.

97. Folkman J. Angiogenesis. Annu Rev Med 2006;57: 1–18.

98. Dome B, Hendrix MJ, Paku S, et al. Alternative vascularization mechanisms in cancer: pathology and therapeutic implications. Am J Pathol 2007; 170(1):1–15.

99. Chaib H, Cockrell EK, Rubin MA, et al. Profiling and verification of gene expression patterns in normal and malignant human prostate tissues by cDNA microarray analysis. Neoplasia 2001;3(1):43–52.

100. El-Gohary YM, Silverman JF, Olson PR, et al. Endoglin (CD105) and vascular endothelial growth factor as prognostic markers in prostatic adenocarcinoma. Am J Clin Pathol 2007;127(4):572–9.

101. Soulitzis N, Karyotis I, Delakas D, et al. Expression analysis of peptide growth factors VEGF, FGF2,

TGFB1, EGF and IGF1 in prostate cancer and benign prostatic hyperplasia. Int J Oncol 2006; 29(2):305–14.

102. Walsh K, Sriprasad S, Hopster D, et al. Distribution of vascular endothelial growth factor (VEGF) in prostate disease. Prostate Cancer Prostatic Dis 2002;5(2):119–22.

103. Lenkinski RE, Bloch BN, Liu F, et al. An illustration of the potential for mapping MRI/MRS parameters with genetic over-expression profiles in human prostate cancer. MAGMA 2008;21(6):411–21.

104. Rasiah KK, Kench JG, Gardiner-Garden M, et al. Aberrant neuropeptide Y and macrophage inhibitory cytokine-1 expression are early events in prostate cancer development and are associated with poor prognosis. Cancer Epidemiol Biomarkers Prev 2006;15(4):711–6.

105. Ruscica M, Dozio E, Motta M, et al. Modulatory actions of neuropeptide Y on prostate cancer growth: role of MAP kinase/ERK 1/2 activation. Adv Exp Med Biol 2007;604:96–100.

106. Ekstrand AJ, Cao R, Bjorndahl M, et al. Deletion of neuropeptide Y (NPY) 2 receptor in mice results in blockage of NPY-induced angiogenesis and delayed wound healing. Proc Natl Acad Sci U S A 2003;100(10):6033–8.

107. Kitlinska J, Abe K, Kuo L, et al. Differential effects of neuropeptide Y on the growth and vascularization of neural crest-derived tumors. Cancer Res 2005;65(5):1719–28.

108. Leach MO, Brindle KM, Evelhoch JL, et al. Assessment of antiangiogenic and antivascular therapeutics using MRI: recommendations for appropriate methodology for clinical trials. Br J Radiol 2003;76:S87–91.

109. Bloch BN, Rofsky NM, Baroni RH, et al. 3 Tesla magnetic resonance imaging of the prostate with combined pelvic phased-array and endorectal coils; initial experience(1). Acad Radiol 2004; 11(8):863–7.

110. Bloch BN, Lenkinski RE, Helbich TH, et al. Prostate postbrachytherapy seed distribution: comparison of high-resolution, contrast-enhanced, T1- and T2-weighted endorectal magnetic resonance imaging versus computed tomography: Initial experience. Int J Radiat Oncol Biol Phys 2007; 69(1):70–8.

111. Rosen Y, Bloch BN, Lenkinski RE, et al. 3T MR of the prostate: reducing susceptibility gradients by inflating the endorectal coil with a barium sulfate suspension. Magn Reson Med 2007;57(5): 898–904.

112. Chon CH, Lai FC, McNeal JE, et al. Use of extended systematic sampling in patients with a prior negative prostate needle biopsy. J Urol 2002;167(6):2457–60.

113. Lopez-Corona E, Ohori M, Scardino PT, et al. A nomogram for predicting a positive repeat prostate biopsy in patients with a previous negative biopsy session. J Urol 2003;170(4 Pt 1):1184–8 [discussion: 1188].

114. Hong YM, Lai FC, Chon CH, et al. Impact of prior biopsy scheme on pathologic features of cancers detected on repeat biopsies. Urol Oncol 2004; 22(1):7–10.

115. Lenkinski RE, Bloch BN, Liu F, et al. An illustration of the potential for mapping MRI/MRS parameters with genetic over-expression profiles in human prostate cancer. MAGMA 2008;21(6)411–21.

Index

Note: Page numbers of article titles are in **boldface** type.

mri.theclinics.com

Printed and bound by CPI Group (UK) Ltd, Croydon, CR0 4YY

03/10/2024

01040348-0011